H.-P. Berlien   P.-P. Schmittenbecher (Eds.)

Laser Surgery in Children

Springer

Berlin
Heidelberg
New York
Barcelona
Budapest
Hong Kong
London
Milan
Paris
Santa Clara
Singapore
Tokyo

H.-P. Berlien
P. P. Schmittenbecher (Eds.)

Laser Surgery in Children

With 143 figures and 15 tables

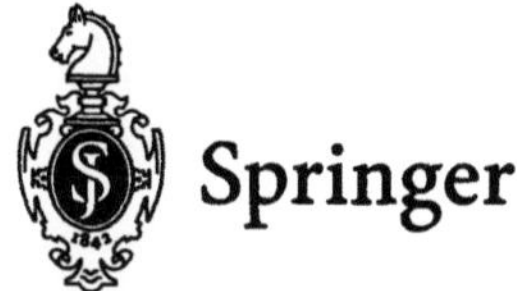

Springer

Professor Dr. med. H.-P. Berlien
Department of Laser Medicine
Hospital Neukölln
Rudower Str. 48
D-12313 Berlin

Dr. med. P. P. Schmittenbecher
Department of Pediatric Surgery
Dr. von Hauners Children Hospital, University of Munich
Lindwurmstr. 4
D-80337 Munich

Library of Congress Cataloging-in-Publication Data

Laser surgery in children / / H.-P. Berlien, P.P. Schmittenbecher
 (eds.).
     p.   cm.
   Includes bibliographical references and index.

   ISBN-13:978-3-642-64331-6   e-ISBN-13:978-3-642-60276-4
   DOI:10.1007/978-3-642-60276-4

   1. Children--Surgery. 2. Lasers in surgery. I. Berlien, H.-P.
 (Hans-Peter) II. Schmittenbecher, P.P. (Peter P.), 1958-
 [DNLM: 1. Laser Surgery--in infancy & childhood. WO 511 L3432
 1998]
 RD 137.L.324   1998
 617.9'8--dc21
 DNLM/DLC
 for Library of Congress   97-18416
                                                    CIP

Typesetting: Michael Kusche, Goldener Schnitt

SPIN: 10087151 24/3135 – 5 4 3 2 1 0 – Printed on acid-free paper

Table of Contents

List of Contributors

BEEK, J. F.
Laser Centre, Academic Medical Centre,
Meibergdreef 9, 1105 AZ, Amsterdam, The Netherlands

BERLIEN, H. P.
Department of Laser Medicine, Hospital Neukölln,
Rudower Str. 48, D-12313 Berlin, Germany

CASELLA, G.
Division of Diagnostic and Surgical Endoscopy,
National Cancer Institute,
Via Venezia 1, I-20133 Milan, Italy

DAL FANTE, M.
Division of Diagnostic and Surgical Endoscopy,
National Cancer Institute,
Via Venezia 1, I-20133 Milan, Italy

DESLOOVERRE, C
ENT Department, University Clinics K. V. Leuven,
Kapucisnenvoer, 33, B-3000 Leuven, Belgium

ENGERT, J.
Clinic of Pediatric Surgery, Ruhr-Universität Bochum
Marienhospital Herne,
Widumerstr. 8, D-44627 Herne, Germany

FEYH, J.
Clinic and Policlinic for Oto-Rhino-Laryngology,
Klinikum Großhadern der Universität Munich,
Marchioninistr. 15, 80377 Munich, Germany

GANS, S. L. (†)
717, North Rexford Drive, Beverly Hills, CA 90210, USA

GIJSBERS, G. H. M.
Laser Centre, Academic Medical Centre,
Meibergdreef 9, 1105 AZ, Amsterdam, The Netherlands

HOGERVORST, W.
Laser Centre, Department of Physics, Free University,
de Boelelaan 1081, 1081 HV Amsterdam, The Netherlands

LEHMANN, R. R.
Vesaliusweg 2–4, D-48149 Münster, Germany

MANCINI, A.
Divison of Diagnostic and Surgical Endoscopy,
National Cancer Institut,
Via Venezia 1, I-20133 Milan, Italy

MANTEL, K.
Division of Pediatric Anaesthesia,
Dr. von Hauners Children Hospital, University of Munich,
Lindwurmstr. 4, D-80337 Munich, Germany

PHILIPP, C.
Department of Laser Medicine, Hospital Neukölln,
Rudower Str. 48, D-12313 Berlin, Germany

POETKE, M.
Department of Laser Medicine, Hospital Neukölln,
Rudower Str. 48, D-12313 Berlin, Germany

SCHMITTENBECHER, P. P.
Department of Pediatric Surgery,
Dr. von Hauners Children Hospital, University of Munich,
Lindwurmstr. 4, D-80337 Munich, Germany

SPINELLI, P.
Division of Diagnostic and Surgical Endoscopy,
National Cancer Institute,
Via Venezia 1, I-20133 Milan, Italy

VAN DER MEULEN, F. W.
Laser Centre, Academic Medical Centre,
Meibergdreef 9, 1105 AZ, Amsterdam, The Netherlands

VAN GEMERT, M. J. C.
Laser Centre, Academic Medical Centre,
Meibergdreef 9, 1105 AZ, Amsterdam, The Netherlands

VON ILLBERG, C.
ENT Department, University Clinics K. V. Leuven,
Kapucisnenvoer, 33, B-3000 Leuven, Belgium

WALDSCHMIDT, J.
Department of Pediatric-Surgery,
University Clinic Benjamin Franklin,
Hindenburgdamm 30, D-12200 Berlin, Germany

WALKER, M. L.
Division of Pediatric Neurosurgery,
Primary Children´s Medical Center,
100 N. Medical Drive, Salt Lake City, UT 84113-110, USA

WELCH, A. J.
Bio-Medical Engineering Laboratory,
Engineering-Science Building 610, Austin, TX 78712, USA

The History of Laser Application in Pediatrics Surgery

P. P. SCHMITTENBECHER

Introduction

Over the past 30 years, the laser has become a helpful instrument in numerous medical specialities, especially in ophthalmology, ENT, dermatology, gastro-enterology, gynecology, urology, and neurosurgery. However, as Gans and Austin mentioned in 1988 [23], pediatric surgery lagged behind in the use of lasers. This statement is correct for all aspects of pediatric medical care.

In a scientific literature search using Medline and the index words "laser" and "child ...", one can find 769 articles in 15 different subspecialities between 1971 and 1996. Up to 25 papers per year from 1971 to 1980 are presented. An increase then took place with a peak of 85 reports in 1985, followed by a decrease to 21 in 1991 (Fig. 1). The majority of the reports is concerned with ophthalmology, followed by papers about dermatology and plastic surgery and about ENT and the tracheobronchial tree (Fig. 2). Ophthalmological laser application was also the earliest routine use of this tool in children starting in the mid-1970s. Around 1980, lasers were introduced into the field of pediatric dermatology and were increasingly used in upper airway obstructions and ENT problems. In

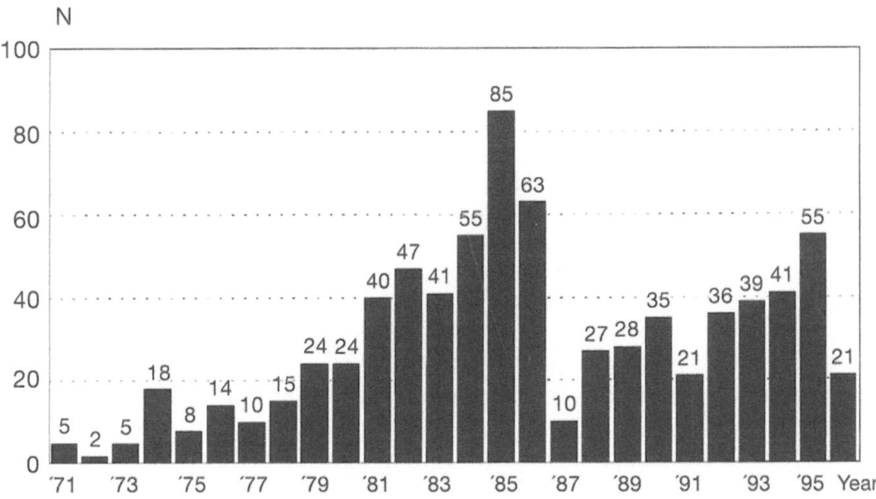

Fig. 1. Papers about "lasers in children," 1971–1996 (n = 769). (According to Medline analysis)

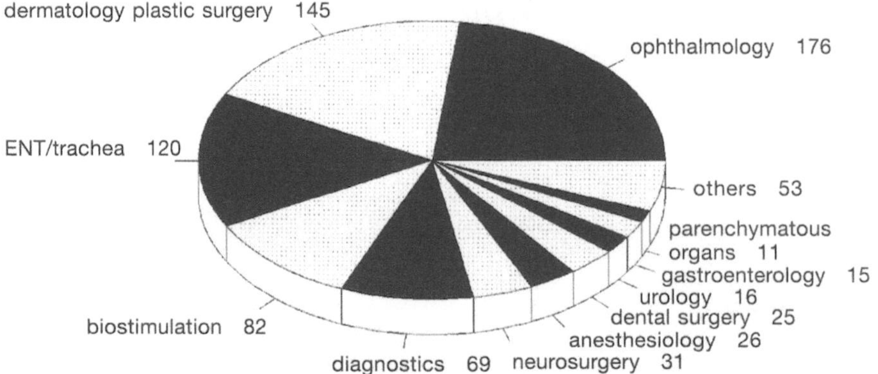

Fig. 2.   Papers about "lasers in children" in different subspecialities, 1971–1996 ($n = 769$). (According to Medline analysis)

the mid-1980s, pediatric neurosurgeons used laser systems, and first attempts were made to resect parenchymatous organs.

In Central Europe, laser use increased in pediatric surgery starting in 1985 when three medical instrument manufacturers together with the local government and university founded the "Laser Medical Center" in Berlin and appointed the pediatric surgeon H. P. Berlien as head of the institute´s medical program. Many pediatric surgeons in Germany and surrounding Central Europe presently work according to the indications, technical procedures, and guidelines for laser use issued by Berlien et al. [11].

However, even today, the laser is not adequately established in pediatric surgery centers. This is astonishing, especially in light of the possibility of operating in combination with the sealing of vessels (less blood loss), lymphatic vessels (reduced edema), and nerves (less pain) accompained by reduced risks of infection. Therefore, laser use is indicated in vascular areas (parenchymatous organs, tongue), vascularized tumors (angiomas, malignant tumors), bleeding conditions (hemophiliac, thrombopenic patients), infected tissues (burn wounds, pilonidal sinus, ingrown toenail, ulcus, gangrenous wounds), and operative procedures with significant blood loss (pectus excavatus, endorectal mucosectomy), as summarized by Gans and Austin [23].

The following sections of the paper will mainly discuss the historical development of laser use in hemangiomas, parenchymatous organs, endoscopic interventions, and, briefly, in some further fields of pediatric surgery.

Laser Application in Hemangiomas and Vascular Malformations

Of the three classical laser systems, the CO_2 laser was first used in children. Initial reports were given by Kaplan et al. [34] from Tel Aviv, Israel, in the excision of hemangiomas in 1973. This group can be considered genuine pioneers in the field of CO_2 lasers. In the following years, Shafir et al. [50] and Ohshiro [44] and

Aronoff [7] confirmed the applicability of the CO_2 laser beam to the excision of hemangiomas, especially in the oral cavity and the lip. Apfelberg et al. [5] (Laser Center, Palo Alto, CA, USA) pointed out the benefits of this modality: it simultaneously cuts and coagulates while reducing postoperative pain and edema. However, so far no one has brought forth an extensive study concerning pros and cons of CO_2 laser application in children, i.e., indications, methods, complications, and results. The undeveloped ability of a flexible laser fiber to transmit CO_2 laser light without articulated arms and mirrors made it complicated to use and restricted applicability to individual cases and special centers.

The argon laser was the second to join the group of instruments for treating vascular malformations. In 1978, Apfelberg et al. [2] established the efficacy of argon laser therapy in the amelioration of superficial lesions and abnormalities. The absorption wave-length of argon near the absorption spectrum of hemoglobin seemed to define the argon beam as an ideal modality in the management of superficial lesions such as capillary angiomas and nevus flammeous or port-wine stains. Apfelberg et al. [3] and Hobby [32] presented the first three and six case reports in capillary angiomas in children, respectively. Indications comprised bleeding, growth, deformation, ulceration, and compromised respiration or vision. The aim was the resolution of bleeding, the cessation of growth, and reduction and involution of surface vascularity. Hobby [33] advised treatment of angiomas at an early stage and when still small as being most effective.

In nevus flammeus, the argon laser revolutionized therapy. However, the first statistical analysis of treatment results showed that children had a worse outcome than adults. Noe et al. [41] found only 41% good, but 58% moderate results, and 25% hypertrophic scarring in 7- to 17-year-old patients. Further more, bad results were correlated with pink color and low blood content as is often seen in children. The supposition of high scarring risk in children was intensively discussed in the following years. Apfelberg et al. [4] assessed "scarring" as a normal result of wrinkle and texture change in natural involution, Dixon et al. [18] emphasized a reduction of the energy dose, and Gilchrest et al. [24] reduced scarring by chilling the angiomas before treatment. Finally Berlien et al. [12], who had been using the argon laser since 1983, presented exact laser parameters for application during childhood (5 W and an exposure time of 0.02 s/single pulse) to minimize heat conduction and exclude coagulation of the irradiated area. Inducing only a thermodynamic reaction within 3–4 weeks, hypertrophic scarring could be avoided.

As Hobby [32] already mentioned in 1983, cavernous components of hemangiomas are least effectively treated by the argon beam. The Nd:YAG laser leads to a diffuse volume reaction because there is no tissue that selectively absorbs laser light of a wave-length of 1060 nm. Rosenfeld and Sherman [49] first used the Nd:YAG laser because of the greater depth of penetration, starting their series in 1979 that included 12 children. The laser parameters were modified from 50–70 W and 0.1 s in the first cases to 20–30 W and 0.2–0.5 s in the later ones. Waldschmidt et al. [56] started treating angiomas with the Nd:YAG laser in 1982. The special application procedure included cooling of the surface and compression of the angioma by ice cubes. Laser power of approximately 50 W was delivered through the ice cube by the continuous wave mode to induce thermic vasculitis without any surface damage. Big caverns were managed by puncturing the angioma, and energy was deposited directly on the endothelium (interstitial therapy). Another interesting aspect of Nd:YAG laser use war supplied by Apfelberg et al. [6] who excised angiomas by sapphire tip technology. In this way, Nd:YAG laser works as in the resection of parenchymatous organs discussed below. Finally, Achauer and Vander Kam [1] completed the possibilities of Nd:YAG laser use by describing treatment modalities in capillary hemangiomas using 9–64 W and continuous wave mode with results better than those of argon laser use.

Lasers in Resection of Parenchymatous Organs

Significant blood loss in the resection of parenchymatous organs may cause numerous problems such as circulation disturbances and shock, especially in neonates and infants. This led to an intensive search for a way of resecting these well-vascularized organs without the above risks.

Laser investigations started when Giler et al. [26] tried to profit from the CO_2 laser in surgery of the spleen. One year later, Karbe et al. [36] used a Nd:YAG laser for liver resections in pigs and kidney upper pole resections in dogs. In pediatric surgery, two postdoctorate studies assessed the effect of Nd:YAG lasers in cuting parenchymatous tissue. First, in 1983 Meier [39] explored the efficacy of Nd:YAG laser light in hemisplenectomy and liver resections, followed by Berlien [10] in 1986, who found the laser to be a practical tool for preparation of split livers in association with liver transplantation in children. In the following years, several indications have been established in pediatric surgery of liver, spleen, kidney, adrenal gland, pancreas, and lung [12, 23]. Either Nd:YAG laser resection in tissue contact with sapphire tips or CO_2 laser cutting represent two main technical possibilities [34, 45].

In this field of pediatric surgery, the laser technique competes with ultrasound dissection, hot knife, water jet, infrared coagulation, and electrical resection. None of the techniques can be named as the method of choice, but each may be helpful in experienced hands in reducing the risks of parenchymatous organ resections in children.

Endoscopic Laser Applications

Laser Use in Laryngotracheobronchoscopy

In former times, most of the obstructive lesions in pediatric airways required tracheotomy followed by an external surgical approach. With the development of adequate instruments, transoral surgery became possible. However, the greatest advance was the introduction of CO_2 laser surgery in the management of upper airway obstructions in children in the 1970s. Laser application was characterized by high precision, excellent hemostasis and visibility, reduced postoperative edema, rapid healing, and minimal scarring [28, 30]. Healy et al. [29] (Department of Otolaryngology, The Children's Hospital Medical Center, Boston, MA, USA) were the first to use CO_2 laser technology and reported indications for its use in the nose (telangiectasia, papilloma, choanal atresia), the oral cavity (papilloma, hemangioma, telangiectasia), the (naso-) pharynx (tonsillectomy, excision of adenoidal tissue), and the larynx (webs, vocal cord nodules, polyps, granulomas, papillomas, neurofibromas, angiomas, membranes, stenosis). They also presented the first results in the fields of choanal atresia, recurrent respiratory papillomatosis, and benign laryngeal tumors [17, 51] followed by experimental studies in the most difficult field, the correction of acquired subglottic stenosis [27]. In subglottic hemangiomas, one (58%), two (29%), or three (13%) laser applications led to patent airways in 94% of the patients, with only two observed complications (6.5%). Ten of the 12 previously cannulated children could be decannulated, and 18 of 19 patients without tracheotomy could be spared such an intervention [31]. At last, even complications of laser interventions were analyzed be the Boston group, as in the 42 pediatric patients treated for respiratory papillomatosis. For example, following 3–60 laser operations, 15 boys and girls (36%) developed commissural, arytenoid, and subglottic webs and scars, with abnormal vocal cord fold movements occurring in five children [17]. Crockett and Strasnick [16] concluded the experience with CO_2 laser use some years later. They showed the pros and cons of the transnasal laser approach in the correction of choanal atresia, discussed whether total removal of laryngeal papillomas is advisable or not considering the risk of vocal cord scars, mentioned the limits of subglottic stenosis excision, and emphasized the safe and effective reduction of subglottic hemangiomas.

Argon laser use in the airways has only been rarely mentioned with regard to pediatric patients. Parkin and Dixon [46] first reported the application of an argon laser in subglottic hemangiomas, Brophy et al. [15] treated laryngeal papillomas with the argon beam, and Azizkhan et al. [9] managed acquired symptomatic bronchial stenosis in infants using an argon laser.

Limitations of CO_2 laser use are mainly due to the lack of flexible laser light transmission. Therefore, applications to tracheal and bronchial lesions are necessarily limited and not easy to perform. Toty et al. [52] described the advantage of flexible Nd:YAG laser application to obstructions of the lower airways. However, the Nd:YAG laser has still not found widespread application in the pediatric population. Mayer at al. [36] compared Nd:YAG and CO_2 laser use in a newborn lamb model of subglottic stenosis. McCaffrey and Cortese [38] reported Nd:YAG laser use in the excision of a subglottic hemangioma. Nowak [43] pointed out the Nd:YAG laser coagulation of semimalignant tumors in children´s airways. In Germany, Nd:YAG lasers were used quite often in the management of upper airway obstructions in children, particularly in the hands of pediatric surgeons. The Nd:YAG laser system is considered as a multifunctional tool in laryngeal, tracheal, and bronchial problems, but only in compliance with special and appropriate application parameters [56].

On the whole, laser procedures are well established in the treatment of airway obstructions in pediatric patients. Choanal atresia or tonsillectomy may be relative indications, but in papillomatosis, hemangiomas, webs, membranes, and scars, CO_2 and Nd:YAG lasers represent the instruments of choice with some variations in single application techniques.

Laser Interventions in the Gastrointestinal Tract

Laser interventions in the upper and lower gastrointestinal tracts are normally related to tumor obstructions or hemorrhages in adults. In children, hemorrhages and benign alterations such as mucosal hemangiomas or polyps can only rarely be managed in this way.

The first report was provided by Ullrich et al. [54] in 1982 when they reported two Nd:YAG laser interventions in stress ulcer bleeding of 10- and 11-year-old girls. In 1988, Noronha and Leist [42] showed that in a boy with mucosal telangiectasia, endoscopy was the only successful diagnostic procedure although subsequently endoscopic laser treatment could be added immediately using a Nd:YAG laser and 50 W of power.

After the endoscopic removal of colonic polyps, bleeding may be an opportunity to intervene by laser application [53]. Recurrent bleeding from mucosal angiomas in vasculocutaneous syndromes may require an extensive endoscopic examination of the upper and lower gastrointestinal tracts. As Spinelli's group demonstrated argon or Nd:YAG lasers are useful in treating bleeding lesions in the stomach and duodenum as well as in the colon and rectum [40]. In addition, Berlien et al. [12] mentioned that laser use can be envisioned in the shrinkage of fistulae and diverticulae or in the canalization of atresias and stenosis of the gastrointestinal tract.

Urological Laser Interventions

Laser use is well established in adult urology. Endoscopically controlled manipulations in pediatric urology are mainly restricted to the urethra and the bladder. Due to the small size of the structures, interventional ureteroscopy or pyeloscopy do not represent methods routinely used.

Therefore, it was not surprising that laser was first used in this field for the ablation of posterior urethral valves. In 1985, Ehrlich et al. [19] started treating six 7- to 20-month-old boys with the Nd:YAG laser, observing no stricture and no postoperative incontinence. They worked in an antegrade direction via the transvesical route with and without direct tissue contact and argued that laser ablation led to reproducible and homogenous tissue necrosis, subsequent reepithelization, less fibrous contraction, and less damage to surrounding tissue. Later, Biewald and Schier [13] resected urethral valves in neonates in retrograde transurethral endoscopy and achieved the same positive results without complications.

The same group also inaugurated the treatment of posttraumatic urethral strictures by retrograde laser recanalization [14]. In 1988, Ritchey et al. [47] presented a case report about pediatric ureteroscopic lasertripsy in a distal ureteral stone. They fragmented the stone with a dye laser beam and extracted the fragments with a basket. Therefore, lasers seem to present an alternative, especially in the management of prevesical ureteral stones that are difficult to treat with extracorporeal shockwave lithotripsy (ESWL).

Other Indications for Laser Use

Neurosurgery was one of the first medical specialities to use laser technology. Rosonoff and Carroll introduced the ruby laser in 1965, Stellar the CO_2 laser in 1970, and Beck the Nd:YAG laser in 1977 [cf. 53]. Beck [9] included patients younger than 12 years old suffering from meningiomas in his report.

In 1982, Epstein and Epstein [20] showed that most benign gliomas in the spinal cord of children could be totally resected using CO_2 laser without exacerbating neurological deficits. Fasano et al. [21] in 1983 compared all three laser types in posterior fossa tumors in children, including medulloblastomas and brain stem tumors. They used the CO_2 laser for incision, cutting, and vaporization, the argon laser for incision and achieving vaporization, and the Nd:YAG laser only for vaporization. The concluded that the main advantages of lasers are seen in radical surgery with relatively few side effects, the possibility of operating near highly functional structures, and reduction of blood loss.

CO_2 laser excision of acute burns should also be mentioned. As long ago as 1974, Fidler et al. [22] presented their experience with 15 excisional procedures using CO_2 lasers in 13 patients who were 17 months to 14 years old. Comparing CO_2 laser excision and conventional scalpel use in similar anatomical locations, the same depth of the burn, and during the same intervention, the authors showed that blood loss was higher in the knife excision by a factor of 3.8 on average, whereas laser excision required a little more time (factor 1.8). Skin grafts survived in either case [22].

Finally, in recent years, discussion has turned to the use of lasers in laparoscopic and thoracoscopic procedures. The efficacy of this modality for the coagulation of mesenteric vessels in appendectomy or for hemostasis in endoscopic lung resection has to be proven in controlled studies [25, 48].

References

1. Achauer BM, Vander Kam VM (1989) Capillary hemangiomas (Strawberry Mark) of infancy: comparison of argon and Nd:YAG laser treatment. Plast Reconstr Surg 84: 60–70
2. Apfelberg DB, Maser MR, Lash H (1978) Argon laser treatment of cutaneous vascular abnormalities. Progress report. Ann Plast Surg 1: 14–18
3. Apfelberg DB, Greene RA, Maser MR (1981) Results of argon laser exposure of capillary hemangiomas of infancy. Preliminary report. Plast Reconstr Surg 67: 188–193
4. Apfelberg DB, Maser MR, Lash H (1981) The argon laser for cutaneous lesions. JAMA 246: 2073–2075
5. Apfelberg DB, Maser MR, Lash H, White DN (1985) Benefits of the CO_2 laser in oral hemangioma excision. Plast Reconstr Surg 75: 46–50
6. Apfelberg DB, Maser MR, Lash H, White DN (1989) Sapphire tip technology for YAG laser excision in plastic surgery. Plast Reconstr Surg 84: 273–279
7. Aronoff BL (1981) The use of lasers in hemangiomas. Laser Surg Med 1: 323
8. Azizkhan RG, Lacey SR, Wood RE (1990) Acquired symptomatic bronchial stenosis in infants: successful management using an argon laser. J Pediatr Surg 25: 19–24
9. Beck OJ (1980) The use of Nd:YAG and the CO_2 laser in neurosurgery. Neurosurg Rev 3: 261–266
10. Berlien H-P (1986) Die orthotope segmentale Lebertransplantation beim Ferkel. Habilitationsschrift, FU Berlin
11. Berlien H-P, Philipp C, Fuchs B, Enegl-Murcke F (1988) Therapeutische Leitlinien zur Laserbehandlung. In: Berlien H-P, Müller G (eds) Angewandte Lasermedizin. ecomed, Landsberg, pp III/2,2/1–57
12. Berlien H-P, Müller G, Waldschmidt J (1990) Lasers in pediatric surgery. Prog Ped Surg 25: 5–22

13. Biewald W, Schier F (1992) Laser treatment of posterior urethral valves in neonates. Br J Urol 69: 425–427
14. Biewald W, Stroedter L (1992) Neodym-YAG-Laserbehandlung der posttraumatischen Urethrastriktur im Kindesalter. Zentralbl Kinderchir 1: 221–226
15. Brophy JW, Scully PA, Stratten CJ (1982) Argon laser use in papillomas of the larynx. Laryngoscope 92: 1164–1167
16. Crockett CM, Strasnick B (1989) Lasers in pediatric otolaryngology. Otolaryngol Clin North Am 22: 607–619
17. Crockett DM, McCabe BF, Shive CJ (1987) Complications of laser surgery for recurrent respiratory papillomatosis. Ann Otol Rhinol Laryngol 96: 639–644
18. Dixon JA, Huether S, Rotering RH (1984) Hypertrophic scarring in argon laser treatment of portwine stains. Plast Reconstr Surg 73: 771–780
19. Ehrlich RM, Shanberg A, Fine RN (1987) Neodymium:YAG laser ablation of posterior urethral valves. J Urol 138: 959–962
20. Epstein F, Epstein N (1982) Surgical treatment of spinal cord astrocytomas in childhood: a series of 19 patients. J Neurosurg 57: 685–689
21. Fasano VA, Lombard GF, Ponzio RM (1983) Preliminary experience with the use of three lasers in posterior fossa tumors in childhood. Childs Brain 10: 26–38
22. Fidler JP, Law E, Rockwell J, Macmillan BG (1974) Carbon dioxide laser excision of acute burns with immediate autografting. J Surg Res 17: 1–11
23. Gans SL, Austin E (1988) The use for lasers in pediatric surgery. J Pediatr Surg 23: 695–704
24. Gilchrest BA, Rosen S, Noe JM (1982) Chilling portwine stains improves the response to argon laser therapy. Plast Reconstr Surg 69: 278–283
25. Gilchrist BF, Lobe TE, Schropp KP, Kay GA, Hixon SD, Wrenn BL Jr, Phillipe PG, Hollabaugh RS (1992) Is there a role for laparoscopic appendectomy in pediatric surgery? J Pediatr Surg 27: 209–212
26. Giler S, Ben-Basset M, Gassner S (1979) The CO_2 laser in surgery of the spleen. An experimental study. In: Kaplan I, Ascher PW (eds) Laser Surgery III. Tel Aviv, Jerusalem Academic Press
27. Healy GB (1982) An experimental model for the endoscopic correction of subglottic stenosis with clinical application. Laryngoscope 92: 1103–1115
28. Healy GB, McGill T, Strong MS (1978) Surgical advances in the treatment of lesions of the pediatric airways: the role of the carbon dioxide laser. Pediatrics 61: 380–383
29. Healy GB, McGill T, Jako GJ, Strong MS, Vaughan CW (1978) The management of choanal atresia with the carbon dioxide laser. Ann Otol Rhinol Laryngol 87: 658–662
30. Healy GB, McGill T, Simpson GT, Strong MS (1979) The use of carbon dioxide laser in the pediatric airway. J Pediatr Surg 14: 735–740
31. Healy GB, McGill T, Firedman EF (1984) Carbon dioxide laser in subglottic hemangiomas. Ann Otol Rhinol Laryngol 93: 370–373
32. Hobby LW (1983) Further evaluation of the potential of the argon laser in treatment of strawberry hemangiomas. Past Reconstr Surg 71: 481–485
33. Hobby LW (1986) Argon laser treatment of superficial vascular lesions in children. Laser Surg Med 6: 16–19
34. Joffe SN, Foster J, Schroder T, Brackett K (1988) Splenic resection with the contact Nd:YAG laser system. J Pediatr Surg 23: 829–834
35. Kaplan I, Ger R, Sharon V (1973) The carbon dioxide laser in plastic surgery. Br J Plast Surg 26: 359
36. Karbe E, Königsmann G, Beck R (1980) Experimentelle Leber- und Nierenchirurgie mit dem CO_2-, CO-, Holmium- und Neodym-Laser. Langenbecks Arch Chir 351: 179–192
37. Mayer T, Matlak ME, Dixon J, Johnson DG, McCloskey D (1980) Experimental subglottic stenosis: Histopathologic and bronchoscopic comparison of electrosurgery, cryosurgery and laser resection. J Pediatr Surg 15: 944–952
38. McCaffrey TV, Cortese DA (1986) Neodymium:YAG laser treatment of subglottic hemangiomas. Otolaryngol Head Neck Surg 94: 387
39. Meier H (1983) Morphologische und funktionelle Untersuchungen sowie erste klinische Anwendungen des Neodym:YAG-Lasers im Gastrointestinaltrakt zum Fistelverschluß und bei Resektionen an parenchymatösen Organen bei Kindern. Habilitationsschrift, University of Erlangen
40. Meroni E, Spinelli P, DelFante M (1989) Laser-Behandlung von Blutungen des Gastrointestinaltraktes bei Kindern. Biotronic 3: 52

41. Noe JM, Barsky SH, Geer DE (1980) Portwine stains and the response to argon laser therapy: successful treatment and the predictive role of color, age and biopsy. Plast Reconstr Surg 65: 130–136
42. Noronha PA, Leist MH (1988) Encoscopic laser therapy for gastrointestinal bleeding from congenital vascular lesions. J Pediatr Gastroenterol Nutr 7: 375–378
43. Nowak W (1988) Die Behandlung semimaligner Tumoren bei Kindern und Jugendlichen mit dem Neodym:YAG-Laser – Indikationen und Abgrenzungen zum operativen Vorgehen. Z Kinderchir 43 Suppl: 30–32
44. Ohshiro T (1981) The CO_2 laser in the treatment of cavernous hemangiomas of the lower lip: a case report. Lasers Surg Med 1: 337
45. Orda R, Wiznitzer T, Bulbis JJ (1982) Hemisplenectomy using a hand held CO_2 laser: an experimental study. J Pediatr Surg 17: 163–165
46. Parkin JL, Dixon JA (1985) Argon laser treatment of head and neck vascular lesions. Otolaryngol Head Neck Surg 93: 211–216
47. Ritchey M, Patterson DE, Kelalis PP, Segura JW (1988) A case of pediatric ureteroscopic laserthripsy. J Urol 139: 1272–1274
48. Rogers DA, Phillipe PG, Lobe TE, Kay GA, Gilchrist BF, Schropp KP, Rao BN (1992) Thoracoscopy in children: an initial experience with an evolving technique. J Laparoendosc Surg 2: 7–14
49. Rosenfeld H, Sherman R (1986) Treatment of cutaneous and deep vascular lesions with the Nd:YAG laser. Lasers Surg Med 6: 20–23
50. Shafir R, Slutzki S, Bornstein SA (1977) Excision of buccal hemangiomas by carbon dioxide laser beam. Oral Surg 44: 347–350
51. Simpson GT, Healy GB, McGill T, Strong MS (1979) Benign tumors and lesions of the larynx in children. Ann Otol Rhinol Laryngol 88: 479–485
52. Toty L, Personne C, Colchen A, Vourc'h G (1981) Bronchoscopic management of tracheal lesions using the Neodymium:YAG laser. Thorax 36: 75–80
53. Ullrich F (1988) Möglichkeiten und Grenzen des Lasers. Klinikarzt 17: 561–566
54. Ullrich F, Nützenadel W, Dietz R (1982) Endoskopische Blutstillung durch Laserkoagulation bei massiver Streßulkusblutung des Magens im Kindesalter. Z Kinderchir 36: 151–153
55. Waldschmidt J, Berlien H-P, Hauck GW, El-Dessouky M (1988) Auswahl verschiedener Lasertypen in der Behandlung von oberflächlichen und tiefen Gefäßanomalien. Z Kinderchir 43: 6–10
56. Waldschmidt J, Schier F, Charissis G (1992) Laserchirurgie an Larynx, Trachea und Bronchien im Kindesalter. In: Berlien H-P, Müller G (eds) Angewandte Lasermedizin. ecomed, Landsberg, pp VI/ 3,8,6/1–5

Laser Physics and Laser – Tissue Interaction

J. F. BEEK, F. W. VAN DER MEULEN, G. H. M. GIJSBERS, A. J. WELCH,
W. HOGERVORST, and M. J. C. VAN GEMERT

Introduction

Application of lasers in medicine is based on the unique properties of laser radiation.

Compared to classical light sources (such as an incandescent lamp), which in general emit light equally distributed in all directions, laser radiation is concentrated in a well-defined, almost parallel beam of high energy. By virtue of its small spot-size diameter, it can be focussed into a fiber and hence be transported by endoscopes to nearly every part of the body through natural or small artificial openings. Being a confined beam of radiation energy, it can be used as an instrument of precision in surgical procedures. Furthermore, short pulses of high energy can cause an acoustic effect which can be used to fragment stones and to remove a postsurgical cataract of the posterior capsular membrane. Secondly, laser radiation can in most cases be regarded as radiation of virtually one wavelength (monochromatic). This monochromaticity can be used, for instance, to induce reactions within certain parts of tissues, thus evoking specific biological responses (e.g., light absorption by hemoglobin, causing selective coagulation in the retina without damage to cornea, lens, or corpus vitrum, or selective coagulation of ectatic vessels of a port-wine stain, without damage to the surrounding dermis). A third difference from light from a conventional light source is that laser light is coherent, i.e., all waves emitted by the laser have the same phase, in contrast to the waves from a classical source which are emitted randomly. This quality is important in special diagnostic applications.

On the basis of these characteristics, the application of lasers in medicine has improved treatment modalities in some fields and has broadened the diagnostic scope in others. To understand currently applied techniques and to be able to follow the development of new ones, a sound understanding of laser physics and dosimetry is indispensible.

Before delving into the principles of laser physics, some concepts and definitions will be elucidated.

Laser radiation is electromagnetic radiation. The spectrum of electromagnetic radiation ranges from radiowave radiation (long wavelength) via microwave, infrared, visible, and ultraviolet radiation of short-wavelength X-ray and gamma radiation. Laser radiation used in medicine ranges from the UV to the far IR (193–10 600 nm). Wavelength is usually expressed in nanometers ($1\ \mathrm{nm} = 10^{-9}\ \mathrm{m}$). This implies that the visible part of the spectrum of electromagnetic radiation is only a part of the spectrum covered by laser radiation. As light

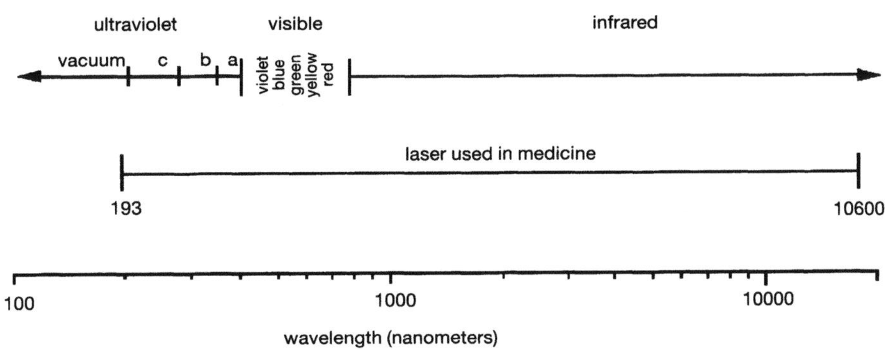

Fig. 1. Wavelength (in nanometers: 1 nm = 10^{-9} m) and color of the electromagnetic spectrum. Visible light is between about 400 nm and 750 nm. The ultraviolet part of the spectrum is subdivided into UV-A, UV-B, and UV-C

in the strict sense is regarded as visible radiation, one should reserve, the term "laser light" for the range of 400–750 nm. However, in practice the terms "laser light" and "laser radiation" are used synonymously (see Fig. 1).

Electromagnetic radiation shows a dual character. On the one hand, the radiation represents packages of energy called photons. A photon is defined as the smallest amount of light energy. On the other hand, light has wave-like properties and thus obeys the physical laws of diffraction. Concerning laser radiation, both aspects are important. Work can be performed with energy, and this is expressed in units of joules. According to Planck, the energy of a photon is dependent on its frequency (f):

$$\text{Photon energy} = h \times f \qquad \qquad \text{[J]} \quad (1)$$

where h stands for Planck´s constant (h = 6.626×10^{-34} J). The frequency of the light determines the wavelength Λ via:

$$\text{Photon wavelength} = \text{velocity of light (m/s)/photon frequency (Hz)} \qquad \text{[m]} \quad (2)$$

The velocity of light in vacuum is 300 000 km/s or 3×10^8 m/s. From Eqs. 1 and 2 it follows that the shorter the wavelength, the more energy a photon contains.

A photon always moves with the velocity of light. A laser beam is merely a very large number of photons that move with the velocity of light in (almost) the same direction. The total amount of energy of all photons (E) that pass by in 1 determines the power P of the laser beam:

$$\text{Power} = \text{energy (J)/time (s)} \qquad \qquad \text{[W]} \quad (3)$$

Power is expressed in watts (W or J/s). Calculation of the amount of energy delivered can be performed by multiplying the power delivered by the duration of exposure:

Delivered energy = power (W or J/s) time (s)   [J]   (4)

Because radiation has wave-like properties, a laser beam can be focussed. A laser beam with a power delivered to an area of 1 cm² will produce a hundredfold intensity increase when concentrated in an area of 1 mm². Power density is defined as the power per area:

Power density = power (W or J/s)/area (m²)   [W/m²]   (5)

and energy density as the energy per area:

Energy density = power (W or J/s) time (s)/area (m²)   [J/m²]   (6)

The terms "power" and "power density" will be discussed of greater length in the section about thermal laser-tissue interaction. Also important in the determination of the impact of laser radiation are the pattern and duration of the light exposure. In some laser systems a constant flux of laser radiation is generated, designated continuous wave (cw). In contrast to this, there is the "pulsed mode"; (peak) pulses of light are evoked, the duration of which may vary from femto- to milliseconds (10^{-15}–10^{-3} s). In the next paragraphs these items will be discussed in more detail.

In the next section the physics of a laser will be explained. Delivery of laser light to the target tissue will be discussed in a separate paragraph, followed by a discussion of processes that influence the light distribution in tissue. Finally, different laser(-light)-tissue interactions will be discussed.

Laser Physics

Introduction

Laser is an acronym for "light amplification by stimulated emission of radiation." The principle of stimulated emission and amplification of radiation was already discussed by Einstein in 1917 in his theory on the interaction of electromagnetic radiation with atoms and molecules. However, it took more than 40 years for developments in physics and technology to become such that the principle of stimulated emission could be demonstrated and applied to the amplification of radiation; this was done for the first time in 1954 with microwave radiation, resulting in the maser (microwave amplification). Townes and his colleagues used a beam of ammonia molecules to demonstrate maser action. In 1960 Maiman succeeded in demonstrating visible maser action, i.e., laser action, in specially prepared ruby crystals illuminated with powerful xenon flashlamps. He observed a strong, red light pulse at a wavelength of 694.3 nm with all of the characteristics of laser radiation. A continuously working laser was built by Javan and coresearchers in 1961 using a mixture of helium and neon gas, thus representing the first gas laser.

Since then, many gas, liquid, and solid-state lasers have become available and a high-tech, billion dollar laser industry has developed. The different types of lasers may be grouped according to emission wavelengths, the mode of operation (pulsed or continuous) and light power or energy. Their characteristics are determined by the laser medium (which usually gives a laser its name) and the physical processes playing a role inside this medium. Pulsed laser radiation may be produced at present large portion of the infrared, visible, and ultraviolet part of the spectrum. The maximum attainable peak power exceeds 10^{14} W. The most powerful cw laser is still the CO_2 laser, which can produce a power of 50 kW, sufficient to cut through a thick steel plate after focussing.

Laser Operation

General Operation

The laser light source consists, with only a few exceptions, of two parts: the active laser medium and the passive laser cavity (Fig. 2).

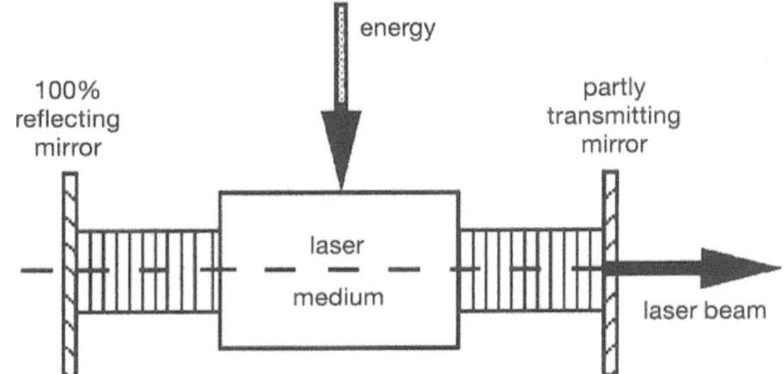

Fig. 2.   A laser, schematically

Energy is supplied to the medium, which subsequently emits its characteristic radiation. This energy may be supplied in various forms. Lasers pumped by electrical energy (such as gas lasers), by energy released in chemical reactions (chemical lasers), and by light energy (e.g., the flashlamp-pumped Nd:YAG laser and the Ar-ion-laser-pumped dye laser). The light produced inside the medium is amplified by stimulated emission and sustained by the cavity. This cavity consists in principle of two highly reflecting mirrors which reflect the emitted light back into the laser medium. With a suitable choice of mirror distance and the support of a continuing supply of energy in between the mirrors, a powerful lightwave may grow. When one of the mirrors is made transmittant, a small part of the light will "leak" out of the cavity in a direction parallel to the axis of the apparatus. This transmitted light in fact is the laser beam. In this picture the laser may be compared with an electronic amplifier which, with a suitable feedback loop in the circuit, starts to work as a transmitter/oscillator. In the "optical amplifier" the mirrors form the feedback loop, resulting in a "laser" oscillator.

The build-up of a lightwave in between the mirrors will continue until equilibrium is obtained between the amount of light energy produced and the amount of light leaking out of the laser cavity. This also determines the efficiency or yield of the laser defined as the ratio of light energy emitted by the laser to the energy supplied to the laser. For most practical lasers the efficiency is not high. An Ar-ion laser has a yield of less than 0.1% (40 kW of electrical power produce about 25 W of light power), while a CO_2 laser and a Nd:YAG laser have efficiencies in the order of a few percent. The wasted energy generates heat that has to be removed by cooling the laser medium.

Stimulated Emission and Amplification of Radiation

The properties of the individual particles in the laser medium (atoms, ions, or molecules) play an important role in the generation of light. In the following discussion only atoms will be considered, but the explanation for laser operation also holds for molecules.

An atom consists of a positively charged nucleus surrounded by a cloud of negatively charged electrons, which together form an electrically neutral particle. When energy is supplied to the atom, the most weakly bound and outermost electron is removed from its regular orbit, the ground state. It is transferred to a more extended orbit with a higher energy; the atom is in an excited state. This is not a stable situation, and after a short time period the atom will decay again to the lower energy level thereby emitting its energy surplus in the form of a lightwave or photon. When the ground state energy is denoted as E_1 and the excited state energy as E_2, then the energy difference $E_2 - E_1$ determines the frequency of the emitted light in the transition via the following relation (see Fig. 3):

$$h f = E_2 - E_1 \qquad\qquad\qquad (7)$$

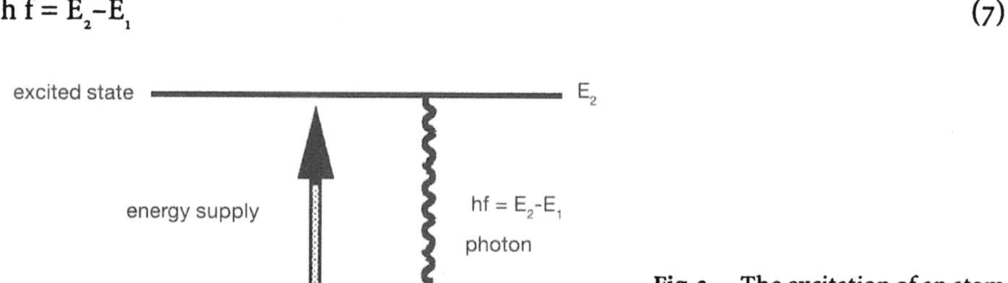

Fig. 3. The excitation of an atom followed by emission of a photon

This decay process, resulting in the, emission of a photon, occurs even in the absence of any external influence and is therefore called spontaneous emission. The photon will be emitted in a completely arbitrary direction (see Fig. 4a). Each type of atom has a number of well-defined energy states and emits radiation that is characteristic for the element (Na: yellow light; Ne: red light, and Hg: among others, ultraviolet light). An excited atom may also be stimulated to emit a photon when it is "hit" by a passing photon with identical frequency. The two photons, the passing one and the one emitted by stimulated emission, move in exactly the same direction and with the same phase (see Fig. 4b).

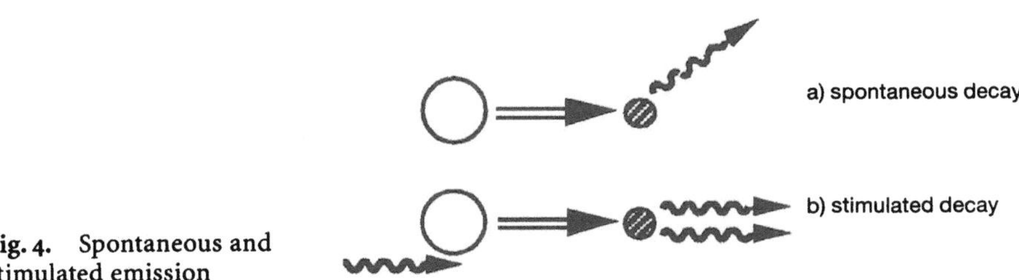

Fig. 4. Spontaneous and stimulated emission

This process of stimulated emission competes with spontaneous emission. When the two identical photons meet two other excited atoms (in a "vessel" filled with many atoms), the stimulated emission process may be repeated and four identical photons moving parallel with the same phase are created. When this process repeats itself many times, a photon avalanche will be produced and a strong light beam grows (see Fig. 5).

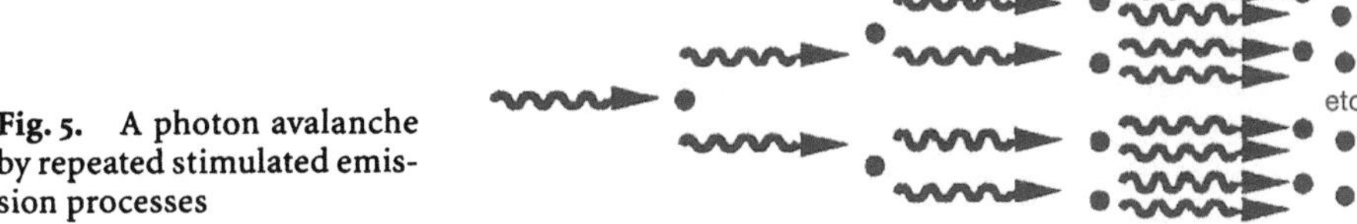

Fig. 5. A photon avalanche by repeated stimulated emission processes

This light amplification is possible only when a sufficient number of atoms is in the excited state and a sufficient number of suitable photons is available to start the avalanche. The latter condition is provided by the optical cavity, which will be treated below. A photon with the correct frequency may pass an atom in its ground state. This atom may absorb the photon, producing an excited state (see Fig. 6).

Fig. 6. The absorption process producing an excited atom

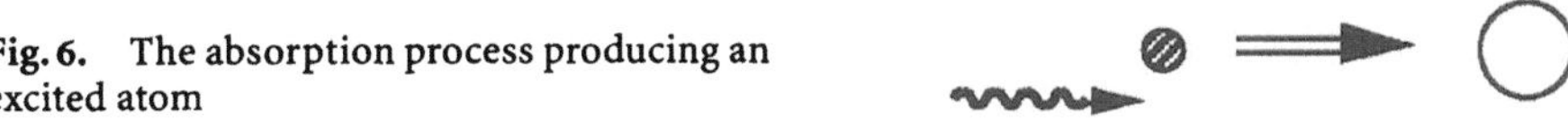

Absorption implies a loss of photons and attenuation of the light beam. The stimulated emission will dominate the absorption process only when the laser medium is active, i.e., when more atoms are in an excited state than in the ground state (population inversion). Only in this case may a net amplification result. Under this condition the medium is transferred with the supplied energy into a state completely different from the normal state (all atoms in their ground state). The necessary condition for laser action is that of population inversion, i.e., more atoms in an excited than in the ground state. The efficiency of the laser will be determined by the competition between absorption, spontaneous, and stimulated emission. It can be shown in a simple way that in an atom with only one excited state, the condition for population inversion can never be fulfilled. The perturbing action of spontaneous emission will prevent the excitation of more than 50% of such atoms; the number of atoms in the excited state at most can be equal to the number in the ground state and net amplification is impossible. Only for atoms with more excited states involved in the laser process may be condition of population inversion be realized. The number of energy levels involved determines whether a laser will operate in a pulsed or continuous mode. In general, three or four energy levels are involved in the laser process. Figure 7 show the possible energy levels or transitions of a three-level system. In three-level lasers, the atom has, in addition to the ground state (level 1), two excited states (levels 2 and 3) with the third level highest in energy. Via the "energy-pump" (e.g., light that fits the transition $1 \rightarrow 3$) atoms are excited to level 3. Level 3 has a short lifetime and rapidly decays to level 2. When level 2 has a long decay time compared to the lifetime of level 3, the lower level 2 will be populated at the expense of level 3 (optical pumping). Because of this optical pumping, after a short time a situation is created with more atoms in level 2 than in the ground state level 1, i.e., population inversion. Within a cavity the process of stimulated emission can now start, and radiation fitting the transition $2 \rightarrow 1$ will be amplified. However, as soon as this process starts, level 2 will be emptied and level 1 filled, population inversion will vanish, and the laser will self-terminale (unless the pump process is extremely quick, i.e., quicker than the laser process $2 \rightarrow 1$). When the pump continues to supply energy, after some time level 2 will be filled again at the expense of level 1 and the process may repeat itself. The laser will fire and quench itself in succession until the energy supply stops. It is extremely difficult to have such a system run continuously; it requires a very powerful energy source. Examples of three-level lasers are the ruby laser and copper- and gold-vapor lasers.

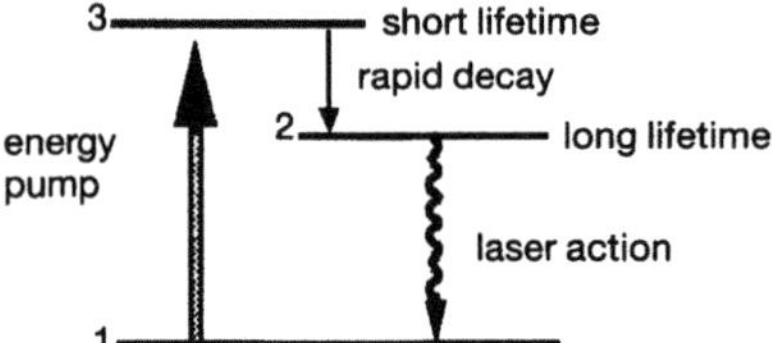

Fig. 7. Three-level laser (example: ruby laser)

From the preceding discussion it is clear that a three-level laser in almost all cases will produce only pulsed light. For pulsed laser action, population inversion that is available intermittently is sufficient. In a four-level system the ground state is not involved in the laser process as initial or final state, and therefore continuous laser action is always feasible, as population inversion can he available constantly. A typical four-level energyscheme is given in Figure 8.

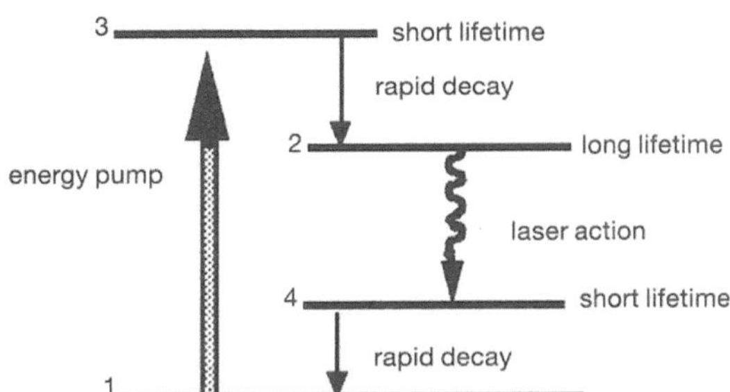

Fig. 8. Four-level laser, for example, Nd:YAG laser

In the pump process the long-lived level 2 again is populated by optical pumping via level 3 from the ground state. When the intermediate level 4 can decay pumping rapidly to the ground state, it is clear that population inversion can be maintained indefinitely between the levels 2 and 4 as long as pump energy is supplied. Such a system can operate both in pulsed and continuous ways and Q switching as well as modelocking is possible. In pulsed operation the four-level system does not produce a train of pulses as in the three-level case. Since constantly available population inversion is a prerequisite, it is considerably more difficult to cover a large wavelength range with continuous lasers. In portions of the infrared (e.g., CO_2 laser at 10.6 µm, Nd:YAG laser at 1064 nm, diode lasers) and in the visible and ultraviolet parts of the spectrum (e.g., Ar- and Kr-ion lasers, dye lasers), continuous laser radiation is available.

The Optical Cavity

The laser cavity or resonator consists of two mirrors mounted parallel and separated by a distance L determining the length of the laser. For the moment it is assumed that the mirrors are flat. One mirror has 100% reflectivity, whereas the other mirror partly transmits to couple some of the light out of the laser (see Fig. 2). The mirrors determine the direction in which the stimulated emission process may start. Only those light waves that are perpendicularly incident on the mirrors will be reflected back in the same direction. The reflected photons will interact again with the laser medium, will be amplified by stimulated emission, will reflect at the other mirror and the process will be repeated. Along the axis an amplified light beam will be generated when the correct interference condition is fulfilled (see hereafter). An obliquely incident wave will leave the resonator after one or more reflections at the mirrors (see Fig. 9), will not take part in the process of amplification, and will contribute to the energy loss of the laser.

A wave reflected parallel to the axis meets the wave incident on the mirror. As in the case of two sound or water waves of the same frequency, light waves may be added or subtracted and can be mutually extinguished. After reflection at both mirrors a light wave will return in itself. Only when the reflected wave and the original wave oscillate in phase does positive interference occur, and the wave will sustain itself. When the reflected wave oscillates out of phase with

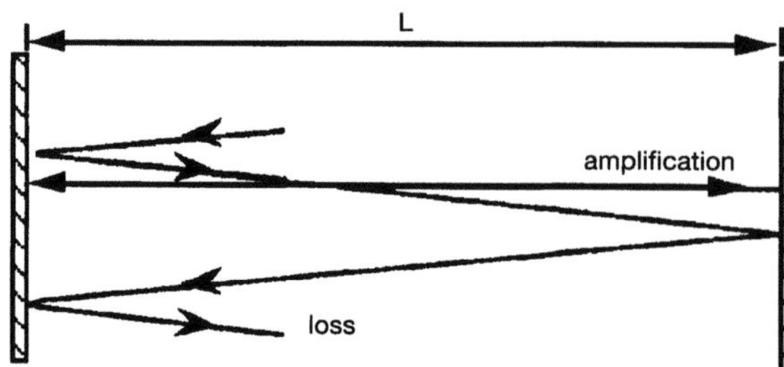

Fig. 9. Light rays within the laser cavity (schematically)

the original wave, they will interfere destructively and the wave will be extinguished. At positive interference, a pattern of standing waves with nodes and antinodes will exist between the mirrors (see Fig. 10), similar to a violin string under tension. Thus, the length of the laser cavity should be n $\times$ $\Lambda/2$, n = 1, 2, 3 ... etc., and is often long because of the amount of laser medium require to obtain population inversion and sufficient power. For a given length of the cavity, generally several wave patterns (..., n-1, n, n+1, ...) may be excited simultaneously within the gain profile of the laser. As these oscillations occur parallel to the optical axis, they are called the longitudinal modes of the laser.

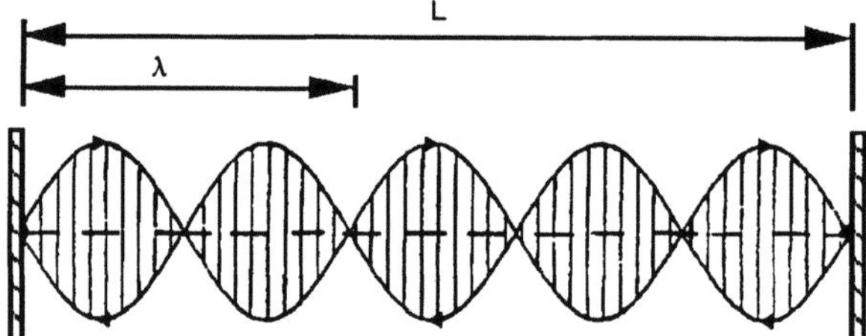

Fig. 10. Positive interference in laser cavity

Due to diffraction a light wave will always show some divergence. The consequence is that wave fronts will never be flat but always show some curvature. In the laser cavity diffraction effects are accounted for by using one or two concave mirrors with suitable radii of curvature (see Fig. 11).

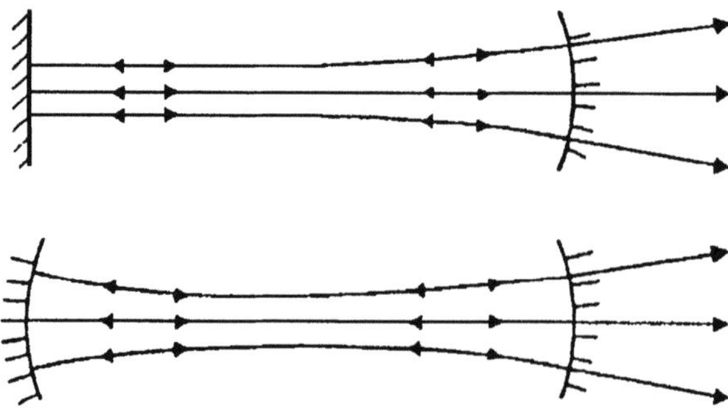

Fig. 11. Stable resonators with diverging laser beams

The curvature of the wave front at the mirror should equal the curvature of the mirror itself, so that perfect reflection of the light beam in itself occurs. In such a cavity modes may also be present that do not oscillate parallel to the optical axis. These transversal modes or transversal electro magnetic (TEM) modes describe the vibrational pattern in the radial direction. This in fact reflects the intensity distribution of the laser beam emitted by the laser in a (transversal) cross section. In these vibrational patterns nodes and antinodes also exist. The simplest intensity distribution is the TEM_{00} mode. Due to diffraction the intensity distribution over the radial beam profile is Gaussian (see Fig. 15). The next transversal mode, the TEM_{01} mode, only exists when the opening angle, mostly limited by the diameter of the laser tube or by a diaphragm, is sufficiently large. In the center of a TEM_{01} mode, there is a node, causing a doughnut-shaped three-dimensional intensity distribution of the laser beam. In Figure 12 the radial intensity distribution of the TEM_{00} and TEM_{01} modes are shown. In Figure 12a the simplest mode is shown, representing a light wave bouncing back and forth along the cavity axis. In Figure 12b the TEM_{01} mode is shown, representing two light waves parallel to the cavity axis.

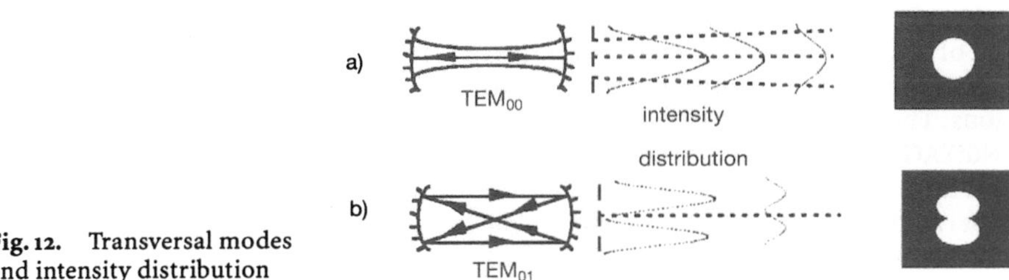

Fig. 12. Transversal modes and intensity distribution

Furthermore, higher-order modes may be observed. The occurrence of these modes increases the losses due to diffraction from the cavity as compared to the TEM_{00} mode. A laser oscillating on more transversal modes can produce considerably more power than a TEM_{00} laser, but optical imaging is complicated.

Examples of Lasers

Solid State Lasers

The first practical laser was the ruby laser. Ruby is a crystal of aluminium oxide (Al_2O_3) with 0.05% chromium oxide (Cr_2O_3) doping. The energy scheme with three levels only allows or pulsed laser action. A powerful flashlamp (a xenon lamp with a flash of about 1 or 2 ms) pumps energy in the system and the laser process repeats itself many times. The laser output shows a train of short, powerful light pulses with a duration of a few nanoseconds (10^{-9} s) at a wavelength of 694.3 nm (red light) as shown in Figure 13.

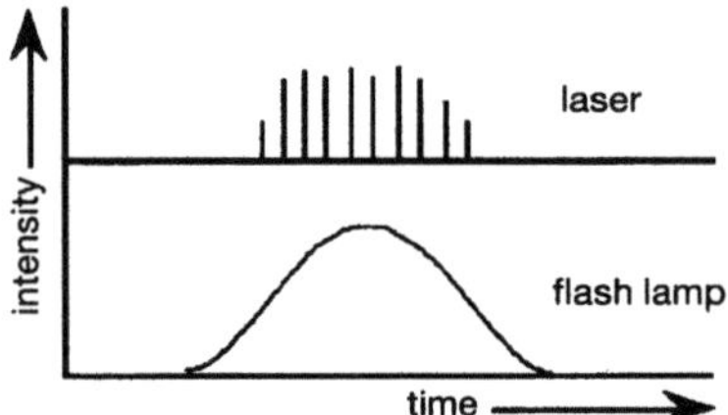

Fig. 13.   Intensity of energy pump and of ruby laser

It is possible to store (in the form of population inversion) all of the light energy from the pump inside the laser medium by preventing the early start of the stimulated emission process. For this purpose the laser resonator is made opaque for red light with an optical shutter. When the shutter is opened at the appropriate time (at the end of the flashlamp pulse), all of the stored energy will be released in one short, gigantic laser pulse, which is called Q switching. With this process, ruby pulses of 10^{-8} s with a peak power of 50 MW have been generated.

An important class of solid-state lasers is based on neodymium (Nd) ions, where by four levels are involved in laser operation. The laser medium is a crystal of $Y_3Al_5O_{12}$ (commonly called YAG after yttrium aluminium garnet), in which some of the yttrium ions are replaced by Nd ions, or just a glass doped with Nd ions. The strongest, most commonly used transition between energy levels in a Nd:YAG laser (selected by the cavity) is that producing 1.06-μm (near-infrared) radiation. Another transition yields 1.32-μm radiation. The Nd lasers can be operated both pulsed and continuously. In pulsed operation, when a powerful flashlamp (xenon lamp with a flash of about 1–2 ms) is used, the system does not produce a pulse train as in the ruby case, but Q switching is just as possible. In continuous operation a high pressure krypton lamp may act as an energy source. In this case short pulses of picosecond duration (10^{-12} s) may be generated using the technique of mode locking. A fast shutter is mounted inside the laser cavity. The shutter is opened at time intervals corresponding to the round-trip time of a photon in the cavity (t = c/2L). Only those waves in phase with the opening of the shutter will participate in laser action and will undergo stimulated emission, thus building up strong but short light pulses. A strong development towards pumping with diode lasers is in process.

An Nd:YAG rod may be 5–20 cm long with a diameter of 5–10 mm (as in the ruby case). Continuous powers up to 150 W from a single rod have been generated, whereas 1 kW could be produced using several rods in an amplifier configuration. In Q switched operation, peak powers of 500 MW are easily generated, more efficiently than in the ruby case. With mode locking, pulses of a few picoseconds have been produced.

Recently, wavelength-tuneable solid-state lasers pumped by fixed-frequency lasers have been introduced. The best-known example is the four-level titanium-sapphire (Ti:Al_2O_3) laser, tuneable in the wavelength range of 700–1000 nm. For pulsed operation it can be pumped, e.g., by the green light of a frequently doubled Nd:YAG laser (see "Non-linear Optical Devices"), whereas for continuous operation pumping with an Ar-ion laser is possible. With a 6-W

Ar-ion laser, about 1 W of continuous power may be generated at the peak of the Ti:sapphire tuning curve (800 nm). In pulsed operation some 100 mJ at a 10-Hz repetition rate have already been realized. Because of its high thermal conductivity, Ti:sapphire can be used in high power amplifier systems. High quality rods of 15 cm in length and 3.5 cm in diameter are presently available. Because of the large tuning range of Ti:sapphire, extremely short pulses may be generated in a mode-locking configuration. Pulses as short as 14 fs (14×10^{-15} s) have been produced.

Gas Lasers

The gas lasers are pumped with an electrical current (continuous or pulsed) through the gas. In the gas an electrical discharge is produced in which free electrons to a large extent provide electrical conduction. These electrons derive their energy from the electric field in the discharge and may excite, ionize, or dissociate atoms and molecules. The excited states decay under the emission of characteristic radiation.

Examples of gas lasers are:

The CO_2 Laser

The CO_2 laser is the most important surgical laser. In the gas discharge of this laser a mixture of CO_2-, N_2- and He gas is used. The precise composition of the gas mixture is determined by the type of laser. Laser action occurs between two ro-vibrational levels in the CO_2 molecule. The addition of the other gases strongly improves laser efficiency. The CO_2 laser is one of the most powerful lasers (a continuous output power of 100 kW has been obtained in a gas dynamic laser) and one of the most efficient (15%–20%). It can be used both pulsed and continuously. Laser action occurs preferentially at 10.6 µm (infrared). The laser may be tuned over several transitions in the wavelength range of 6–9 µm.

The Excimer Laser

In the excimer laser, light amplification takes place in a rather special two-atom molecule, a so-called excimer (excited dimer). These molecules are of the type in which only the excited state is stable, albeit for an short period of time only. When such a molecule decays to its ground state under the emission of a photon, it breaks apart and two free atoms remain. Important excimer lasers are those where a noble-gas atom (such as Ar, Kr, or Xe) in excited state binds with a halogen atom (such as F or Cl). These are the noble-gas-halogen excimer lasers. Examples are ArF (193 nm), KrF (248 nm), XeCl (308 nm), and XeF (355 nm), all producing ultraviolet light in short pulses. Pulse durations are in the order of 10^{-8}–10^{-6} s and averagy, output powers around a few hundred Watts, and pulse repetition frequencies up to 1 kHz are obtained with an efficiency of about 1%.

Argon and Kr-Ion Lasers

The argon laser operates at several wavelengths. The strongest lines are the 488 (blue-green) and 514.5 nm (green) transitions. Commercial lasers deliver a power of up to 25 W at all lines, whereas in the laboratory 200 W of continuous power have been produced. In the ultraviolet wavelength region around 350 nm, with special optics 3–7 W of power are currently available. It is possible to mode-lock the argon laser, and short pulses of about 200 ps may be produced.

The Kr-ion laser may also oscillate at several lines in the visible region. The strongest line is at 647 nm (red) and about 5 W are available. These lasers have a rather low efficiency of about 10^{-3} and thus consume a great amount of electrical power (up to 40 kW in commercial systems).

Copper- and Gold Vapor Lasers

The best-known metalvapor laser is the Cu laser. It produces light at 510 nm (green) and 578 nm (yellow). Average powers of 40–60 W at a repetition rate of 20 kHz have been obtained at the green line. The Cu laser is the most efficient green laser developed thus far. The Au laser emits at 628 nm (red) with an average power of 10 W at a repetition rate of 20 kHz, too. These lasers operate only in a pulsed way as the system is self-terminating as in the ruby case (see above).

Liquid Lasers (Dye Lasers)

The medium of a liquid laser is a solution of an organic molecule such as rhodamine 6G (xanthene dye) with, e.g., ethylene glycol as solvent. These soluble organic dyes strongly absorb light in the ultraviolet or visible part of the spectrum. After excitation with light of a suitable wavelength, they fluoresce intensely in a broad spectral band shifted towards longer wavelengths. The dye laser may be tuned over this broad fluorescence band.

The dye solution is injected into the laser cavity. Energy is supplied with light that fits the maximum in the absorption curve. Flashlamps (flashlamp-pumped dye lasers), pulsed lasers (excimer, Nd:YAG, and N_2 lasers), and continuous lasers (Ar-ion and Kr-ion lasers) may be used. To prevent dye heating in the intense pump light, the dye solution is pumped around. In order to cover the visible wavelength region, some 20 dyes are required. Wavelength tunability is achieved by tuning the optical elements inside or changing the length of the cavity over the fluorescence band of the dye. Modelocking of dye laser pumped by Ar-ion lasers is possible, and extremely short light pulses in the femtosecond can be generated. The shortest pulse produced is 6 fs. Using optical amplifiers, high peak powers may be generated.

Semiconductor Laser (Diode Laser)

In semiconductor materials laser action occurs in a slightly different way. In atoms or molecules the properties of the individual particles and their excited states play an important role. In semiconductor materials the possible, energy states and the material properties of the complete crystal have to be considered. Often the crystal itself acts as a cavity. When it is cut along a crystalaxis, two parallel endfaces are created. These endfaces are sometimes coated with a reflective layer, but this is not always necessary as the crystal endfaces themselves have a considerable reflectivity. Tuning of the laser is possible by temperature change of the diode or by variation of the electrical current through the diode. Current changes also induce temperature changes. In practice the tuning range is fairly limited.

In the most important class of diode lasers use is made of the semiconductor material $Ga_{1-x}Al_xAs$ (a GaAs crystal in which a fraction x of the gallium atoms is replaced by aluminium atoms). A higher percentage of Alatoms results in a shorter laser wavelength. This type of laser typically produces 20–30 mW of continuous output power at room temperature, and a wavelength region of 670–860 nm may be covered. Extension to still shorter wavelengths is being pursued. These lasers may be mode-locked, and light pulses as short as 5 ps have been produced. Higher output powers of up to the order of 20 W are continuous available with laserdiode arrays. An array is a row of adjacently grown coupled diodes each generating 20–30 mW. Higher peak powers have already been obtained in pulsed operation (microsecond pulses).

Nonlinear Optical Devices

In classical optics, the response of a medium to a weak beam of incident light is proportional to its intensity I while the frequency spectrum is unchanged (in the absence of atomic or molecular transitions). However, this no longer holds for strong (collimated or focussed) laser beams, and the response of the medium becomes nonlinear. As a result new frequencies may be generated inside the medium that are related to the incident frequency (nonlinear frequency conversion). When, e.g., a beam of monochromatic laser light of fixed frequency f enters a nonlinear crystal cut at a well-defined orientation angle a beam of light with frequency 2f may be generated with an intensity proportional to I^2 (frequency doubling). The crystal is nonlinear because along two different axes, different refractive indices exist (birefringence). Different refractive indices are required to fulfill the conservation laws of physics in the frequency doubling process (conservation of energy and conservation of momentum).

When two laser beams with the frequencies f_1 and f_2 enter a crystal a beam of light with the frequencies $f_1 +$ or f_2 or f_1 may be produced (sum- and difference frequency generation prospectively).

These nonlinear frequencyconversion techniques are now widely used to extend the wavelength ranges of existing laser systems into regions otherwise inaccessible, and more and more nonlinear crystals are becoming available for this purpose. Best-known is the frequency doubling of the 1064-nm infrared radiation from a Nd:YAG laser in a KTP crystal producing intense green light at 532 nm. Using both the 1064-nm and the 532-nm radiation in a sumfrequency scheme with another

KTP crystal, 355-nm ultraviolet radiation may be generated, whereas frequency doubling of the green light results in even shorter wavelength radiation at 266 nm. These techniques may also be applied to tuneable laser systems to produce, e.g., tuneable ultraviolet radiation. In the latter case a complication is that the crystal orientation is wavelength dependent and must be adjusted when tuning the lasers (angletuning). In some crystals these adjustments can also be made by changing the temperature of the nonlinear material (temperature tuning).

To conclude this section, a new nonlinear optical device will be discussed which holds promise in replacing pulsed dye lasers in the near future in many applications. This device is the optical parametric oscillator (OPO). As an example using the nonlinear crystal BBB (beta-barium borate) pumped by 355-nm UV light from an Nd:YAG laser, fairly broadband, tuneable radiation covering the complete wavelength range from 410 nm to 2.65 μm can be produced with only three sets of cavity mirrors and rather high pulse powers. In an OPO the opposite process of sumfrequency generation is realized. An incident photon with a frequency f is split in the nonlinear crystal into two frequencies f_1 and f_2 in such a way that $f = f_1 + f_2$. The frequencies of the two beams thus generated (highest frequency beam is called signal, lowest frequency beam is called idler) are determined by the orientation of the crystal that matches the incident wave with the generated waves. By rotating the crystal the frequencies can be tuned smoothly. In the example mentioned above, the signal beam can be tuned from about 410 nm to 710 nm; the idler beam then changes wavelength from 2.65 μm down to 710 nm. Signal and idler beam have the same wavelength at the degeneration point of 710 nm. To enhance conversion efficiency, the crystal is placed inside a cavity which in its simplest form involves only two plane mirrors (see Fig. 14), but more elaborate configurations such as a three-mirror ring cavity are also used. The cavity may be designed to be resonant for signal or idler beam (determined by the coatings on the mirrors of the cavity). In this way it is possible, when pumping a BBO-OPO with 300-mJ pulses from a 355-nm Nd:YAG laser, to generate tuneable radiation with pulses of at least 50 mJ in the signal beam.

OPOs based an different nonlinear materials such as BBO, LBO, and KTP have been designed and made operational. The BBO-OPO is the most promising candidate to replace the pulsed dye laser in the entire visible range.

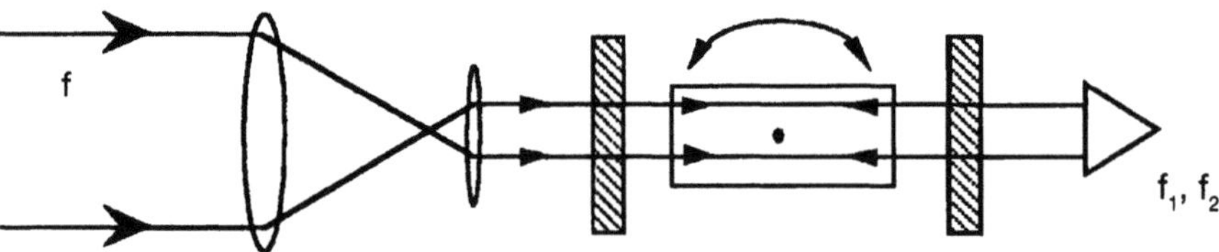

Fig. 14. An optical parametric oscillator. *f, f1,* and *f2* are frequencies

Summary and Survey

In Table 1 a survey is given of the properties and performances of some of the lasers of interest for medical applications. These properties are changing rapidly, so reliable specifications are hard to provide. In the table only some general characteristics are reported, which might only be correct as far as the order of magnitude is concerned. The table shows the large wavelength region in which lasers are available as well as the large variation in performance. Output powers

Table 1. Lasers and specifications

Laser type duration	Pulsed (P) Continuous(C)	Wavelength (nm)	Average power (W)	Peak power (kW)	Pulse (s)
Ruby	P	694.3	1	10	10^{-3}
	P, Q-switched		1	5×10^4	10^{-8}
	P, modelock		1	2×10^6	10^{-11}
Nd:YAG	P	1064	400	10	10^{-3}
	P, Q-switched		400	5×10^4	10^{-8}
	P, modelock		400	2×10^6	2×10^{-11}
	C		150	–	–
	C	1320	10	–	–
HeNe	C	632.8	15×10^{-3}	–	–
Cu	P	510	60	150	3×10^{-8}
	P	578			
Au	P	628	10	25	3×10^{-8}
Ar$^+$	C	514.5	10	–	–
	C	488	10	–	–
	P, modelock	514.5	2	0.1	2×10^{-10}
Kr$^+$	C	647	5	–	–
	C	413	1	–	–
	P, modelock	647	2	0.1	2×10^{-10}
HeCd	C	441		–	–
	C	325		–	–
CO$_2$	C	10 600	10^{-3}	–	–
	P	10 600		10^9	10^{-8}
Excimer			400		
	P	193			$10^{-7}–10^{-8}$
	P	248			$10^{-7}–10^{-8}$
	P	308			$10^{-7}–10^{-8}$
	P	351			$10^{-7}–10^{-8}$
Dye	C + P	400–900	0.13	100	10^{-13}–cont.
Ho:YAG	P	2100			4×10^{-4}
Er:YAG	P	2900			4×10^{-4}
GaAlAs	C	690–860	0.05	–	–
	P	640–860	0.05	10^{-3}	$10^{-11}–10^{-12}$

from a few milliwatts up to many tens of kilowatts may be continuously produced. Peak powers of 10^{14} W are available, and pulses as short as 10^{-14} s have been generated. This enormous variety in laser types provides extensive opportunities for many applications.

Beam Delivery

Introduction

Once laser radiation has been generated it has to be directed to the tissue to produce the required laser-tissue interaction. In principle laser radiation can be delivered to tissue in one of four different ways:
1. By direct illumination
2. By means of a fiber, with or without a special fiber tip
3. By means of an articulated arm containing mirrors
4. By means of a special setup or device consisting of optical components such as lenses, mirrors, fibers, beam splitters, etc.; the Hexascan for the treatment of port-wine stains is such an example

The following paragraphs describe the behavior of a TEM_{00} laser beam which is the best collimated beam available, the behavior of such a beam when passing through a lens, and the handling of a laser beam by means of optical fibers, and a brief description of an articulated arm and some devices for light delivery is given.

The Properties of a TEM_{00} Laser Beam

Most lasers, but certainly not all, emit their beam in the so-called TEM_{00} mode. TEM refers to the standing electromagnetic waves in the resonant cavity and stands for "transverse electric and magnetic" mode. The TEM_{00} mode is the lowest order mode and has a smooth cylindrical Gaussian distribution (see also above). Although a laser beam can possess the highest degree of collimation possible in nature, it always has some divergence, and the TEM_{00} mode laser beam has the lowest divergence. Higher modes like TEM_{01} or TEM_{11} exhibit more peaks in the intensity distribution and larger divergence. The following will only take the TEM_{00} mode into account. The radial cross section of a TEM_{00} beam has a Gaussian profile (see Fig. 15).

A Gaussian bell has no distinct boundary. By convention the radius of the beam is defined as the radius at which the intensity is $1/e^2$ times (13.5%) the maximum at radius zero. This radius is denoted by w. Every TEM_{00} beam is characterized by a beam waist where the radius w has a minimum denoted as w_0. Here the wave front is completely flat. Often w_0 is found at the exit of the laser. Due to diffraction the wave fronts start to curve, leading to an increase in the radius w (divergence); therefore the radius is a function of the distance z along the optical axis (see Fig. 16).

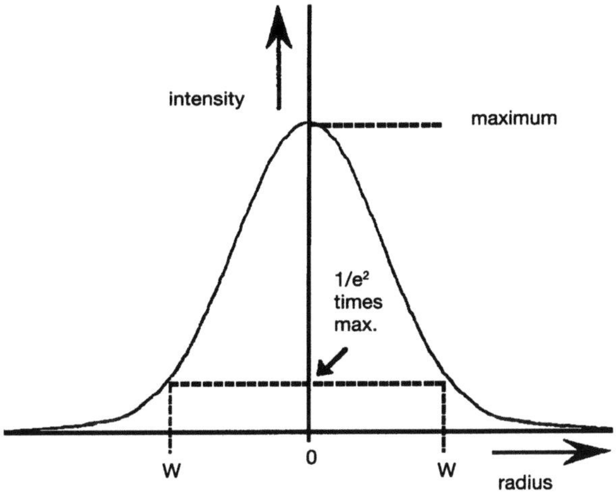

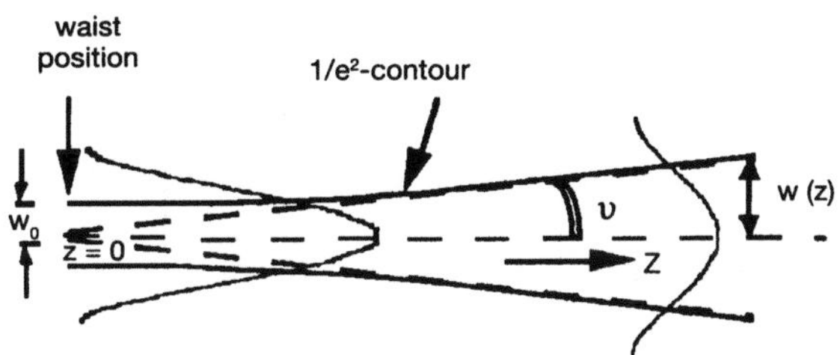

Fig. 15. The distribution of the laser power as a function of the distance (radius) from the optical axis at radius o. The radius *w* of a laser beam is defined as the position where the intensity has fallen to $1/e^2$ times (13.5%) the maximum on the optical axis

Fig. 16. At the beam waist a TEM00 beam has a minimum radius w_0. Due to diffraction the beam spreads after passing the waist position, and the radius w increases. While the beam travels along the z-axis, the intensity cross section remains Gaussian. The $1/e^2$ contour gradually approaches a cone with an angle Δ the divergence angle of the beam

It is stressed that the energy distribution retains its Gaussian shape and only the radius w increases. The contour w(z) has a hyperbolical shape, meaning that the beam far away from the waist position can be considered as a cone with a half angle D. Usually the waist is located at the front near the exit aperture of the laser beam. The divergence of a TEM_{00} beam can be small indeed. For example, an argon laser emitting a single-line (one wavelength) TEM_{00} beam at 514.5 nm (green) has a waist radius of typically 1 mm; the divergence angle is 0.009 deg. This is hardly observable; indeed such a laser beam looks like the ultimate light ray. Only at very large distances can the spreading be seen. For instance, the radius w at a distance of 100 m has become 16 times larger and is 1.6 cm.

For small waist diameters the divergence angle Δ can be quite large. A small waist can be obtained by focussing a laser beam using a lens. Essentially a lens transforms one waist to another. This will be treated later.

Therefore, although a laser beam may seem very collimated, the extent of the beam divergence is dependent on the waist diameter. A measure of the degree of collimation is the so-called waist length L. The waist length L is defined as the distance along the optical axis at which the initial waist w_0 increases to a waist

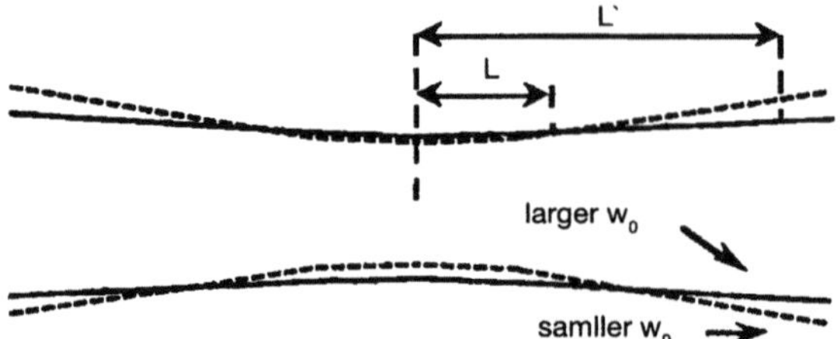

Fig. 17. Comparison of two TEM_{00} beams of equal wavelength. The beam with the smallest waist radius *(smaller w_o)* has a larger divergence and shorter waist length L than the beam with the larger waist radius *(smaller w_o)* has a larger divergence and shorter waist length L than the beam with the larger waist radius *(larger w_o, waist length L)*

w of w_0 times $\sqrt{2}$. Figure 17 shows how the waist length, divergence, and waist radius are related.

The waist length for the argon beam as treated above is 6.1 m. Applications by illumination directly from the laser cavity are quite rare in medicine. In most cases, for practical reasons or reasons of dosimetry, optical components (such as lenses, fibers, etc.) are used for projection of the laser radiation on tissue.

The Behavior of a TEM_{00} Beam Through a Lens

The behavior of light from a conventional source through a lens is described by the well-known lens formula (see Fig. 18a):

$$\frac{1}{d_1} + \frac{1}{d_2} = \frac{1}{f} \tag{8}$$

Where d_1 is the distance from the object to the lens, d_2 the distance of the image to the opposite side of the lens, and f the focal length of the lens. The magnification is d_1/d_2. Here an object is imaged by the lens.

A laser represents something similar. Here a waist is transformed to another waist (see Fig. 18b), and the divergence and waist length of the beam behind the lens are determined by the new waist radius w'_o.

The waist-to-waist projection can be described by a similar equation as the lens formula. However, here d_1 and d_2 must be substituted by the so-called complex radii of curvature of the wave fronts q_1 and q_2 at the front and back of the lens.

The concept of a complex radius follows from the mathematical analysis of the Maxwell equations but goes far beyond the intent of this treatise; however, these concepts are necessary to reach the proper result for a waist-to-waist projection.

Usually one wants to focus a laser beam to a small spot, for instance, in order to couple the energy in a light guide or optical fiber.

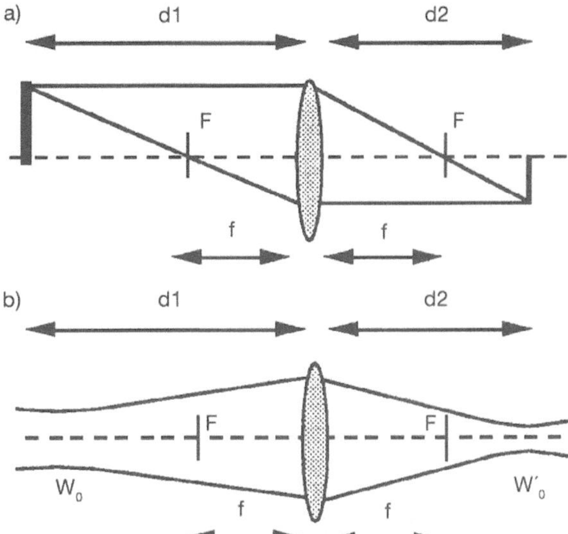

Fig. 18. **a** The imaging of an object by a lens. d_1 and d_2 are the distances from object and image to the lens. F denotes the focal points, f is the focal length. **b** The waist-to-waist transformation of a TEM00 beam by the same lens. d_1 and d_2 are the distances of the original and new waists to the lens

As seen above, a beam can have a long waist length and is nearly collimated. If one stays well within the waist length, the beam can be considered to be parallel and the beam diameter is 2 w$_0$. Mathematically this means that the waist length L is much larger than d_1–f (see Fig. 19).

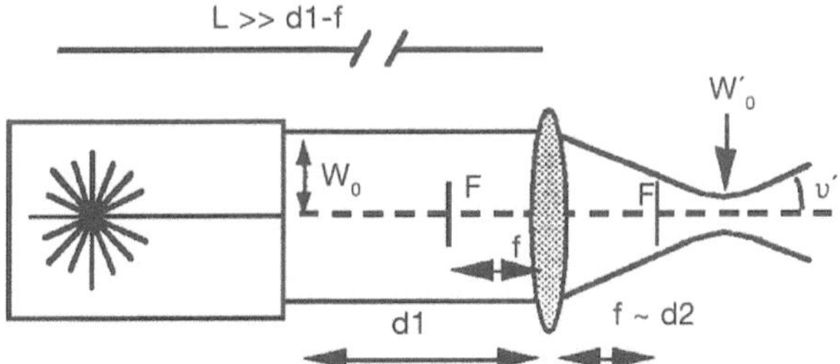

Fig. 19. The focussing of a TEM$_{00}$-collimated beam. The lens is placed well within the waist length of the beam ($L \gg d_1$-f); therefore the beam radius is (nearly) equal to the waist radius w_0. A new, very small waist is formed at the focal point behind the lens. Behind this new waist the beam is much more divergent with angle υ

Under these conditions for a collimated laser beam, the waist after focussing is located at approximately the focal point of the lens. Thus extremely small spot sizes can be obtained when focussing a laser beam. In this case the new waist radius is given by

$w_0' = f\lambda/(\pi w_0)$, the divergence angle υ´ is given by υ´ = w_0/f.

A note of caution has to be made: high power laser beams might destroy objectives because of the unavoidable residual absorption in the material that glues together the separate lenses constituting the objective (a rule of thumb is that one has to avoid powers beyond 20 W). A very reasonable alternative is the use of so-called laser singlets. These are single lenses optimized for a minimum of spherical aberration. Using an optimized single lens, the spot size is only some 30% larger than the theoretical limit. These lenses can handle high laser powers and are supplied by all major optical companies.

Fiber Delivery

Many applications in medicine are performed using optical fibers. By employing optical fibers, it is possible to direct the major part of the energy of a laser beam to sites such as vessels and internal organs which it would otherwise never reach without surgery. Essentially, an optical fibre is a thin, flexible glass or quartz rod in which light, when trapped inside, is transported along the total length. This length can be very great, such as the distance between Europe and America (plans for a fiber optic communication link). The principle of light being confined is depicted in Figure 20. The glass or quartz rod (the core) is surrounded by a cladding with a lower index of refraction than the rod. From basic optics it follows that when light is incident on this core-cladding interface at angles greater than a critical angle, the light is totally reflected. This critical angle is dependent on the difference of the indices of refraction between core and cladding. Once totally reflected, the light is reflected totally every time it hits the boundary. Thus the light stays in the fiber. The fibers can be made so thin that

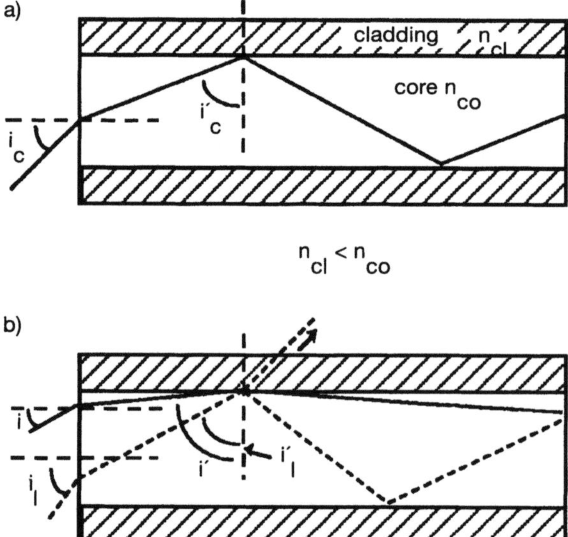

Fig. 20. The entrance end of an optical fiber. The indices of refraction of the core and of the cladding are n_{co} and n_{cl} with $n_{cl} < n_{co}$. a i'_c is the critical angle for total reflection. **a, b** The rays drawn as *solid lines* enter the fiber at angles smaller than or equal to i_c and will be reflected totally in the fiber. The *dotted line* depicts a ray entering at an angle i_I. The ray will partially be transmitted through the cladding and will eventually leak out of the fiber. So only light entering in a cone determined by i_c will be transported through the fiber.

they can easily be bent to a small radius without breaking. In a bend the angles at which the light hits the boundary can change so that part of the light is incident below the critical angle. In this way part of the light can escape from the fiber. However, in most applications this loss is negligible, and the majority of light is emitted through the fiber. One has to bear in mind that some light might be lost by absorption into the fiber material. As will be clear from Fig. 20, at the entrance of the fiber only light that is incident in a cone at angles smaller than i_c will be totally reflected inside the fiber.

This is the acceptance cone of the fiber. Light incident at larger angles is not totally reflected in the fiber and will leak gradually out of the fiber. The acceptance cone is usually given by the numerical aperture (N.A.) which is defined as:

$$N.A. = \sin i_c \tag{9}$$

From Snell´s Law it follows that:

$$N.A. = \sqrt{n_{co}^2 - n_{cl}^2} \tag{10}$$

Here the properties of a TEM_{oo} beam and optical fibers meet. As described above it is possible to focus the beam to a small spot that can be positioned at the flat end of a fiber (see Fig. 21).

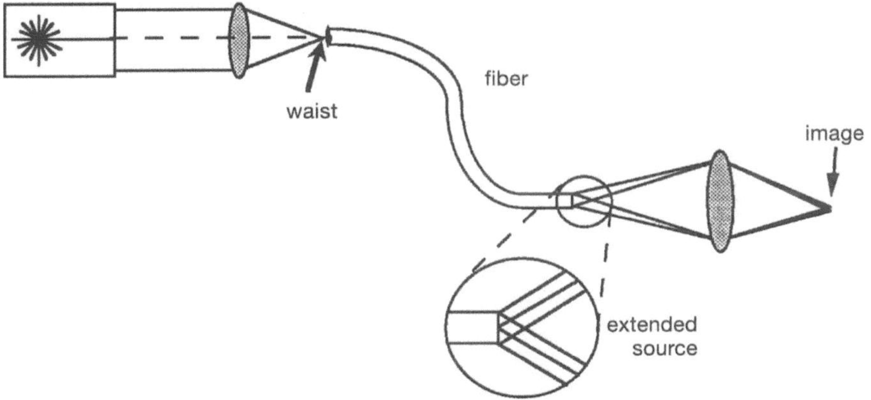

Fig. 21.   A laser beam is coupled into a fiber by focussing a waist within the acceptance cone of the fiber onto the entrance face. At the exit face these light is emitted in all directions within the numerical aperture at all points of the core. Thus, the exit face has become an extended source. This means that the focussing of light energy from this source obeys the "normal" lens imaging properties.

If the divergence angle υ (or better: convergence angle in this case) falls within the acceptance cone of the fiber then all of the light power (apart from reflection which is in the order of 4%) is trapped in the fiber and will be transported to the other end.

In telecommunication fibers with core diameters of a few micrometers are used. These are so-called monomode fibers that preserve the TEM_{00} properties of the laser beam. However, these fibers are not able to withstand the high laser powers necessary in most medical applications. Therefore, in most medical applications fibers with core diameters of about 100 μm to 1 mm are used to guide the laser light. As seen above, it is no problem to focus the spot to a spot that falls completely in the core area. State-of-the-art fibers are clear enough to be able to transport several hundreds of watts.

At the exit (distal) end of the fiber, the light is emitted in the same cone determined by the N.A. Usually the light is incident at the entrance (proximal) side in a cone smaller than the N.A. When a fiber is completely straight and optically clear, and the entrance and exit faces are completely flat, the exit cone is equal to the entrance cone. However, due to bending of the fiber and unavoidable impurities present in the core, the exit cone is usually completely filled up to the N.A. Very important is the phenomenon that partly due to bending and imperfections but also due to the large diameter of the fiber core compared to the wavelength, the light is redistributed in the fiber. Because of this, the diameter of the core is completely filled with light. Every point within the core diameter at the exit face emits light in a cone determined by the N.A. This means that the exit face becomes an extended source (as opposed to the collimated beam of a laser that can be considered a point source), and the TEM_{00} properties are lost. It also means that the light cannot be considered to originate from a single point. Therefore it is not possible to focus the light to such a small spot as can be done with the original beam. Depending on the bending and the quality of the coupling of the laser, the output is more or less (usually less) Gaussian in distribution.

So, although optical fibers are very convenient for transporting laser light, it is not possible to obtain the initial power density from the original laser beam. Nevertheless, the light from a fiber can be completely imaged into a spot as depicted in Fig. 21. A rule of thumb is that practically a one-to-one imaging is the best that can be obtained with a well-designed optical system. For example, a widely used fiber is a quartz fiber with a core diameter of 600 μm. Assume the fiber end which emits 10 W of light is imaged one-to-one using a singlet lens with a focal length of 20 mm. Therefore the diameter of the spot is also 600 μm (0,6 mm). The area of the spot is 0.28 mm². Therefore the power density is:

$$\frac{10\ W}{0{,}28\ mm^2} = 35{,}7\ W/mm^2 \tag{11}$$

This is about 5000 times less than can be obtained by focussing the unspoiled TEM_{00} beam by the same lens.

Optical fibers can be used to deliver light to skin or eye, to all tissues than can be reached through natural orifices by endoscopes and through small artificial openings to vessel walls (laser angioplasty) and internal organs (in minimal invasive surgery such as laparoscopic surgery). Furthermore, a fiber can be positioned within the tissue through a needle. Often a so-called bare fiber is used. The fiber tip of a bare fiber has not been modified in any way. A fiber tip can be modified by mounting a special cap on the fiber tip, or by reshaping the tip itself. Caps of various shapes and materials have been used, such as metal, quartz, and sapphire. In a metal tip the laser energy is absorbed, thus giving a hot tip without any light distribution within the tissue. By using translucent materials of different shapes and indices of refraction or by reshaping the fiber tip itself, one can influence the light distribution coming from the fiber. Examples are sapphire tips which are used as a laser scalpel, and cylindrical diffusers which used in interstitial and photodynamic therapy (see below). The energy delivered to tissue by means of a cylindrical diffuser is expressed in Joules per diffuser length (J/cm).

All applications in which laser light is incident on an air-tissue interface are examples of noncontact irradiation. An example of contact irradiation is light application through a fiber that is held against the tissue surface. If the fiber is positioned inside the tissue, one speaks of interstitial light delivery. Figure 22 gives different examples of light application.

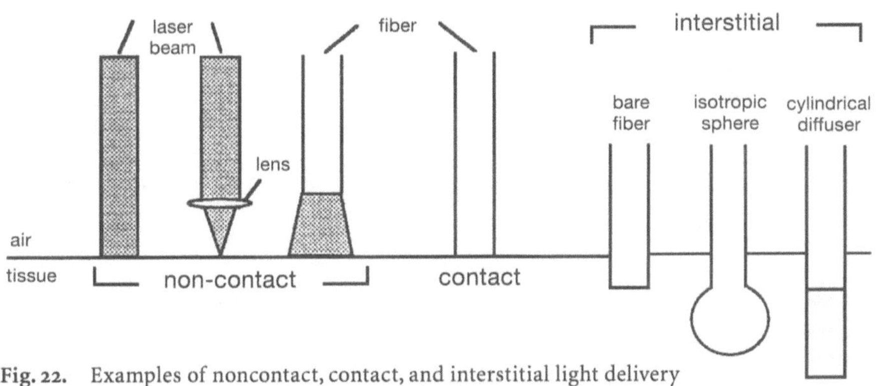

Fig. 22. Examples of noncontact, contact, and interstitial light delivery

Articulated Arm

At some wavelengths or at high power densities, it is not possible to use a fiber because absorption of the core material is too large at that wavelength or because dielectric breakdown occurs in the fiber material which may damage the proximal fiber end. Alternatives such cases are rigid articulated optical arms with various mirrors or hollow wave guides. Figure 23 shows an articulated arm as is used for a CO_2 laser. Fibers that can be used in combination with a CO_2 laser have been developed recently. The brittleness of these experimental fibers is still a problem in routine clinical use.

Devices for Light Delivery

For some applications special devices have been developed. These devices consist of optical components such as lenses, fibers, prisms, beam splitters, etc., in

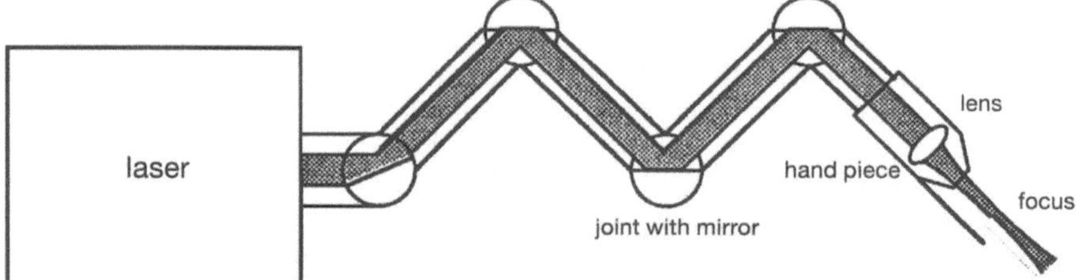

Fig. 23. An articulated arm as used for a CO_2 laser

combination with computer control. Various types of these devices are available for the treatment of port-wine stains in adults and children. An example is the Hexascan, a device that can be used in combination with various lasers. An example that is used in ophthalmology is the fully computerized cornea shaping device which utilizes a 193-nm ArF excimer laser beam able to ablate the cornea in a very controlled way.

Absorption, Scattering, and Light Propagation in Turbid Media

Introduction

The above section discussed how laser light is transported from the laser to the biological target. When laser light is incident perpendicularly on tissue in air (noncontact irradiation), about 4% of the incident intensity (called irradiance) is reflected directly due to a mismatch in refractive index (Fresnel reflection). The remaining 96% will be either absorbed or scattered.

If tissues were only absorbing, nonscattering media, the spatial light distribution in response to laser irradiation could be described by simple exponential attenuation. Actual light distributions in tissue, where scattering is important, can be substantially different from those estimated when scattering is neglected. As tissues are turbid media for wavelengths between about 250 nm and 1200 nm, light scattering has to be considered. Scattering of light in tissue can cause a photon to pass several times through the same location, thus enhancing the probability of absorbtion of that photon by a tissue molecule relative to a nonscattered photon that passes only once. For strongly scattering tissues, this implies that more photons are available for absorption within the tissue than based on the incident intensity. At wavelengths at which absorption is relatively low (in many tissues between (600 nm and 1500 nm), this increase in available light may have a factor of 2 or 3. Even larger ratios (4 to 7) may occur for a hollow organ such as the bladder. Also, scattering extends the available light beyond the lateral dimension of the incident beam. After one or more scattering events, photons might be scattered out of the tissue. The sum of the direct reflection and the photons that are scattered out of the tissue in the direction of the source is called the remittance. The magnitude of the scattering effects and their importance depend

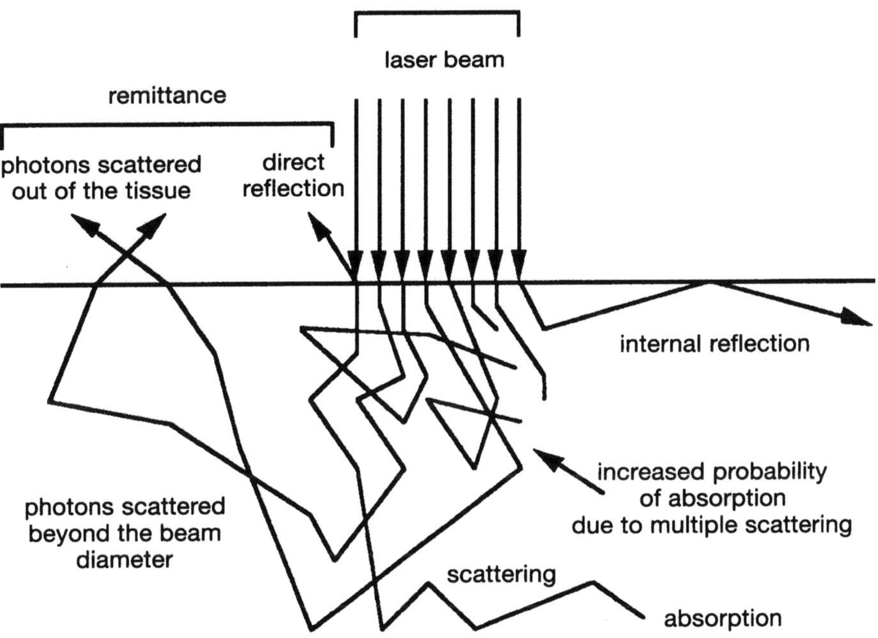

Fig. 24.   Light transport within tissue

strongly on the scattering and absorbing abilities of the tissue, the refractive index of the tissue, and the diameter of the laser spot. Figure 24 gives examples of
scattering and absorption in tissue.

The ability of tissues to absorb (laser) light and to convert light energy into
heat is the essence of thermal laser-tissue interactions (see below) such as
coagulation or vaporization. The rate of heat production in the tissue is the
product of absorption and the available amount of light energy. Tissue absorption can vary strongly over the wavelength range of clinical laser medicine
(from 193 nm to 10–600 nm). In the ultra-violet region (< 300 nm), the cell proteins and nuclear acids primarily are the absorbing chromophores in the tissue,
causing high tissue absorption coefficients. Absorption in the visible and near
infrared (400–1200 nm) is primarily due to the presence of chromophores
such as hemoglobin, flavins, cytochromes, and carotenoids. In the infrared
(> 1200 nm), water becomes the main absorbing element within the tissue spe-
cies. These various endogenous chromophores are responsible for the wide variability of tissue absorption at various wavelengths.

In contrast, tissue scattering is greatest at shorter wavelengths and decreases monotonically with increasing wavelength. However, the net light distribution in tissue depends strongly upon the ratio of scattering to absorption.
An example is that the Nd:YAG laser (1064 nm) for nonpigmented tissues is
known to result in deeper tissue effects than the argon laser (488 and 514.5 nm).

However, scattering is greater at the argon wavelengths than at the Nd:YAG wavelengths. The reason for the greater penetration at 1064 nm is that the ratio of scattering to absorption is greater at 1064 nm than at 488 or 514.5 nm.

It is the purpose of this chapter to demonstrate the effect of scattering upon the distribution of light in tissue. Some mathematical definitions will be presented.

Definitions

Absorption and Scattering Parameters

A tissue consists of different scattering particles that probably are not randomly distributed, as tissue is an organized structure. The scattering coefficient, as it is defined for tissue optics, simplifies tissue to a medium with randomly distributed scatterers with a minimum distance between these scatterers of at least three times their average radius of the particles apart. Furthermore, it is assumed that scattering occurs with reference to intensity only (and not polarization and/or amplitude). Thus any kind of interference is ignored. Given these assumptions, the scattering coefficient represents the probability that a photon travelling a certain infinitesimal distance is scattered, which is expressed by μ_s. Similarly, the absorption coefficient represents the probability that a photon travelling a certain infinitesimal distance is absorbed. The absorption coefficient is expressed by μ_a. Both the absorption and scattering coefficients are expressed in units of reciprocal length (e.g., cm^{-1} or mm^{-1}). The reciprocal of μ_a or μ_s represents the average distance that a photon travels without being absorbed or scattered (mean free path of absorption or scattering).

Scattering is generally assumed to depend only on the angle O between incoming and outgoing directions of the scattered photon. Such an assumption neglects the fact that some tissues (such as striated muscle) have a preferred scattering axis. The probability of scattering over the angle O can either be constant (isotropic scattering) or depend on O (anisotropic scattering). Human and animal tissues are now known to scatter strongly forwards. A measure of the degree of anisotropy in scattering is the anisotropy factor g, with $g = 1$ meaning totally forward scattering and $g = 0$ meaning isotropic scattering. Mathematically, g is defined as the average cosine of the scattering angle O over all possible angles. For in vitro tissues, g turns out to be between about 0.7 and 0.99.

Optical Depth, Albedo, and Penetration Depth

From the optical depth and the albedo of a tissue, the absorption and scattering coefficients can be derived.

The optical depth τ is defined as a distance (z) times the sum of the absorption and scattering coefficients:

$$\tau = (\mu_s + \mu_a)z \tag{12}$$

If the optical properties of a slab of tissue are considered, the optical depth can be given as the optical thickness of that slab, in which case the distance (z) is substituted by the thickness (d) of the slab. An optical depth of is sometimes referred to as a mean free path. A mean free path is the average distance a photon will travel before interacting with the tissue through either absorption or scattering. The optical depth is dimensionless.

The albedo is the ratio of scattering to absorption and scattering:

$$a = \frac{\mu_s}{(\mu_s + \mu_a)} \qquad (13)$$

If the albedo is 0 (i.e., $\mu_s = 0$), all of the light that interacts with the medium is absorbed and none is scattered. Conversely, when the albedo is 1 (i.e., $\mu_a = 0$), no light is absorbed by the medium. This is called conservative scattering. The albedo gives the fraction of light scattered as it travels one optical depth (a mean free path). Note that the albedo is dimensionless as well. Dimensionless optical parameters are advantageous because they combine related quantities to make one parameter.

For example, being told that the scattering coefficient is 1 mm⁻¹ provides little useful information without supporting knowledge of the absorption coefficient. If the absorption coefficient is 10 mm⁻¹, the medium is strongly absorbing; if the absorption coefficient is 0.1 mm⁻¹, then the medium is strongly scattering. One must know the characteristic dimensions of the object being studied. Dimensionless parameters provide all the information of in two numbers – the albedo and the optical depth.

The penetration depth has to be distinguished from the optical depth. The penetration depth is defined as that depth in the tissue at which the incident irradiance I_0 decreased by a factor of 1/e (to approximately 36.8% of the incident irradiance).

Irradiance and Fluence Rate

The light that is incident on the air-tissue boundary is called the irradiance, the light present within the tissue is called the fluence rate.

The irradiance (E) at a given point on the air-tissue boundary is the radiant power incident on an infinitesimally small surface element around that point, divided by the area of that surface element. E is expressed in watts per area.

The fluence rate (ϕ) at a given point (in the tissue) is the total power that passes through the surface of an infinitesimally small sphere, centered around that point and divided by the cross paragraphal area of the sphere. Fluence rate is expressed in watts per area. The spatial distribution of the fluence rate in tissue is the key to the thermal use of lasers in medicine because the local volumetric heat production (Q) is equal to the product of (local) absorption coefficient $\mu_a(r)$ and (local) fluence rate $\phi(r)$. Q is expressed in watts per volume, and r denotes the location in the tissue:

$$Q(r) = \mu a(r)\, \phi(r) \qquad (14)$$

The above equation is the source term for heat production in the bioheat equation for calculation of temperature distributions in laser irradiated tissue.

Transport Equation

The equation of radiative transfer is generally assumed to be the golden standard for light propagation in turbid media. The equation originates from the photon energy balance of the radiance incident upon a cylindrical volume with infinitesimal cross section and infinitesimal length. The radiance represents the (local) power density flowing in a certain direction and confined within an infinitesimal solid angle. The transport equation is an integrodifferential equation, and analytical solutions for situations of interest in clinical laser medicine are generally not available. Recently, numerical Monte Carlo codes have become available that produce solutions to the transport equation under clinical laser conditions.

Absorption and Scattering Properties of Tissues

Experimental results clearly show that
a) tissues are strongly forward-scattering materials,
b) that scattering is stronger at shorter wavelengths, and
c) that tissues can have strongly varying absorption depending on wavelength.

Figures 25 and 26 show the absorption coefficient of blood and water, respectively.

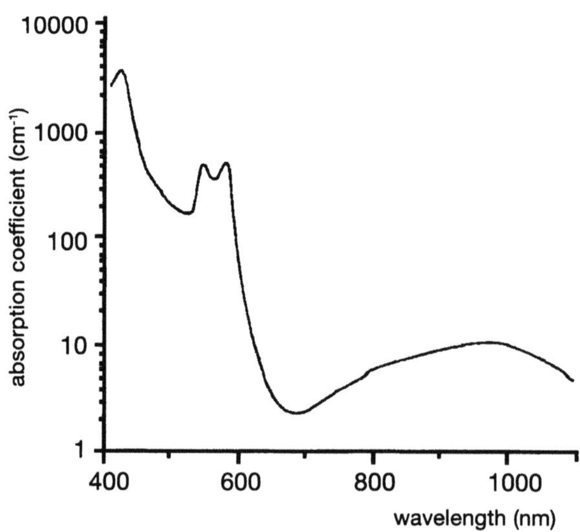

Fig. 25. Absorption coefficient of oxyhemoglobin in whole blood as a function of wavelength

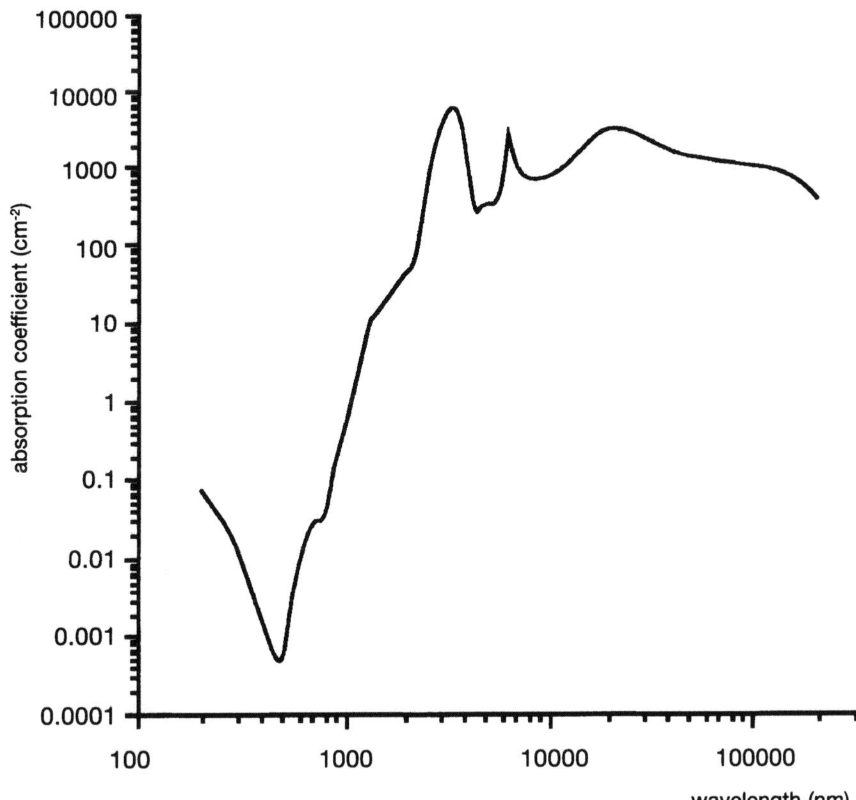

Fig. 26. Absorption coefficient of water as a function of wavelength

Figure 25 explains the hemostatic properties of the Nd:YAG laser at 1064 nm and of the Ar frequency-doubled Nd:YAG laser (using a KTP crystal) at 488/514.5 nm and 532 nm respectively (high absorption coefficient for oxyhemoglobin at 488/514.5 nm and 532 nm and relatively high coefficient at 1064 nm). Figure 26 explains the shallow penetration depth of the CO_2 laser at 10 600 nm (high absorption coefficient for water at 10 600 nm).

Figure 27 shows the estimated penetration depth in tissue as a function of wavelength.

Dependence of the Fluence Rate on the Beam Diameter

Figure 28 shows the dependence of the fluence rate on the beam diameter at 476 nm.

In this case human aortic tissue at 476 nm is modelled. The index of refraction is 1.5. The optical coefficients are $\mu_a = 0.6$ mm^{-1}, $\mu_s = 41.4$ mm^{-1}, $g = 0.91$. The fluence rate on the center line of a flat beam, normalized to the incident irradiance, in-

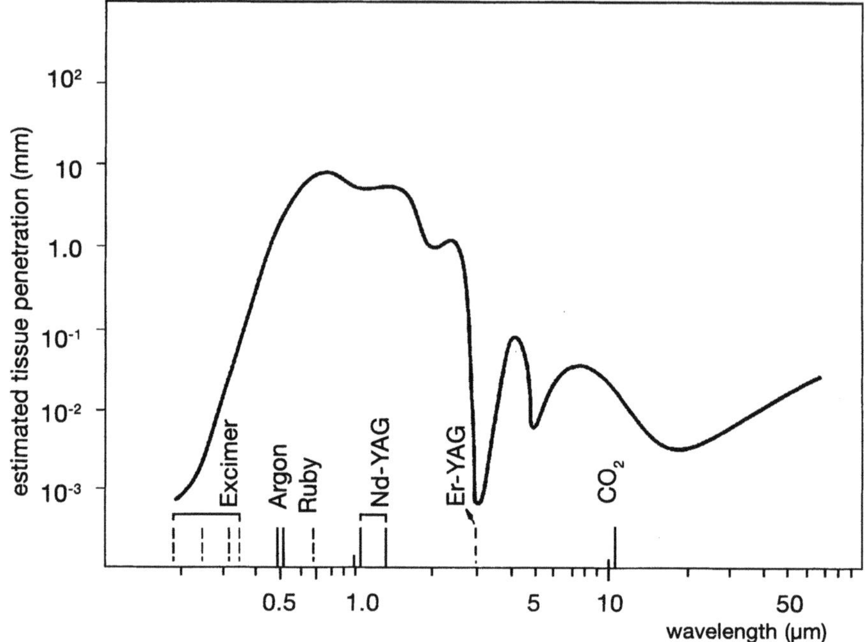

Fig. 27. Estimated penetration depth in tissue as a function of wavelength [penetration depth defined as that depth in the tissue at which the incident irradiance I_o has decreased by a factor of 1/e (to approximately 36.8%) of the incident irradiance]

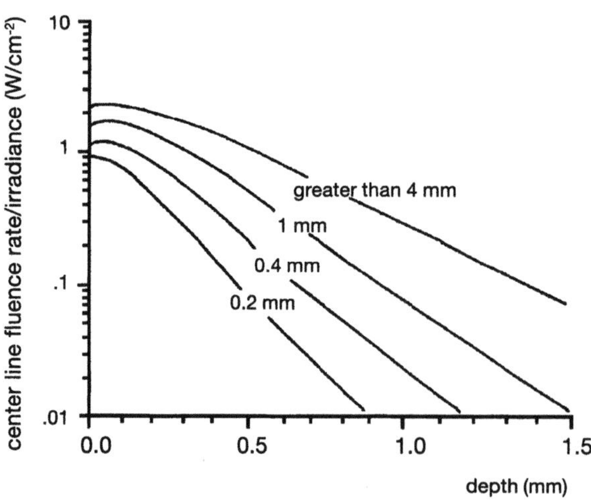

Fig. 28. Center line fluence rate/irradiance as a function of tissue depth for various values of the beam diameter. Optical properties used are: $\mu_a = 1.32$ mm⁻¹, $\mu_s = 41.4$ mm⁻¹, $g = 0.91$ which represent human aortic tissue at 476 mn. μ_a, absorption coefficient; μ_s, scattering coefficient; g, anisotropy factor

creases with beam diameter because light is scattered from the rest of the beam onto the center line. As the beam diameter increases, more light is available for scattering, and the fluence rate on the center line increases. However, once the beam reaches a diameter of about 4 mm, further increases in beam diameter cannot affect the center line fluence rate because light is absorbed before reaching the center line. Thus, in this tissue, once the beam diameter is larger than 4 mm, the fluence rate on the center line can be predicted with a one-dimensional model.

Laser-Tissue Interactions

Interaction of Laser Light with Tissue

In the previous chapter the phenomena describing the distribution of light in tissue were discussed. The interaction between laser light on the one hand with its characteristics such as wavelength, power density, duration, and exposure (pulsed, continuous wave) and the tissue with its biological composition and the presence of "chromophores" on the other will determine the possible effect of laser radiation.

Six laser-tissue interactions will be distinguished in this chapter:
1. A thermal interaction where by the absorbed light is converted into heat.
2. A photochemical interaction during which light absorbed by a photosensitizer-like hematoporphyrin derivative induces a chemical reaction.
3. A mechanical interaction with light producing stress or shock wave.
4. A photoablative interaction in which ultraviolet light energy is assumed to break chemical bonds, thus creating gaseous debris; the tissue is removed by the expansion of this gas.
5. Biostimulation or low level laser therapy during which light stimulates tissue healing by a mechanism yet unknown.
7. Fluorescence where by light is absorbed by some of the tissue molecules and reemitted at a longer wavelength.

Thermal Laser-Tissue Interaction

Introduction

Most laser applications in medicine today are based on thermal laser-tissue interaction. This interaction involves four distinct phenomena: conversion of light into heat, temperature rise as a function of time and position, tissue damage, and the late biological wound healing response. Except for the latter phenomenon, they can be modelled.

Temperature Ranges

Which tissue alterations can be induced by this conversion of light energy to heat? One can distinguish several ranges of temperature with various types of tissue damage.

41°–44°C. Such a moderate temperature increase for several minutes causes irreversible damage to malignant tissue and reversible damage to healthy tissue. This interaction is called (photo)hyperthermia. When interstitial fibers are used to establish this effect, one speaks of interstitial laser hyperthermia (ILH). The action mechanism of hyperthermia is based on the thermosensibility of cells, which in the S phase differs from that in other phases.

45°–60°C. During short expositions (a few seconds) no tissue damage occurs. However, a temperature increase to a temperature of 45°–60°C for 10–30 s causes irreversible damage to healthy and malignant tissue by loosening of membranes, denaturation of proteins (e.g., enzymes) and cell death. In tissue welding, denaturation of tissue proteins is used to reanastomose vessels, tubular structures, nerves, and skin.

60°–100°C. A temperature increase for 0.5–30 s causes irreversible damage by denaturation of proteins. The reaction of collagen important is these structures loosen the trihelical configuration and shrink, as can clearly be observed in the tissue just beside the laser impact. This coagulation reaction in the collagen of blood vessels accounts for part of the hemostatic activity of the thermal lasers. Additionally, hemostasis is also stimulated by shrinkage of perivascular collagen due to heat conductions. Secondary intravascular thrombosis completes the process.

100°C. At this temperature water turns into steam. Once it is reached, further thermal energy delivered will be used to evaporate the tissue. When water is being converted into steam, it shows a substantial increase in volume. As a consequence the cell explodes and steam and cellular particles are launched into the air, the latter being burnt when caught in the incident laser beam. Once all of the water is vaporized, some cell debris remains.

300°–500°C. By continuous heating the desiccated cell remnants described above will be carbonized. The carbonized material will be further heated by the absorbed light and will be partly evaporated and partly burnt. The latter process will act as an additional heat source.

>500°C. Left-over tissue particles will be further burnt and evaporate.

Temperature Response Versus Tissue Penetration

Different thermal lasers have different temperature responses, depending on their absorption characteristics for the tissue. In this section it is assumed that the laser light is incident on a tissue surface in air.

The rate of change of local temperature rise $d\Delta T/dt$, that is the temperature rise per second, is approximately equal to the product of
a) the absorption coefficient of tissue of the tissue for the wavelength, and
b) the (local) intensity of the laser light:

$$\frac{\delta \Delta T}{\delta t} = \text{absorption coefficient light intensity} \qquad (15)$$

Although this relation is not exact as the influence of heat conduction is neglected, it is nonetheless instructive to apply it to the comparison of different lasers as follows.

Choose a constant light intensity for all lasers to be considered here. We will not specify this value as we wish only to compare $d\Delta T/dt$ for various lasers. Then, with the estimated absorption coefficients of the CO_2, Nd:YAG, and frequency-doubled Nd:YAG lasers, we can predict the early temperature effects according to Eq. (see Table 2).

Table 2. Some absorption coefficients and their effect on tissue response

Laser	Wavelength	Estimated absorption coefficient (mm^{-1})	Tissue response
CO_2	10.6 μm	~ 50	Fast, shallow
Nd:YAG	1064 nm	~ 0.1 "white"	Slow, deep
		~ 0.2–0.3 "red"	Less slow, less deep
		~ 50* "black"	Fast, shallow
Frequency-doubled Nd:YAG	532 nm	~ 0.2 "white"	Moderately slow and deep
		~ 0.4–40 "red"	Variable, depending on tissue redness
		~ 50* "black"	Fast, shallow

* Absorption coefficients of carbonized tissue are not accurately available; for simplicity they are assumed equal to the estimated value of the CO_2 laser for any soft tissue.

For example, a laser wavelength with a very large absorption coefficient such as that of the CO_2 laser (approximately 50 mm^{-1}) produces a relatively large product of absorption coefficient and light intensity, and hence a large rate of temperature change $d\Delta T/dt$. In other words, the CO_2 laser produces a relatively fast temperature rise. In addition, a large absorption coefficient also implies a shallow tissue penetration. Thus Eq. 14 couples fast temperature response to shallow penetration. In contrast, a Nd:YAG laser at 1064 nm wavelength has a small absorption coefficient for "white" tissue Equation 14 then predicts a "slow" temperature rise, and a deep tissue penetration. It is important to realize that the Nd:YAG laser wavelength shows selective absorption for blood. Hence, "red" tissue responds faster than "white" tissue. In addition, once the tissue has carbonized, the absorption is greatly increased, and the temperature rise is "fast and shallow" again. The third laser wavelength discussed in Table 2 is the frequency-doubled Nd:YAG laser at 532 nm. This green wavelength is strongly absorbed by blood, and hence shows "strongly red dependent" tissue responses.

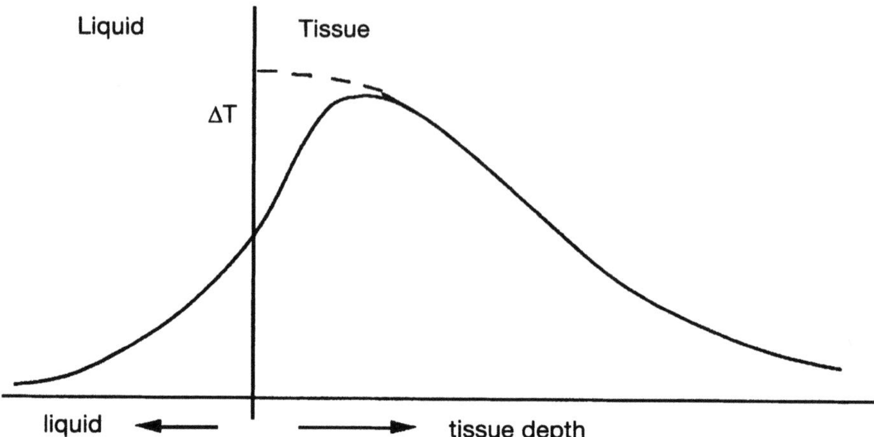

Fig. 29. Temperature distribution around the liquid-tissue interface when the tissue is heated by a laser. The temperature at the tissue surface is lower than inside the tissue. *Dashed line* indicates ideal temperature rise in air

Popcorn Effect

Soft tissue irradiated by laser light sometimes "explodes." The classical example is a Nd:YAG laser irradiating soft tissue under liquid. The temperature rise versus tissue depth is (qualitatively) shown in Figure 29.

After laser irradiation of about 1 s or more, cooling of the liquid-tissue interface by the liquid produces a maximum temperature inside the tissue. When this maximum temperature is more than 100°C, steam will be produced, resulting in a pressure increase and an "explosion""(the popcorn effect).

In air, the temperature rise is, ideally, as indicated by the dashed line in Figure 29. Under such circumstances, a temperature maximum cannot occur inside the tissue; however, it has been shown that the popcorn effect also occurs in irradiated air-tissue surfaces, although not as often as in liquid-tissue surfaces. This may be due to a subsurface maximum in the light fluence rate in the case of major-diameter beams (see also Chap. 4), but most likely, the popcorn effect for an air-tissue interaction is due to evaporation of tissue water at the surface which causes cooling of this surface. This also leads again to a maximum inside the tissue; however, this effect is not yet well understood.

Selective Laser Photo Thermolysis

The selective destruction of benign skin constituents such as ectatic dermal blood vessels in port-wine stains (PWS), dermal pigments in tattoos, or epidermal or dermal melanin pigmented cells in pigmented lesions (Fig. 30) is a topic that is of interest for clinical as well as scientific purpose. A change of the abnormal skin color to a (virtually) normal color is the goal of all of these treatments, and selective destruction of the "excess pigment" without injury to the rest of the skin is the goal to be achieved.

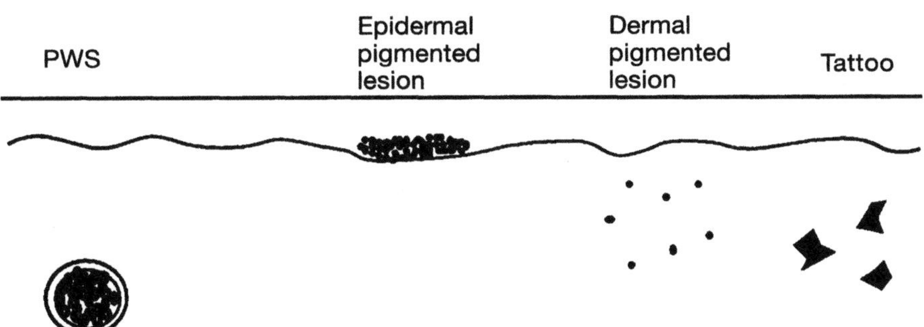

Fig. 30.   Anatomy of various benign skin lesions. *PWS*, port-wine stains

The laser parameters that are varied to optimize these laser treatments are:
1. laser wavelength,
2. pulse duration, and
3. spot size diameter. Each lesion requires, in principle, different sets of laser parameters.

The spot size diameter is chosen large enough to produce the deepest tissue penetration of the light fluence rate per unit of irradiance. For skin and for visible light, 3–5 mm is considered optimal for reaching deep dermal lesion chromophores (red blood cells in PWS and melanin in incontinent dermal pigmented lesions). However, for epidermal pigmented lesions, large beam diameters are not required for deep dermal injury.

The laser pulse duration is chosen sufficiently short to confine the laser-produced tissue injury to the volume of the chromophore unit that constitutes the lesion (ectatical venule for PWS, an ink particle for tattoos, and a melanosome for pigmented lesions), but at the same time sufficiently long to injure the whole chromophore unit.

For PWS, the red blood cells, are the target chromophores for laser light absorption but the laser pulse duration should be sufficiently long to injure the vessel wall transmurally by conduction of heat from the hot red blood cells. This ideally requires a few milliseconds for a wall thickness of 3–6 μm. For pigmented volumes (tattoos as well as melanosomes), the pulse duration must be in the order of a few hundred nanoseconds.

"Subtile Surgery," or the Influence of the Laser Pulse Repetition Frequency

Laser with Shallow Tissue Penetration

Benign lesions of the vocal folds, treated by the CO_2 laser, are a clinical example in which "subtile surgery" is required. Vocal folds are a delicate part of the body where the density of the tissue determines the uniqueness of a person´s voice. Treatment of a benign lesion by a laser ideally requires vaporization of the lesion without producing any injury to the distal underlying tissue. In other words, it requires a laser for vaporization that only very shallowly penetrates the tissue, and a laser pulse repetition frequency that is so low that laser-heated tissue cools completely before the next laser pulse arrives. This can be achieved by a superpulsed CO_2 laser. However, experimental work in our group has indicated that after more than 0.1 s after a single CO_2 laser pulse, there is still some temperature increase in tissue. Consequently, super pulse CO_2 lasers should have very low pulse repetition frequencies (of less than 10 Hz) to prevent temperature accumulation and thermal damage because of this effect.

Laser with Deep Tissue Penetration

Although super pulse Nd:YAG lasers are commercially available, it seems unclear at the moment what the clinical advantage is over a cw Nd:YAG laser. The cooling rate for this laser is, because of its deep penetration, in the order of seconds, so with any practical pulse rate there will always be a considerable temperature accumulation, where as a pulsed laser is meant to reduce this effect.

Photochemical Interaction

In this kind of interaction the radiation is absorbed by a compound present in the tissue either by nature or by administration. Absorption of energy leads to activation of the compound and hence to the induction of chemical processes. An example of photochemical interaction is found in photodynamic therapy (PDT). Interaction of light with the before-mentioned compounds will sometimes lead only to the reversible process of fluorescence. This will be dealt with below.

PDT is an experimental treatment modality for malignant disease. In short, tumor destruction by PDT is based on the light activation of an administrated photosensitive drug which is preferentially retained in malignant tissue. In practice the photosensitizer is given intravenously, and after about 48 h illumination of the tumor is carried out with (laser) light of a suitable wavelength. The activated drug induces several processes that eventually result in tumor destruction.

At the beginning of the century the toxic activity of some dyes activated by light was already known. However, it was not until the 1970s that Dougherty and co-workers brought forward a breakthrough of this therapeutic modality with their animal studies, biochemical research, and clinical investigations.

The photosensitizers most widely applied in the clinic today are the hematoporphyrin derivates (HpD) and, as a more purified substance, dihemats porphyrin ether (DHE). In fact, both drugs consist of a mixture of different porphyrins, the latter containing a higher percentage of the active component. After intravenous injections these porphyrins bind preferentially to or me more selectively retained in malignant tissue. However, they appear to also accumulate in normal liver, kidney, spleen, and normal skin. This explains the phenomenon of skin photosensitivity observed in patients injected with ten hematoporphyrins: exposure to (sun) light can cause serious skin burns up to 4–8 weeks after injection. Sometimes the hypersensitivity shows an even more prolonged duration. A part from the photosensitivity, no toxic side effects of the drug have been reported. Within the tumor tissue the porphyrins appear to be concentrated mainly in the vascular stroma and in the reticulo-endothelial components i.e., cells and macrophages. Within the cells there is an mast association with the mitochondria and nuclear membranes as shown by in vitro studies. The exact mechanisms of retention in tumor tissue are yet to be elucidated. There are indications that binding of HpD to hydrophobic structures, such as mitochondria, nuclear material, and those lipoproteins present in cell membranes, plays a role. Twenty-four hours after injection the "selective" retention of HpD is completed, the non localized porphyrins having been removed. With the usual dose of sensitizer of 2–3 mg/kg bodyweight intravenously, illumination should be performed from the second day to 1 week after injection. Activation of porphyrins can be induced by light of several wavelengths. However, 625–630 nm is used because this wavelength shows the optimal combination of light penetration in (tumor) tissue and absorption by the sensitizer. Light activation of porphyrins leads to the formation of toxic substances such as singlet oxygen, which causes occlusions of vessels and vascular damage with extravasation of blood cells. On the cellular level membrane damage has been detected by in vitro studies. As a result the tumor becomes necrotic and sloughs off in the week following PDT treatment. As may be clear PDT can only take place in aerobic circumstances. During illumination the power density of the radiation should not exceed 200 mW/cm^2 order to prevent a direct hyperthermic effect on the tissue. Therefore, in contrast go thermal interactions, photochemical treatment requires low power densities and thus long exposure times. According to the site of treatment and the tumor various light doses are applied, in most cases varying between 30 and 200 J/cm^2. Treatment of superficial lesions, for instance, on the skin, can be carried out by conventional light sources (with filters) able to produce radiation of the desired wavelength and power density. However, in endoscopic procedures (lungs, GI tract, bladder) light has to be transported by fibers, and hence the laser as a light source is indispensable. In practice this means that for PDT treatment nearly always lasers will be used. Laser types used are the argon dye laser, the gold vapor laser, or the frequency-doubled Nd:YAG laser (532 nm) pumping a dye laser. The penetration depth of 625–630-nm radiation in tissue amounts to 5–10 mm. This implies that only superficial tumors less than 10 mm thick can be treated by surface or external irradiation (directly or endoscopically). For the management of more bulky tumors fibers can be placed into the tumor tissue and thereby interstitial irradiation carried out. Sometimes several cylindrical diffusing fibers have to be implanted into the mass. With irradiation of 500 mW/cm^2 an effective illumination can be established. Crucial in PDT treatment is the knowledge of what happens with the light in the (tumor) tissue, so dosimetry is of prime importance for this kind of treatment. Clinically, PDT is presently gaining in various fields of treatment, for instance, in early lung cancer, early bladder malignancies, and superficial skin and mucosal tumors, notwithstanding the fact that much energy has still to be put into optimizing PDT and into developing better sensitizing drugs. Ideally, the optimal sensitizer should be nontoxic, present a high tumor-to-healthy-tissue ratio and should be activated by light of a wavelength that allows deep penetration into tumor tissue. Another field of investigation deals with the topical application of sensitizers, a method that would offer the advantage of overcoming the problem of photosensitivity. Currently much research is being carried out all over the world to improve this interesting mode of treatment.

Mechanical Effects

Electromechanic Effects

An intense light flux concentrated upon a small surface using a laser with an irradiation time on the order of nano- and picoseconds can create a plasma. At the proximal side between the ionized plasma and the external medium, a pressure gradient induces the propagation of a shock wave. It is the expansion of this shock wave that provokes the destructive effects. The plasma and shock wave are produced, for instance, by an Nd:YAG laser with nanosecond or picosecond irradiation (Q-switched). At present these laser pulses can only be transported by means of mirrors.

Thermomechanic Effects

When the laser irradiation is short (micro-to milliseconds), heat has no time to diffuse away from its "primary" source. If thermal rise is considerable, important mechanical forces are produced which generate mechanical effects. At present, this effect is achieved with a dye laser emitting in the green part of the spectrum with pulses of 1 µs. The advantage of thermomechanical interactions over electromechanical ones stems from the possibility of transmitting the microsecond laser beams via an optic fiber.

Application of Mechanical Effects

The mechanical effects are applied in ophthalmology to intersect thin intraocular membranes and in endoscopy to fragment renal or bile stones. In ophthalmology, essentially nanosecond pulsed lasers are used, even though picosecond lasers still maintain their supporters. In this discipline it is not considered an insurmountable disadvantage that the laser beam is transported with mirrors. In endoscopy, transmission by optic fibers is obligatory, which explains the use of microsecond dye lasers.

Photoablative Effects

Photoablation is usually associated with the use of UV-pulsed lasers, primarily excimer lasers such as the ArF laser (193 nm), the KrF laser (248 nm), and the XeCl laser (308 nm). The UV photons are thought to be capable of breaking chemical bonds. The thereby created gas expands, and the resulting explosion ejects the surrounding tissue. Although the creation of gas has been observed, excimer lasers also have been found to vaporize tissue water, and we assume that tissue removal is a combined effect of gas and water vapor expansion. In this respect, photoablation is very much similar to ablation by short-pulsed IR lasers, such as Ho:YAG (2.1 μm) and Er:YAG (2.9 μm) lasers, whose ablative action is entirely based upon the rapid heating of the tissue water. However, the thermal damage of the surrounding tissue may be less when using an excimer laser rather than an IR laser since in excimer lasers, part of the laser pulse energy is used for bond breaking instead of heating.

Biostimulation or Low Level Laser Therapy

Biostimulation or low level laser therapy is a laser-tissue interaction that is still controversial. In medicine milliwatt lasers are used as a therapy for instance, for pain relief, crural ulcers, and rheumatoid arthritis. Especially in dentistry, biostimulation is used as a therapy for pain and wound healing. Although widely practiced, only a few studies on biostimulation are reported in literature. Most of these studies claim that light stimulates tissue healing and releaves pain by a mechanism yet unknown. Further research is needed before biostimulation will be generally accepted as a worthwhile therapeutic modality.

Fluorescence

Fluorescence is a process of absorption followed by emission of photons of longer wavelengths (see Fig. 31). The shift of the fluorescence spectrum to longer wavelengths than those of the absorption spectrum is caused by a deexcitation of a molecule to lower vibrational levels whose energies are still higher than the ground state from which the molecule was excited by absorption of the incoming photon.

Fluorescence is used as a method of diagnosis of diseases. This method is based on differences in concentrations of fluorescent substances in, for instance, carcinomas in situ or tumor and healthy tissues. These fluorescent substances can either be natural (such as the difference in NADH in tumor and healthy tissues) or be introduced artificially. An example of the latter is a difference in concentration of HpD after i.v. injection of HpD for photodynamic diagnosis (PDD).

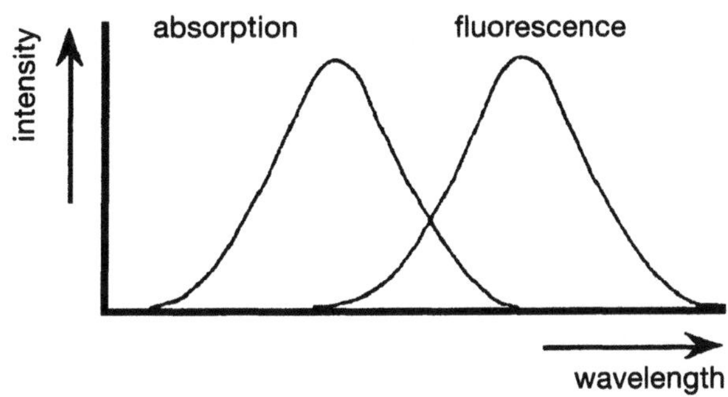

Fig. 31.   Absorption and
fluorescence spectrum

Electron Microscopic Investigations After Laser Radiation

R. R. Lehmann

Microscopic Evaluation

The primary concern of microscopy is the description of structure and organization of cells, tissues, and organs. It is also concerned with the functions of cells, tissues, and organs, for it is primarily from function that structure derives meaning. Furthermore, knowledge of molecular biology is essential to microscopic studies, for the biochemical reactions characterizing life take place on the numerous surfaces and interfaces that cellular and tissue structure provide.

Limitations in the Use of Light Microscopy

Most tissues do not retain sufficient color to make them and their components visible under a bright field microscope. It is therefore expedient to add colors to tissues by staining them with the proper dyes. The hematoxylin and eosin stain (H&E) is the most commonly used stain for ordinary histologic work. The advantages are a clear staining of cell nuclei and an easy handling. H&E is perhaps the best general histologic stain; however, its usefulness has limits. Although H&E is commonly used in histology of laser irradiated tissues, other staining techniques (Table 1) have proved to be more useful in recognizing the type and extension of tissue injury after laser irradiation.

For example, the AZAN method (azocarmine, aniline blue, orange G) stains collagen fibers damaged by laser irradiation brilliant red instead of blue [5–7].

Table 1. Comparison of some characteristics of light and electron microscopic techniques

Method	Type of section	Thickness of section	Standard staining methods
Light microscopy	Paraffin section	8–10 μm[a]	Hematoxylin/eosin, AZAN stain, Masson Trichrome stain, van Gieson stain
Light microscopy	Semithin section	0.5–1.0 μm[a]	Toluidine blue, methylene blue
Transmission electron microscopy	Ultrathin section	60–70 nm[a]	Uranyl acetate, lead citrate

[a] 1 mm = 1000 μm; 1 μm = 1000 nm.

In Contrast, the same staining turns from red to blue in laser irradiated muscle tissue. Comparable changes of the normal staining pattern are seen using Masson trichrome stain or van Gieson staining. With increasing distance from the laser treated surface, the staining of the tissue first turns to a kind of mixed color and then to normal. However, this does not mean that the normal stained tissues are not injured by laser irradiation or other stress factors. The staining behavior of relatively uninjured tissues remains almost unchanged as revealed by comparative light- and electron microscopic studies [5]. Therefore, light microscopy alone always leads to an incomplete evaluation [7] of the true dimensions of tissue damage.

Furthermore, obtaining a clear and detailed image depends on the resolving power of the light microscope. Since the resolving power of the best light microscope is approximately 0.2 µm (= 200 nm), cell membranes having a thickness of 7.5 nm and all cellular structures formed by such membranes can never be observed in the light microscope. Almost all cellular structures remain a secret to the light microscopist. If one wishes to detect more in tissues after laser irradiation than loss of material, carbonization, coagulation, necrosis, or endematous changes, electron microscopy becomes the method of choice.

Significance of Electron Microscopic Studies

Transmission electron microscopy – a widely used tool today – gives deeper insights into structural and functional interrelation of cells and tissues exposed to various stress factors. Of major importance are the integrity, number, and distribution of the membrane-delimited cell organelles (mitochondria, rough and smooth endoplasmic reticulum, Golgi apparatus, lysosomes, peroxisomes, secretory granules, and other vesicles) and the components of the cytoskeleton (microfilaments, microtubules, intermediate filaments). These structural proteins not only determine the form and shaping of cells but also play an important role in cytoplasmic and cellular movement. The cell membrane functions as a selective barrier that regulates the passage of certain materials into and out of the cell. The nuclear envelope plays a similar role. A decision as to whether the plasmalemma of a cell or its nuclear envelope is still present, injured or missing after being exposed to laser radiation can only be made by means of the electron microscope. The same holds for a reliable evaluation of extracellular matrix components.

Another important point is that blood and lymph capillaries can hardly be seen in light microscopic images because of the relatively large shrinkage effect of the usual paraffin embedded material. Shrinkage is minimized if objects are embedded in epoxy resin commonly used for semithin and ultrathin sectioning. Although capillaries and lymphatic gaps may be visualized in semithin sections, further details such as endothelial pinocytotic and transport vesicles, fenestrae, intercellular junctions, and the basement lamina can only be identified in the electron microscope.

There is considerable interest in determining the effects of laser irradiation on the various intracellular structures and extracellular matrix components [6, 7, 14, 18–21]. Relying solely on light microscopic findings would mean ignoring a considerable amount of information. Our own electron microscopic studies have revealed that cytologic injury of intra- and extracellular components roughly extends twice as far from the laser exposed surface as could be distinguished in the light microscope [5–7].

Alterations of structural elements are always related to functional and molecular events. For example, collagen is not only a structural element of connective and other tissues as well as the most abundant protein of the human body, but also an important constituent of the extracellular matrix involved in controlling gene expression [11]. The role of the extracellular matrix has received particular emphasis due to its well-known effects on cell adhesion, proliferation, migration, and differentiation [17]. The significance of electron microscopic studies is further emphasized by the fact that several human and animal diseases are related to altered cellular components that cannot be identified in the light microscope (Table 2).

Table 2. Significance of electron microscopy in recognizing altered cellular elements related to disease

Cellular component	Morphological alteration	Disease
Mitochondria	Increase in size and number	Mitochondrial cytopathy
Cilia	Atypical number of microtubuli doublets	Chronic sinusitis
Desmosomes	Increase in desmosomes	Keratoacanthoma

Application of Electron Microscopy

A careful preparation of tissue specimens is an essential prerequisite for the quality of electron microscopic images. Obviously, even with the best technique available and the greatest possible care, not all artifacts can be excluded. However, method-related artifacts are relatively constant and can therefore be largely neglected. However, additional artifacts caused by careless handling of the tissue specimens are a variable factor leading to confused, inconsistent, and even false results. In view of the high resolution afforded by the electron microscope, greater care is necessitated in fixation in order to preserve ultrastructural details. This requirement is best met by perfusing the tissue with the fixative via blood vessels. If fixation by perfusion is not applicable (e.g., most human material), the most critical point for avoiding artifacts is the size of the tissue specimens and the time between sampling of the tissue and the beginning of fixation. The specimens should not be thicker than 1 mm and put into the fixative as quickly as possible. Although the volume of such tissue samples seems to be relatively small compared to pieces of tissue prepared for light microscopy, 1 mm of tissue would yield approximately 15 000 ultrathin sections. To further illustrate the different dimension between light and electron microscopy, one should imagine that a 10-µm paraffin section could be cut into about 140 ultrathin sections (Table 1).

The Immediate Tissue Response

Four zones have been described in the damaged tissue immediately after laser radiation:
1. a carbonized zone, in which no cellular detail can be distinguished;
2. a zone where cell contours but no intra- and extracellular structures are visible;
3. a zone characterized by homogenization and/or vacuolization of cell organelles;
4. a zone with persisting filamentous structures [12].

Comparative electron microscopic studies from our laboratory have been aimed at describing and understanding the various cytological changes that occur in biopsy material and under experimental conditions. In the following sections, examples are taken from clinical and experimental laser applications mainly related to pediatric surgery.

Differential Response of the Laser-Treated Surfaces

Laser treatment may or may not result in a carbonized surface layer. Various alterations of tissue surfaces directly exposed to laser radiation are depicted in Figure 1a–d. The carbonized surface of a laser-resected teratoma is interspersed with numerous vacuoles of different sizes, yet smaller and less frequent at the very surface (Fig. 1a). No structural elements can be recognized. This is also the case for the surface material of a laser-re-sected spleen cyst (child Nd:YAG 1064 nm). Here the tissue is characterized by irregular spaces (Fig. 1b). It corresponds to a less carbonized surface than in Figure 1a. In Figure 1c carbonization was avoided (Nd:YAG 132 nm). Although the shape and stratification of the keratinized epithelium can still be recognized, the cellular proteins are swollen and coagulated. The spaces represent the extended intercellular fissures. Even better preserved are the keratinized layers of the human skin 16 h after argon laser irradiation (Fig. 1d). The underlying cells of the stratum granulosom are disintegrated into differently shaped vacuolized material.

Experimental Work Using the Rat Esophagus

Electron microscopic studies from our laboratory have been directed toward describing and understanding the various cytological changes that occur in biopsy material and under experimental conditions immediately, 2 days, and 14 days after laser treatment of the rat esophagus.

The rat esophagus was chosen as an animal model for the study of laser treatment of the inborn esophagotracheal fistula. The more one works with animal models, the more apparent it becomes that a model is rarely found that is satisfactory in all respects. If one wishes to study basic aspects of ultramorphologic alterations of laser irradiated tissues, such as the endoderm – derived epithe-

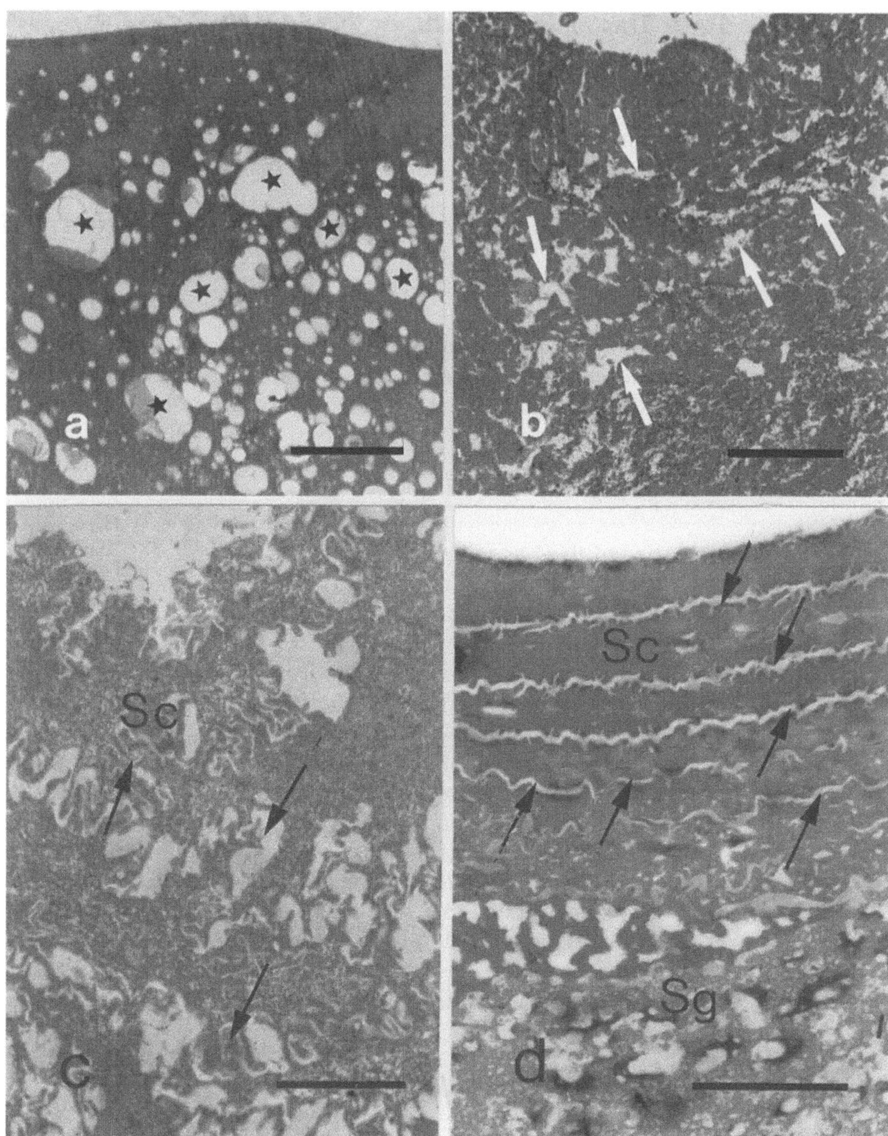

Fig. 1a–d. Damaged tissue surfaces after differential laser radiation. **a** Nd:YAG 1064 nm, 40 W, continuous wave (cw); human teratoma; *stars* indicate vacuoles. **b** Nd:YAG 1064 nm, 75 W, cw, human spleen cyst; *arrows* indicate irregular spaces. **c** Nd:YAG 1320 nm, 5 W, 8 s; rat esophagus; *arrows* indicate remnants of cellular interdigitations. **d** Argon laser, 4.5 W, 249 shots, 0.02 s; human skin; *arrows* indicate fissures between adjacent keratinized layers. **a–c** Immediate effect, **d** 16 h after exposure to laser irradiation. *Sc*, stratum corneum; *Sg*, stratum granulosum; *bar* = 2 μm

lium, loose connective tissue, and smooth and striated muscle cells, then the rat model may contribute valuable information. These studies are supplemented by autoradiographic experiments in which the nuclei of regenerating cells were labeled with [³H]-thymidine [8, 9] which is incorporated into the cell for DNA synthesis. As early as 90 min after laser irradiation, many cell nuclei of fibroblasts and epithelial and endothelial cells situated beyond the damaged zone were radioactively labeled, indicating initiation of proliferation.

The esophagi were cannulated orally with a glass fiber. Its tip was equipped with a radial applicator designed to ensure a radial symmetrical distribution of light and irradiation of a definite circumferential volume of the esophageal wall [14, 18, 19]. Segments most affected by laser irradiation are referred to as the laser center. Additionally, segments are examined at a distance of 2 and 4 mm from the laser center immediately, 2 days, and 14 days after laser irradiation, respectively. The parameters of the lasers used are summarized in Table 3.

Table 3. Application of laser in the experiments described

Type of laser	Wavelength (nm)	Power (W)	Time of radiation	Mode
Nd:YAG	1064 nm	7.5	20	cw
Argon	514 nm	2.5	12	cw

cw, continuous wave.

Since most of the following description of tissue response to laser irradiation concerns the results of our experimental work, it seems appropriate to briefly describe the normal structure of the rat esophagus. The esophagus of the rat is composed of a lumen surrounded by a wall of four principal layers; the mucosa, the submucosa, the muscularis externa, and the adventitia. The mucosa is composed of a stratified squamous keratinized epithelial lining, a lamina propria of loose connective tissue rich in blood and lymph capillaries, and the lamina muscularis mucosae consisting of smooth muscle cells. The submucosa is composed of loose connective tissue with many blood and lymph capillaries and a submucosal nerve plexus. The muscularis externa consists of striated muscle cells and contains the myenteric nerve plexus.

Epithelium

The unaffected striated squamous epithelium lining the rat esophagus is composed of several layers of flattened nonnucleated keratinized cells (Fig. 2a). They consist only of fibrillar and amorphous proteins and clearly thickened plasma membranes. The cells of the underlying stratum granulosum are characterized by electron-dense keratohyalin granules (Fig. 2a). Immediately after laser irradiation this structural pattern is converted into a filamentous network (Fig. 2b). The sites of the former interdigitations between the keratinized cells are still indicated.

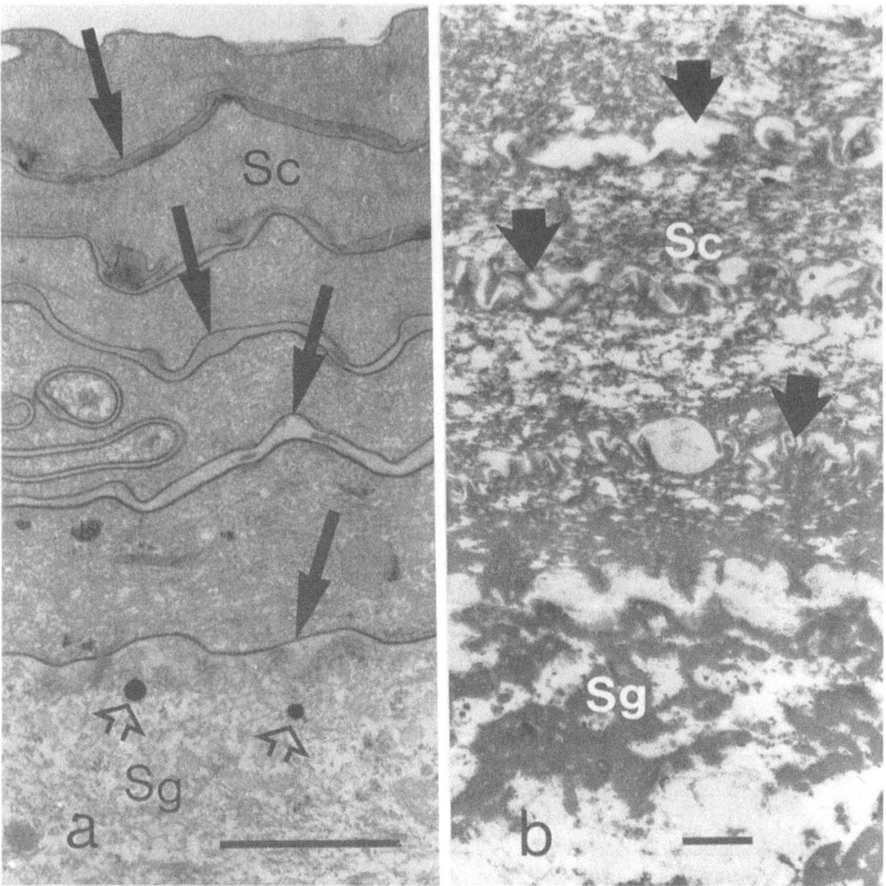

Fig. 2a, b. Comparison of uninjured (a) and irradiated (b) stratum corneum *(Sc)* and stratum granulosum *(Sg)* of the epithelium of the rat esophagus immediately after argon laser treatment (514 nm, 12 s, 2.5 W). **a** *Small arrows* indicate keratohyalin granules, *large arrows* indicate thickened plasma membranes. **b** *Arrows* indicated former interdigitations; *bar* = 1 μm

The uninjured stratum basale consists of a single layer of columnar cells resting on the basal lamina (Fig. 3a). It separates the epithelium from the connective tissue of the lamina propria. Desmosomes in great quantity bind the epithelial cells in their lateral and upper surfaces. Hemidesmosomes, found in the basal plasmalemma, help bind these cells to the basal lamina. Immediately after laser irradiation, none of the cellular components described above can be recognized in the basal epithelial layer (Fig. 3b). Furthermore, irradiation is accompanied by a considerable loss of material not observed to such an extent in the keratinized layers (Fig. 2b). The irradiated lamina propria, clearly separated from the remnants of the epithelial lamina basale, consists mainly of coagulated collagen microfibrils (Fig. 3b).

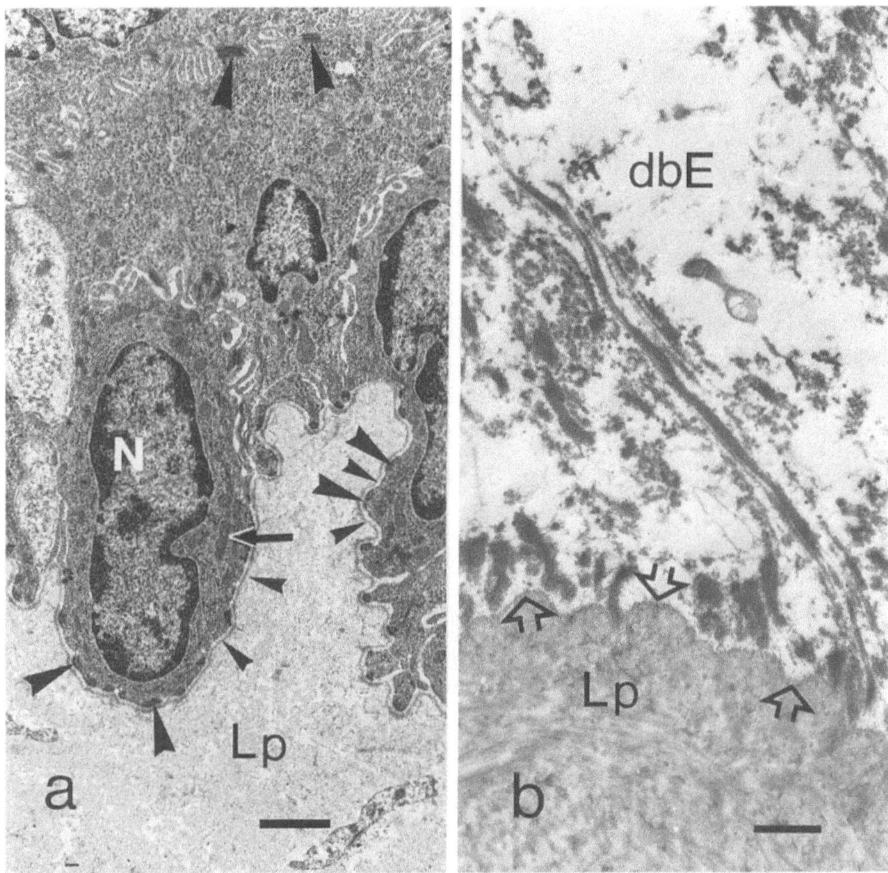

Fig. 3a, b. Comparison of uninjured (**a**) and irradiated (**b**) stratum basale of the epithelium of the rat esophagus immediately after argon laser treatment (514 nm, 12 s, 2.5 W). **a** *Arrow* indicates mitochondrium, *large arrowheads* desmosomes and hemidesmosomes, *small arrowheads* basal lamina. **b** *Arrows* indicate junction between epithelium and lamina propria. *dbE,* destroyed epithelium, *Lp,* lamina propria; *N,* nucleus; *bar* = 1 µm

The destroyed epithelial layer was more than twice as thick as in the normal epithelium [14]. At a distance of 2 mm from the laser center, the epithelial layers nearly presented the same damaged appearance, whereas at a distance of up to 4 mm, the epithelial structure changed to normal.

Connective Tissue Components

The loose connective tissue of the esophageal wall is mainly distributed within the lamina propria, lamina submucosa, and lamina adventitia. Figure 4a, b com-

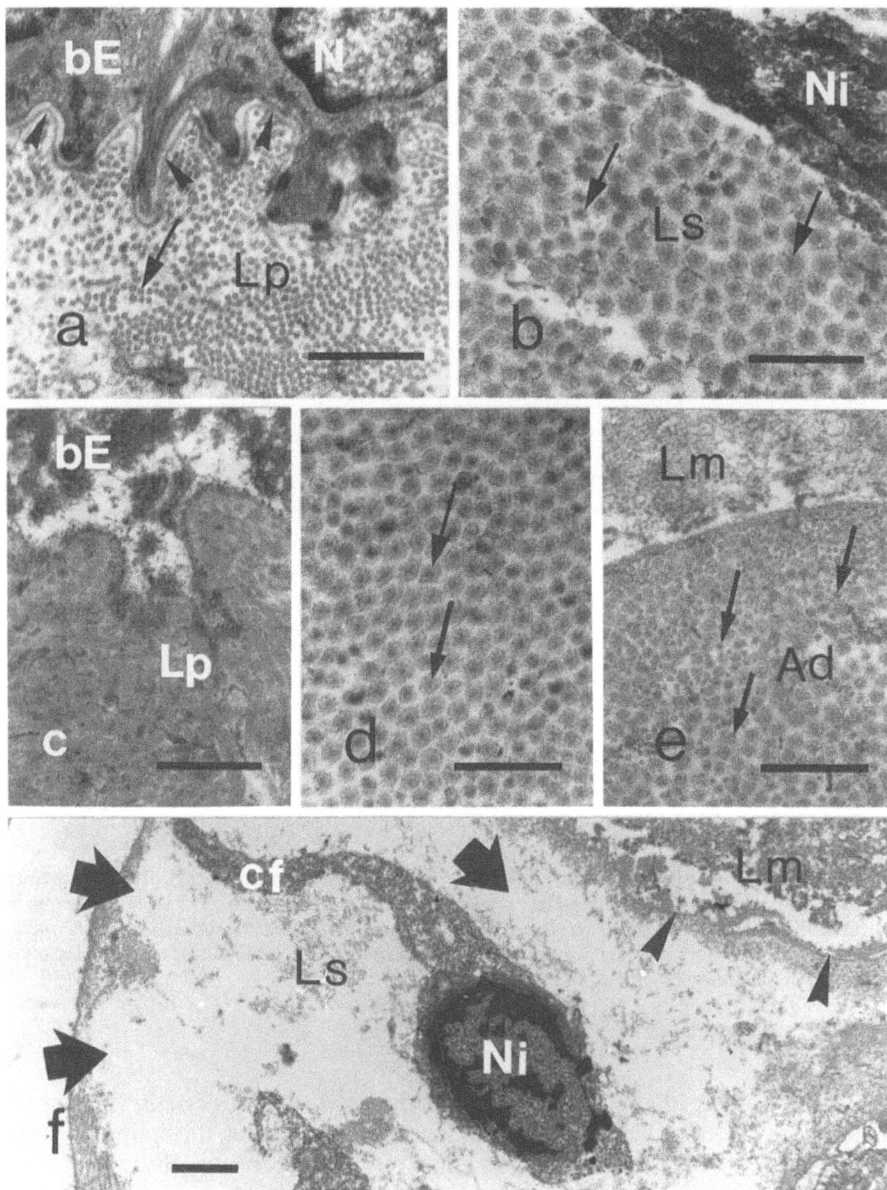

Fig. 4a–f. Cross-sectioned collagen microfibrils of the normal lamina propria (**a**) and the lamina submucosa (**b**). **c–e** Lamina propria, submucosa, and adventitia of the same section. **f** Lamina submucosa *(Ls)* adjacent to the lamina muscularis *(Lm)*. **b–f** Immediately after laser irradiation. **b, c** Argon laser, 514 nm, 12 s, 2.5 W. *Arrowheads* indicate basal lamina, *thin arrows* individual collagen microfibrils, *thick arrows* submucosal spaces. *bE,* basal epithelium; *Lp,* lamina propria; *N,* nucleus; *Ni,* injured nuclei; *cf,* cytoplasmic filament of a destroyed fibroblast; *bar* = 1 μm

pares the cross-sectional appearance of normal and laser irradiated collagen microfibrils of the lamina propria. The irradiated microfibrils have a significantly greater diameter than the injured microfibrils. The clear demarcation between adjacent microfibrils disappears. The swollen microfibrils seem to be linked to each other by a filamentous network (Fig. 4c). With increasing distance from the most damaged zone, the structural changes decrease (Fig. 4c–e). The differing diameters of the cross-sectioned microfibrils in the adventitia are interpreted as an uneven injury.

In the submucosa of the Nd:YAG (1064 nm)-treated material, some structurally normal microfibrils appeared [19]. In contrast, large intercellular spaces often occur after irradiation which contain an undefined fuzzy material (Fig. 4f). Unlike the epithelial layer, cell nuclei are visible within the connective tissue. The overall appearance of the chromatin is more electron-dense than in normal cell nuclei, and it is coarsely granulated with increased portions of heterochromatin. The nuclear envelope is no longer present in these functionless nuclei. The cytoplasm of the former fibroblasts consists of a granulated material. No cell organelles or other intracellular structures can be identified.

At a distance of 2 mm from the laser center the connective tissue exhibits the same tissue lesions as shown above [14, 19]. However, at a distance of 4 mm the cytologic structure of connective tissue components does not markedly differ from the regular structure.

Smooth Muscle Cells

The difference between the structure of normal smooth muscle cells (Fig. 5a) and laser irradiated smooth muscle cells (Fig. 5b) in the rat esophagus is evident. All cell organelles, other intracellular structures, and the plasma membrane are completely destroyed. The diameter of the cells has increased to more than double. The cytoplasm exhibits irregularly shaped vacuoles filled with a weak electron-dense material. Remnants of chromatin mark the site of the former nucleus. There are no spaces between adjacent cells. However, the basal lamina, although thicker than normal and with a loosened-up structure, can still be recognized. At a distance of 2 mm, the smooth muscle cells are less injured than in the laser center (Fig. 5c). At a distance of 4 mm, the smooth muscle cells exhibit the normal fine structure, except for large vacuoles occasionally seen.

Striated Muscle Cells

There is a striking difference between normal (Fig. 6a) and laser-treated (Fig. 6b) striated muscle cells of the lamina muscularis externa. The regular pattern of sarcomeres formed by thick myosin and thin actin filaments adhered to the so-called Z-line (Fig. 6a) is reflected in irregular more or less electron-dense stripes. The degraded and expanded proteins remain in the primary position, resulting in stripes of differential electron density (Fig. 6b). It is of particular interest that the overall damage of striated muscle cells seems to exceed the laser-induced changes

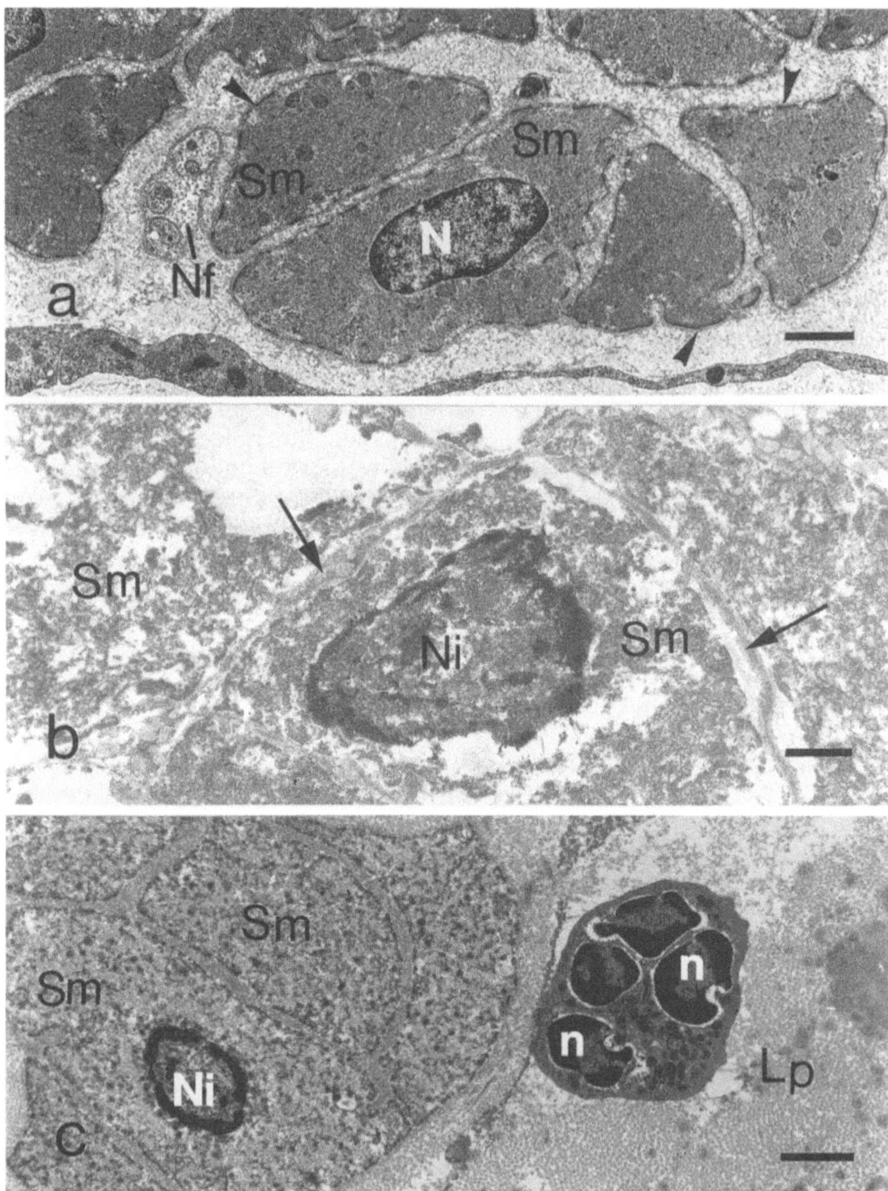

Fig. 5a–c. Portions of the lamina muscularis mucosae of the rat esophagus. **a** Cross-sectioned smooth muscle cells *(Sm)* of the normal lamina muscularis mucosae; *arrowheads* indicate dense bodies associated with the basal lamina. **b** Destroyed smooth muscle cells *(Sm)* immediately after laser irradiation; *arrows* indicate remnants of the basal lamina. **c** Injured smooth muscle cells *(Sm)* 2 mm from the laser center. **b, c** Argon laser, 514 nm, 12 s, 2.5 W. *Lp,* lamina propria; *N,* nucleus; *n,* lobulated nucleus of a neutrophil; *Nf,* unmyelinated nerve fiber; *Ni,* destroyed nuclei; *bar* = 1 μm

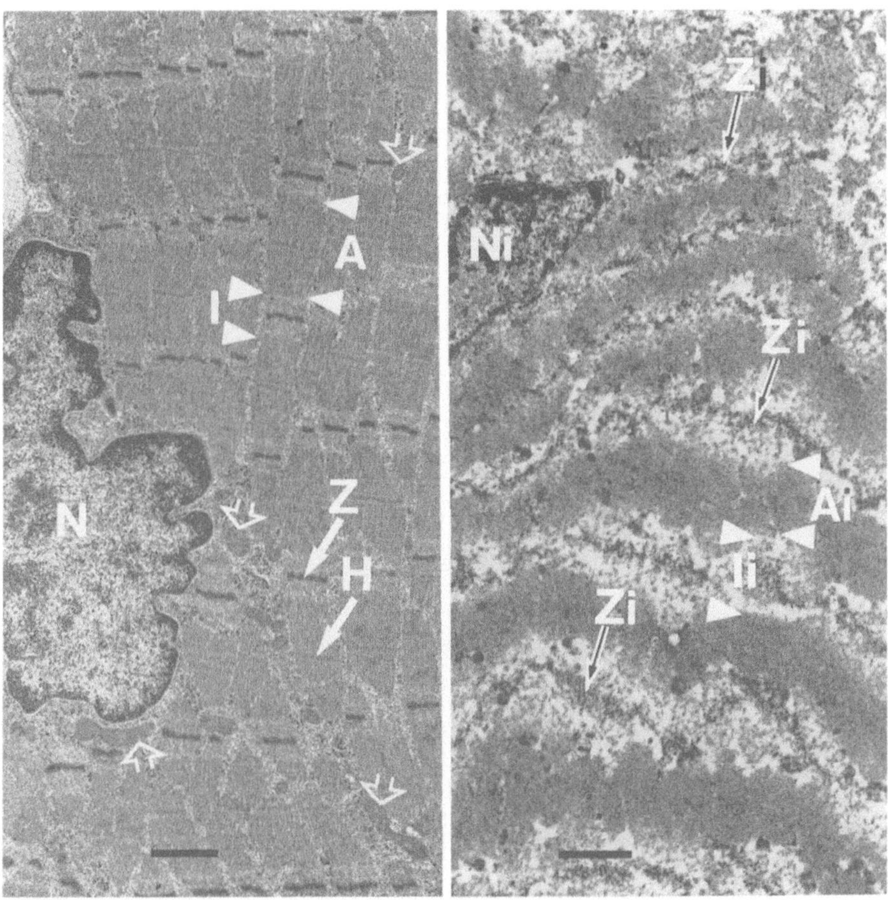

Fig. 6a, b. Portions of longitudinal sections of the lamina muscularis of the rat esophagus. a Normal striated muscle cell; *small thin arrows* indicate mitochondria. b Striated muscle cell immediately after radiation (argon laser, 514 nm, 12 s, 2.5 W). Note the same magnification of a and b. *A,* A band; *Ai,* destroyed A band; *H,* H band; *I,* I band; *Ii,* destroyed I band; *N,* nucleus; *Ni,* destroyed nucleus; *Z,* Z line; *Zi,* destroyed Z line; *bar* = 1 μm

in the smooth muscle cell layer of the lamina muscularis mucosae. Even at a distance of 4 mm from the laser center, injured striated muscle cells were found. Striated muscle cells seem to be more sensitive to the laser irradiation used than other tissue components, as confirmed by Viehberger et al. [22].

Blood Capillaries

Normal capillaries in the lamina propria are of the continuous type. They are approximately 8 μm wide, running in close proximity to the basal epithelium

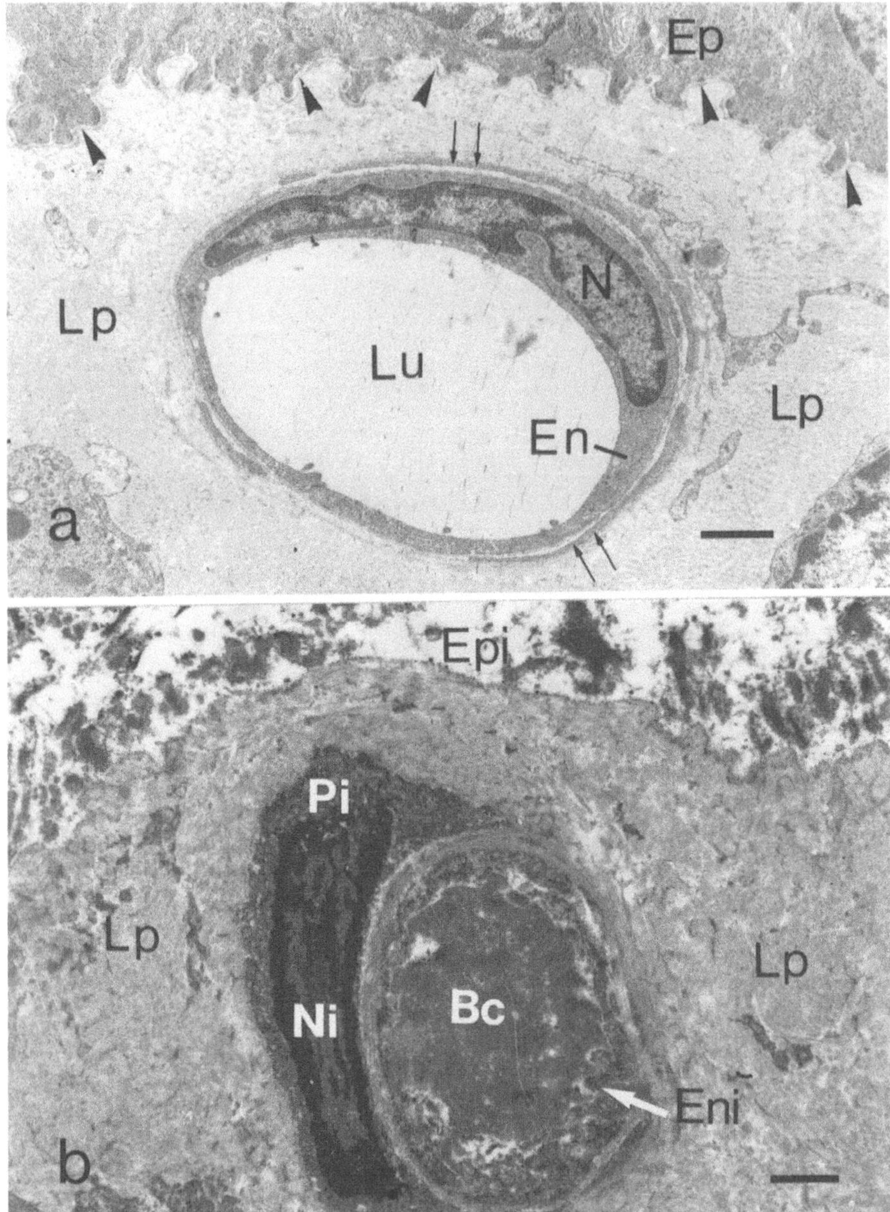

Fig. 7a, b. Capillaries within the lamina propria *(Lp)* of the rat esophagus. a Normal structure with open lumen *(Lu); arrows* indicate processes of perivascular cells, *arrowheads* basal lamina, *white arrow* destroyed nucleus. b Immediately after irradiation (argon laser, 514 nm, 12 s, 2.5 W), lumen occluded by a blood clot *(Bc). En,* endothelial cell; *Ep,* basal epithelium; *N,* nucleus; *Eni,* destroyed endothelial cell; *Epi,* destroyed basal epithelium; *Ni,* destroyed nucleus; *Pi,* destroyed perivascular cell; *bar* = 1 μm

(Fig. 7a). The nucleus causes the cell to bulge into the capillary lumen. The cytoplasm tapers towards the margins. The endothelial cell is partly surrounded by cytoplasmic processes of perivascular cells. They are enclosed in their own basal lamina, which may fuse with that of the endothelial cells. After irradiation their living structures are completely destroyed. The lumen is occluded by coagulated blood plasma intermingled with fractions of blood cells (Fig. 7b).

The Long Term Effect

Electron microscopy is not only important for assessing the strength and extension of cell injury immediately after laser irradiation, but even more so for assessing the late response of the tissue. How is the injured tissue removed? Which cell types are involved? Where do these cells come from? Are all tissue layers and cell types capable of regenerating? When and where can newly synthesized matrix components first be recognized? Do the regenerated tissues differ morphologically from normal tissues?

Leukocytes and Other Cells

Neutrophils are the most common leukocytes and account for about two thirds of the white cells in human blood. They are short-lived end cells with one main function, which is phagocytosis, and one main physiological role, which is to protect the host tissue against invading microbes. Migration of neutrophils into the laser-injured tissue begins immediately after laser treatment. They are first seen in the less damaged region in a distance of 2 mm from the laser center. Subcellular structures other than granules are relatively scarce in the cytoplasm of the mature neutrophil. The dense masses of heterochromatin are distributed on the inner surface of the nuclear envelope. Portions of less condensed euchromatin are mainly located in the center of the nucleus (Fig. 8a, b). The neutrophils reach the injured zone using two different paths. On the one hand, they move inside the damaged capillaries (Fig. 8a), on the other hand they find their way through the mass of coagulated collagen microfibrils (Fig. 8b). Guided by chemotaxis, the neutrophils may cross the wall of either uninjured or injured capillaries. It is well known that neutrophil proteinases degrade fibrinogen, elastin, structural collagen, and elastin [1]. The activity of neutrophil leukocytes can still be observed 14 days after laser irradiation.

Two days after irradiation, neutrophil leukocytes, lymphocytes, and macrophages can be observed. Although macrophages occur throughout the damaged tissue, they belong to the frequently seen living cells in the injured endomysium of the irradiated striated muscle layer (Fig. 9a). Highly active macrophages are still seen 14 days after laser irradiation (Fig. 9b). Small bundles of newly synthesized collagen microfibrils are surrounded by extensions of the cell surface. It seems that the initially produced collagen is again replaced by new collagen microfibrils, probably achieving a higher order of the intercellular matrix. Generally, the constituents of the extracellular matrix are continually synthesized

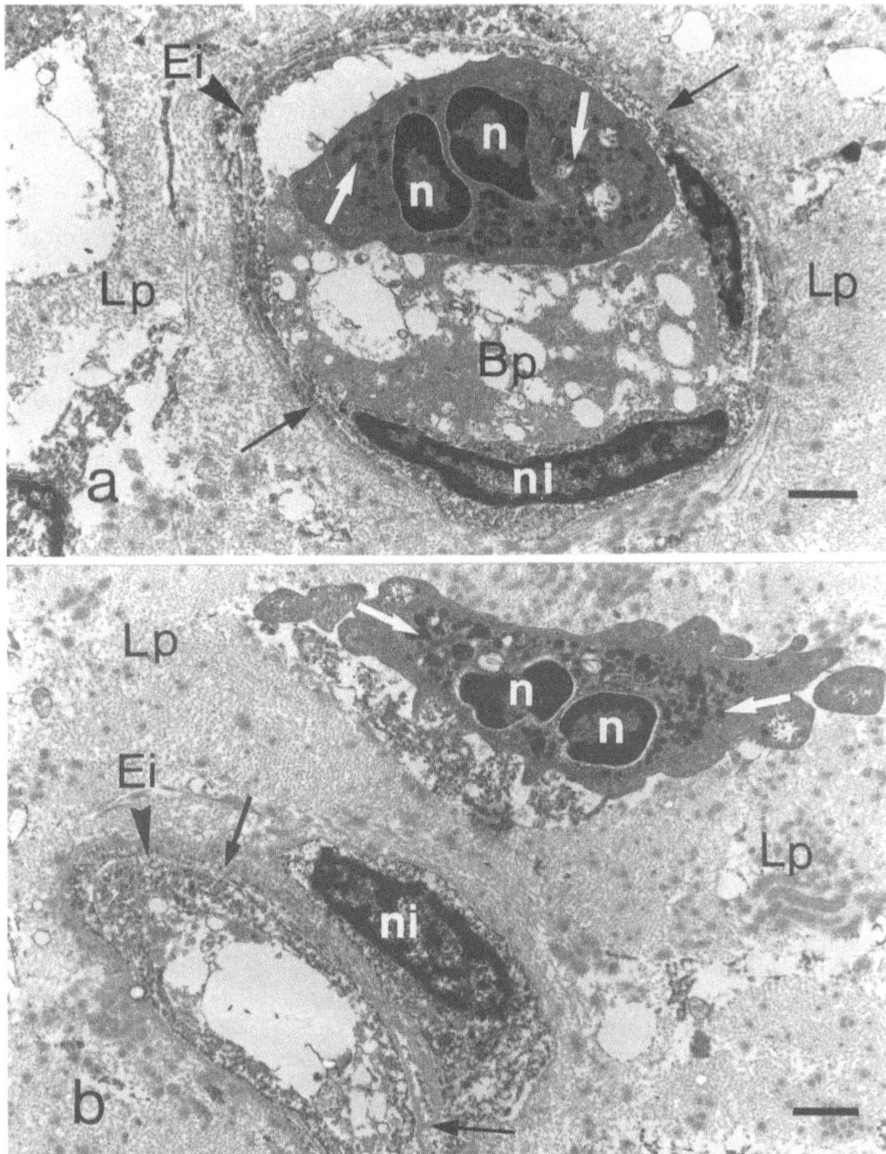

Fig. 8a, b. Neutrophils within differential regions of the irradiated rat esophagus. **a** Within a destroyed capillary of the lamina propria 2 mm from the laser center 90 min after irradiation (argon laser, 514 nm, 12 s, 2.5 W). **b** Adjacent to a destroyed capillary of the lamina propria *(Lp)* 2 mm from the laser center 90 min after irradiation (argon laser, 514 nm, 12 s, 2.5 W). *Black arrows* indicate injured basal lamina; *white arrows* lysosomes, *arrowheads* injured endothelium. *Bp,* coagulated blood plasma; *Ei,* injured endothelium; *Lp,* lamina propria; *n,* lobulated nuclei of neutrophils; *ni,* injured nuclei; *bar* = 1 µm

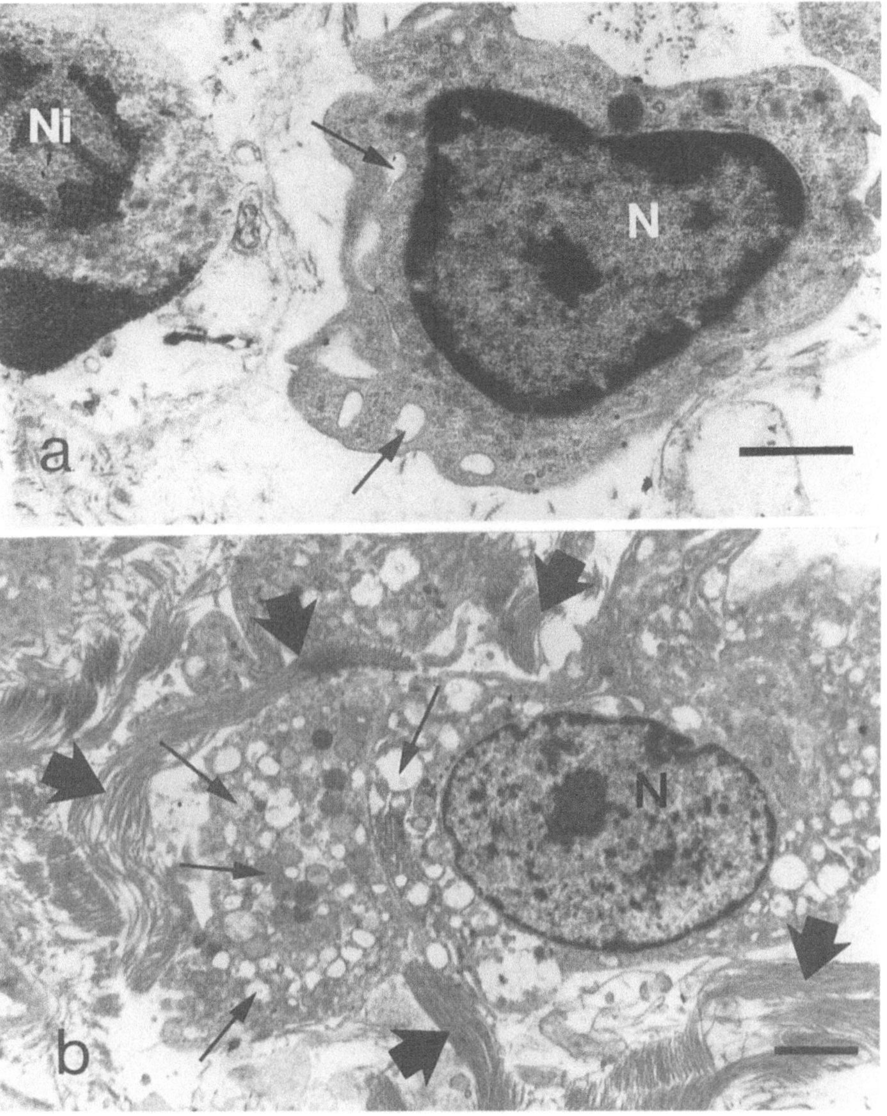

Fig. 9a, b. Macrophages 2 days (**a**) and 14 days (**b**) after irradiation (Nd:YAG laser, 1064 nm, 12 s, 7.5 W). **a** Within the endomysium of the destroyed lamina muscularis; *bar* = 1 μm. **b** Highly active macrophage in the regenerating lamina propria. Vacuoles indicated by *thin arrows; thick arrows* show irregular bundles of collagen microfibrils; *bar* = 2 μm; *N,* nucleus; *Ni,* injured nucleus

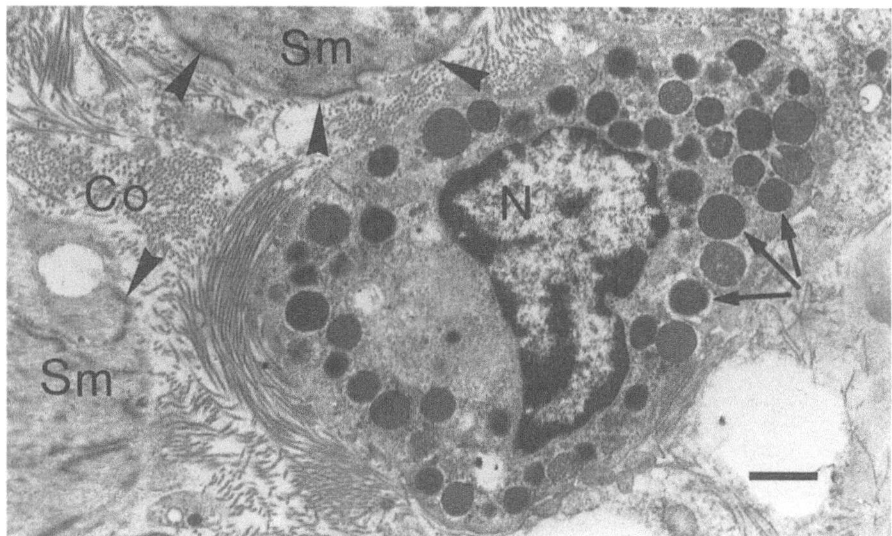

Fig. 10. Mast cell in close proximity to smooth muscle cells *(Sm)* 14 days after irradiation (Nd:YAG laser, 1064 nm, 12 s, 7.5 W). *Arrows* indicate granules, *arrowheads* dense bodies. *Co,* collagen microfibrils; *N,* nucleus; *bar* = 1 μm

and degraded. However, their rate of turnover during regeneration seems to be considerably increased compared to uninjured tissue.

Mast cells are regular constituents of the mucosal and submucosal loose connective tissue. Unlike most other cells of inflammation they maintain a permanent residence in the connective tissue. Fourteen days after laser irradiation, they appear in close proximity to the smooth muscle cells of the lamina muscularis mucosae (Fig. 10). Their cytoplasm is densely packed with electron-dense, basophilic granules. Mast cells have been shown to produce and store heparin, histamine, and serotonin, and they also participate in the synthesis of collagen microfibrils and hyaluronic acid. Their significance in the secretion of specific mediators of the inflammatory response is generally recognized [4].

New Connective Tissue Components

As early as 2 days after laser irradiation, new, activitated fibroblasts are seen within the lamina propria (Fig. lla). The damaged tissue material has been removed by macrophages and other cells. Within the empty spaces, newly formed collagen microfibrils are laid down. The proliferation of the connective tissue has been studied autoradiographically by incorporation of [³H]-thymidine, an integral building block of DNA specifically incorporated during the S phase of the cell cycle [8]. Fourteen days after irradiation, formation of large bundles of collagen microfilaments in the submucosa is completed (Fig. 11b). Fibroblasts in this area are still characterized by abundant profiles of the rough endoplasmic reticulum, indicating continual protein synthesis.

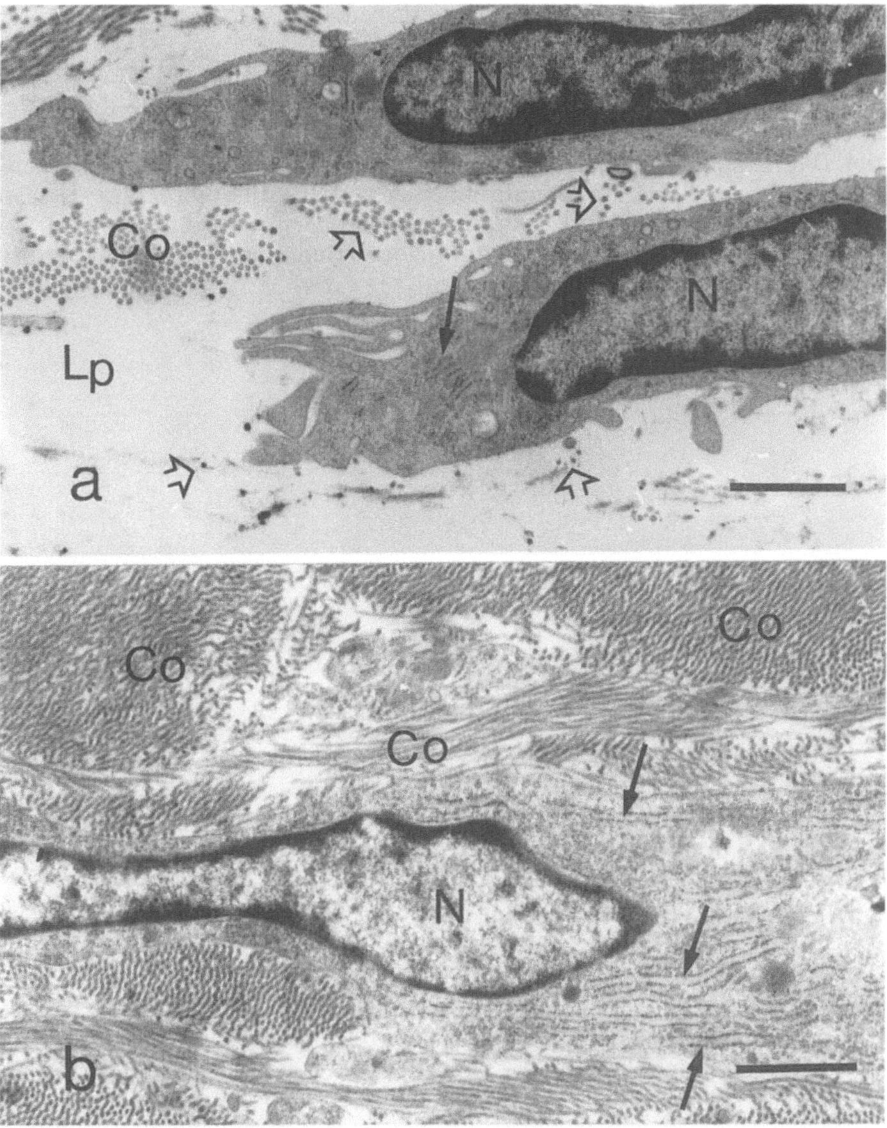

Fig. 11a, b. Regenerating connective tissue components after irradiation by Nd:YAG laser, 1064 nm, 12 s, 7.5 W. **a** Two fibroblasts migrate into the damaged lamina propria *(Lp)*, 2 days after irradiation; *short arrows* indicate newly synthesized collagen microfibrils. **b** Abundant bundles of collagen microfibrils *(Co)* have been synthesized 14 days after irradiation; *long arrows* indicate rough endoplasmic reticulum. *N*, nucleus; *bar* = 1 μm

Regeneration of the Epithelium

The epithelial layer regenerates from the margin of the damaged zone. The new epithelial cells migrate as a continuos sheet underneath the damaged epithelial layer. Numerous cell divisions can be observed even 14 days after laser irradiation (Fig. 12b). In the most damaged epithelium, several layers of the stratum corneum and the stratum granulosum (Fig. 12a) and all other layers are seen. The proliferation behavior of the epithelium has been studied in detail [8]. The relatively high epithelial capability of regeneration after laser irradiation has been reported by several authors [2, 3].

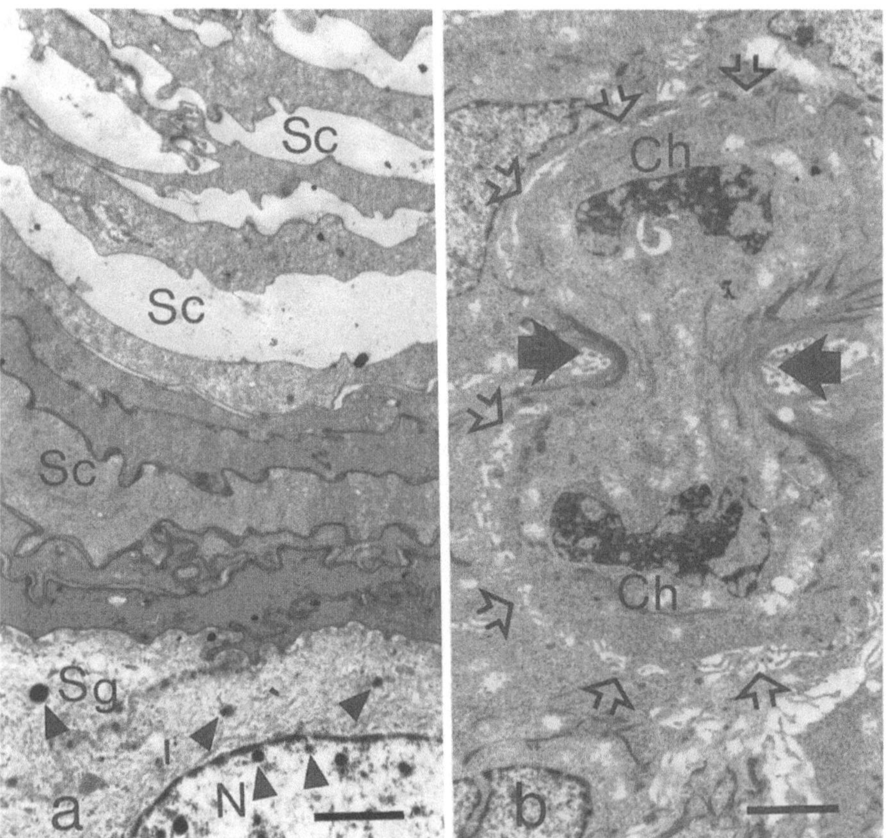

Fig. 12a, b. Regeneration of the stratified keratinized squamous epithelium 14 days after laser irradiation (Nd:YAG laser, 1064 nm, 12 s, 7.5 W). **a** Portions of the stratum corneum *(Sc)* and underlying stratum granulosum *(Sg); arrowheads* indicate keratohyalin granules. **b** Late anaphase/early telophase of the proliferating stratum basale; *large arrows* indicate cleavage furrow, *small arrows* interdigitations with adjacent cell surfaces. *N*, nucleus; *Ch*, transformation of chromosomes into daughter nuclei; *I*, coagulated intercellular matrix; *bar* = 2 μm

Smooth Muscle Cells

There was no continuous layer of smooth muscle cells in the regenerated esophageal wall [14, 18]. Smooth muscle cells were absent in extended regions, resulting in a continual transition from the lamina propria to the lamina submucosa. Only occasionally could single smooth muscle cells be recognized, especially in the 2-mm zone.

Regeneration of Striated Muscle Cells

Fourteen days after laser irradiation, striated muscle cells have fully regenerated at a distance of 2 and 4 mm from the laser center respectively. In the laser center, however, regeneration of striated muscle cells is not yet completed (Fig. 13). A variety of stages of incomplete sarcomeres are seen in the cytoplasm of newly formed muscle

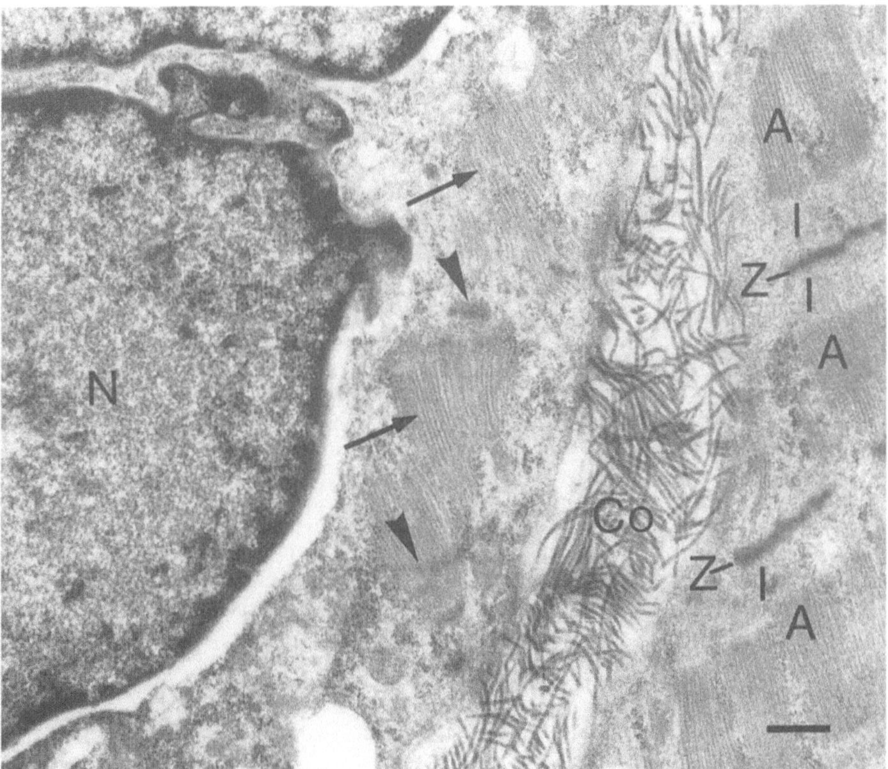

Fig. 13. Regeneration of the lamina muscularis 14 days after laser irradiation (Nd:YAG laser, 1064 nm, 12 s, 7.5 W). The formation of sarcomeres is still incomplete *(center)*; new Z line indicated by *arrowheads*, newly synthesized thick myosin filaments are marked by *arrows*. The adjacent striated muscle cell *(right)* shows new sarcomeres with A bands *(A)*, I bands *(I)*, and Z lines *(Z)*. *Co*, collagen microfibrils of the renewed endomysium; *N*, nucleus; *bar* = 1 μm

cells. Mester et al. [10] stated that the histologic picture after laser-induced muscle injury resembles the arrangement of myoblasts in early embryonic development. The regeneration of the striated muscle cell layer may derive either from regeneration of partly damaged striated muscle cells or from sarcoblasts deriving from dividing satellite cells [15, 16].

Conclusion

The various examples described above have been selected to emphasize the need for more fundamental knowledge of biological structures and their functions after laser irradiation. One basic question is: How is the organization of cellular function influenced by laser irradiation? The evaluation of laser treated tissues is often limited to the light microscopic descriptions of vaporization, carbonization, coagulation, and necrosis. Surely, these types of tissue damage are evident, and the most obvious sign of cell damage is necrosis. The electron microscope has greatly enhanced the possibility of assessing cell damage by alterations in the ultrastructure. Some of the altered structural signs are reversible; others are the inevitable prelude to cell death. Electron microscopy allows the investigator to find out variations occur in the more than a dozen cellular compartments or organelles and in the extracellular matrix following laser irradiation.

Acknowledgements.   The author is indebted to Dr. Katalinic for providing the human skin specimens, Dr. K. Schaarschmidt for conducting the rat experiments, Dr. U. Stratmann for preparing the rat material and contributing to the microscopic evaluation.

References

1. Baggiolini M (1980) The neutrophil. In: Glynn LE, Houck JC, Weissmann G (eds) The cell biology of inflammation. Elsevier/North-Holland, Amsterdam, p 179 (Handbook of inflammation, vol 2)
2. Gaster RN, Binder PS, Coalwell K, Berns M, McCord RC, Burnstein NL (1989) Corneal surface ablation by 193 nm excimer laser and wound healing in rabbits. Invest Ophthalmol Vis Sci 30: 90–98
3. Godlewski G, Rouy S, Dauzat M (1987) Ultrastructural study of arterial wall repair after argon laser micro-anastomosis. Lasers Surg Med 7: 258–262
4. Lagunoff D, Chi EY (1980) Cell biology of mast cells and basophils. In: Glynn LE, Houck JC, Weissmann G (eds) The cell biology of inflammation. Elsevier/North-Holland, Amsterdam, p 179 (Handbook of inflammation, vol 2)
5. Lehmann RR (1990) Laser: Bedeutung morphologischer Untersuchungen. Klinikarzt 19: 280–289
6. Lehmann RR, Willital GH (1990) Morphological alterations following laser resection of abdominal tumors in children. Lasermedizin 10: 25–35
7. Lehmann RR, Meier H, Willital GH (1990) Electron microscopic observations following Nd:YAG laser resection of tumors in children. In: Waidelich W, Waidelich R (eds) Laser optoelectronics in medicine. Springer, Berlin Heidelberg New York, pp 45–48
8. Lehmann RR, Stratmann U, Schaarschmidt K, Hellweg PC, Willital GH, Maragakis M (1991) ³H-thymidin autoradiographie: Untersuchung am Ösophagus der Ratte nach Laserbestrahlung. In: Waidelich W, Waidelich R, Hofstetter A (eds) Laser in medicine. Springer, Berlin Heidelberg New York, pp 343–346

9. Lehmann RR, Stratmann U, Schaarschmidt K, Hellweg PC, Willital GH (1994) Proliferation von Epithel- und Bindegewebe im Ösophagus der Ratte nach Nd:YAG-Laser-Bestrahlung. Eine autoradiographische Untersuchung. Lasermedizin 110: 168–178

10. Mester E, Korényi-Both A, Spiry T, Tisza S (1975) The effect of laser radiation on the regeneration of muscle fibers. Z Exp Chir 8: 258–262

11. Piez KA (1975) The regulation of collagen fibril formation. In: Slavkin HC, Greulich RC (eds) Extracellular matrix influences on gene expression. Academic, New York, pp 231–236

12. Rainoldi R, Candiani P, de Virgilis G, Bini M, Sideri M, Mauri L, Garsia S, Remotti, G (1983) Connective tissue regeneration after laser-CO_2 therapy. Int Surg 68: 167–170

13. Riedel HH, Stamer U, Mecke H (1987) Methoden elektronenmikroskopischer Untersuchungen am Uterushorn des Neuseeländer Kaninchens nach Anwendung von 4 verschiedenen Koagulationstypen. Zentralbl Gynaekol 109: 1345–1349

14. Schaarschmidt K, Stratmann U, Lehmann RR, Heinze H, Willital GH, Unsöld E (1992) The rat esophagus: ultrastructure and radiological aspects of tissue response after 1320 mm Nd:YAG laser radiation. Exp Toxicol Pathol 44: 239–244

15. Schmalbruch H (1985) Skeletal muscle. In: Oksche A, Vollrath L (eds) Handbook of microscopic anatomy, vol 2/6, 2nd edn. Springer, Berlin Heidelberg New York, pp 280–296

16. Snow MH (1978) An autoradiographic study of satellite cell differentiation into regenerating myotybes following transplantation of muscles in young rats. Cell Tissue Res 186: 535–540

17. Solursh M (1989) Extracellular matrix and cell surface as determinats of connective tissue differentiation. Am J Med Genet 34: 30–34

18. Stratmann U, Schaarschmidt K, Lehmann RR, Heinze A, Willital GH, Störmann J, Wessling G (1991) Light and electron microscopic study of the rat esophagus following intraluminal argon laser radiation. Acta Anat (Basel) 141: 85–89

19. Stratmann U, Schaarschmidt K, Lehmann RR, Willital GH, Wessling G, Kessler T (1993) Die Gewebeantwort des Rattenösophagus nach intraluminaler Bestrahlung mit Nd:YAG-Laser (1064 nm) zu unterschiedlichen postoperativen Zeitpunkten: Eine licht- und elektronenmikroskopische Studie. Ann Anat 175: 95–100

20. Stratmann U, Schaarschmidt K, Lehmann RR, Willital GH (1995) The interaction of laser energy with ureter tissues in a long-term investigation. Scanning Microsc 9: 805–816

21. Stratmann U, Schaarschmidt K, Lehmann RR, Schürenberg M, Willital GH, Berens A (1995) The morphological tissue response of the piglet oesophagus to experimental irradiation by ND:YAG laser treatment J Anat 187: 661–670

22. Viehberger 6, Fischer R, Kyrle P, Plenk H (1979) Ultrastructure of skeletal muscle after CO_2-laser incision. Res Exp Med 176: 69–7

Clinical Features and Classification of Congenital Vascular Disorders

M. Poetke, C. Philipp, and H. P. Berlien

Introduction

The two basic types of congenital vascular disorders (CVD) are based on aberrances of embryonic angiogenesis. Although not fully understood, there seem to be types that are present at birth with mostly constant size and others that develop during the first weeks of life and later present phases of growth and sometimes involution. In most cases, the first type is classified as vascular malformation, while the latter is classified as hemangioma (Fig. 1) [3, 6]. The differential diagnosis of a hemangioma may prove difficult, whereby the medical history provides important information. Relaying on the clinical aspects alone can lead to a false diagnosis [7].

Hemangioma	Vascular malformation
• Capillary • Tuberous	• Capillary • Arterial • Venous • Lymphatic • Mixed

Fig. 1. Classification of congenital vascular disorders (CVD)

Hemangiomas

Clinical Features and Morphology

Between 2% and 3% of newborns develop a hemangioma [5]. The hemangioma is a vascular tumor that usually starts to grow in the first weeks of life. Acute progression and a spontaneous involution, are both possible.

Hemangiomas are usually not seen at birth. Prodromal phases appear quite often that occasionally still exist at birth; however, they are often misinterpreted [6]. The following prodromal phases are possible:
1. The white spot
2. Central vessel in spite of the presence of a vascular spider
3. Telangiectatic vascular spreading
4. Port-wine stain-like lesion

Hemangiomas often grow intensively, causing the parents of such children to become concerned.

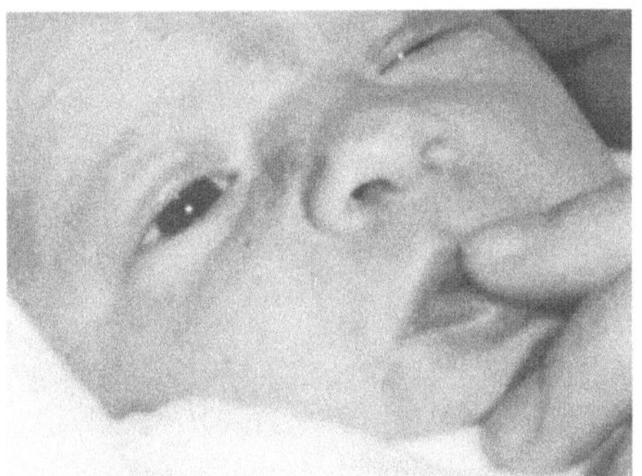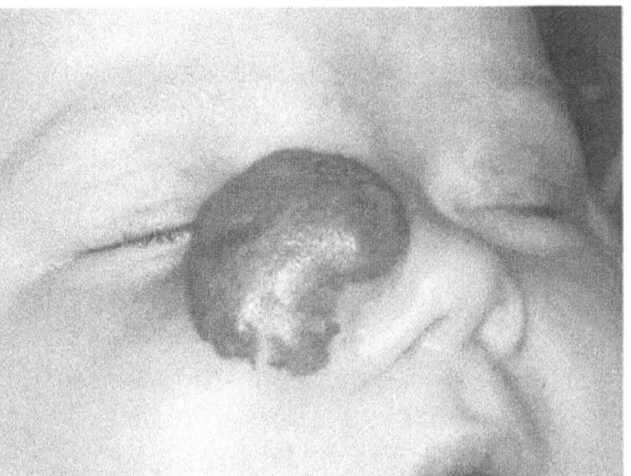

Fig. 2a, b. **a** Newborn child with a port-wine stain-like lesion of the nose. **b** At the age of 6 months a hemangioma causing astigmatism

There are two forms: capillary and tuberous. Capillary hemangiomas often appear in a pale skin area (white spot) in which a vascular mark shows up days or sometimes weeks later, often misinterpreted as a spider nevus. Highly perfused skin areas considered to be port-wine stains or "birthmarks" should be observed for growing tendencies during the first days and weeks of life, as tuberous hemangiomas can present this type of prodromal state (Fig. 2). Once growth is observed, it must be assumed that a hemangioma has started to develop, yet the duration of the growth period and termination remain unpredictable.

The color intensity of hemangiomas essentially depends on their depth and spread and the lumina of the vessels involved, but there may be fluctuation due to localization, state of excitement, and temperature.

Localization

Though all regions of the body can be affected by hemangiomas, 70% of them are localized on the head. Typical sites are the eyelids, base and tip of the nose, the lips, and the forehead and hairy head. Hemangiomas are also often observed at the extremities, on the trunk and in the anogenital region. Here ulceration and bleeding accompanied by a superinfection are possible as a result of urine and stool soiling or friction of diapers or clothing edges.

Hemangiomas are not only found on the skin. They also appear in soft tissue, organs, and bones. A multiple appearance is frequent.

Follow-up

In the course of a few months, growth termination can be observed, followed by a spontaneous involution that can continue for a few months or often several years. Several phases can be distinguished in the spontaneous course:
1. Prodromal state at birth

2. Proliferation phase up to the age of 1 year
3. Phase of early involution at the age of 1–5 years
4. Phase of late involution up to adolescence

The infiltrating and partially destructive growth of these benign vascular tumors is the main problem.

Initially, in the phase of early involution growth stops. The spontaneous regression process covers several years and is individually very variable. In 30% of hemangiomas, regression is incomplete, with cosmetically and functionally unsatisfactory residuals which have to be corrected in subsequent operations. An additional 20% of hemangiomas do not regress, nor can the regression tendency be predicted. However, spontaneous regression is no guarantee for a satisfactory cosmetic result as is often presumed. Complete healing presents very differently, with de- or hyperpigmentation, telangiectasia, dermatochalasis (cutis laxa), atrophia, or scarring. The best cosmetic regression can be seen in plane hemangiomas. If skin changes occur, remaining changes of the skin may correspond to the largest size of the hemangioma. Scarred changes can also be observed during spontaneous regression, which appears within previous ulceration of the hemangioma with hypertrophic thickened parts. Tuberous hemangiomas, though, often show continuous enlargement and tend to include larger vessels in their development.

Often there is a dissociation in the proliferation phase, especially in combined cutaneous and subcutaneous hemangiomas. While the cutaneous part of a hemangioma may stop growing, the subcutaneous part can continue to grow and reach a considerable size.

Besides cutaneous residuals, there are often irrevocable functional defects due to the location. Hemangiomas of the eyelid can obstruct the eye. Within a short time, loss of eyesight is possible when the eye becomes amblyopic. Scars after spontaneous regression of hemangiomas of the lip can negatively influence the normal development of speech and of the jaw by dentoalveolar distortion.

Vascular Malformations

Clinical Features and Morphology

Vascular malformation can be characterized by the following: It is present at birth, but sometimes not in full size. The process grows proportionally to natural growth; the volume can change. There is no spontaneous involution, but there is often enlargement due to the pathologic flow of blood.

In some cases, the vascular malformation remains preformed and latent and grows as a result of a lesion, trauma, or a hormonal effect. This can happen during adolescence or even during adulthood.

Vascular malformation is based on a disturbance of the vessel architecture. There are truncular and extratruncular forms [1]. Often one can find a combination of both. The truncular form of a vascular malformation is fundamentally based on an obstruction, dilatation, arteriovenous communication, or a combination of these different forms. A malformation with an obstruction shows either agenesis, aplasia, hypoplasia, or hyperplasia of vessels. An irregular structure of the vessel wall, position anomaly as a result of an irregular origin and course, or a persistent fetal vessel can be the reason for this. Often there are arteriovenous microshunts or a hemolymphatic anastomosis. Vascular malformation shows vessels that are of capillary, arterial, venous, lymphatic, or mixed origin.

Localization

Vascular malformations are often localized on the extremities. They can infiltrate the skin but can also appear in soft tissue, muscle, bones, and structures of the organs.

Particularly venous malformations are often well compressible. In the case of truncular malformations, hypo- or hypertrophy of bones and soft tissue is often present. When comparing the two sides, one can see a difference in the length and the circumference of the extremities.

Follow-up

In contrast to the hemangioma, there is no proliferation of the vessel wall in vascular malformations (Figs. 3, 4). Especially through a lesion, an operation, and hormonal effects such as appear in pregnancy, deterioration and further enlargement are possible.

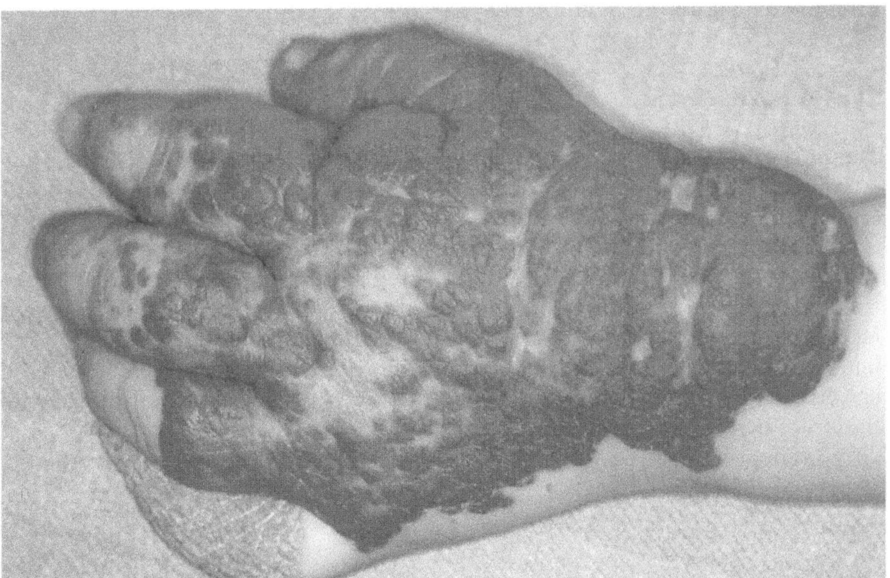

Fig. 3. Four-month-old child with a vascular tumor of the hand which appeared shortly after birth and grew rapidly: a hemangioma

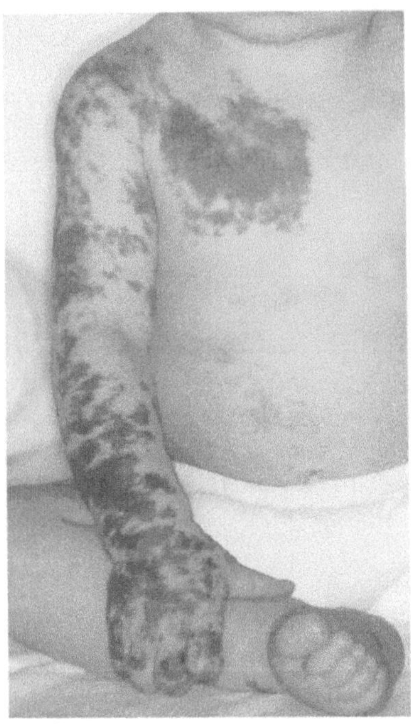

Fig. 4. One-year-old boy with a diffuse vascular birthmark of upper and lower extremity present since birth and enlarging proportionately: a vascular malformation

There is no chance of spontaneous involution.

The Port-Wine Stain

The port-wine stain is a special form of vascular malformation and is based on a congenital dilatation of the capillary vessels. No vascular proliferation is found. These cutaneous capillary malformations appear at an incidence of 0.3% in newborns [5]. The stain´s glowing red color is noticeable and stands apart sharply from the remaining skin. With increasing age the so-called tuberous transformation with outpouching of vessels and outward bulge of the skin surface develops. The color of the port-wine stain can change to dark red or livid blue. As often described, it is not the question of hemangiomas as an independent disease but as an aftereffect of an aging port-wine stain. Therefore, early initiation of therapy is required.

The congenital port-wine stain in particular is frequently observed with other structural defects.

Lymphatic Malformation

The lymph vessels can also show a malfunction or predisposition in the sense of a vascular malformation. The primary lymphedema caused by an aplasia or hypoplasia of the lymph vessels is a well-known example. In addition, course abnormalities can be described that are comparable to the arterial or venous form. There are also lymphangiectasias that manifest themselves as the so-called lymphangioma, a lymphatic malformation [6].

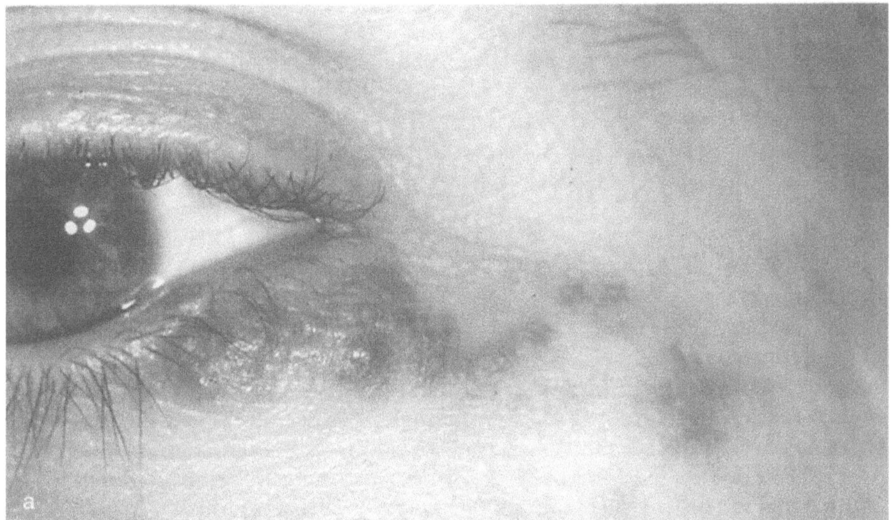

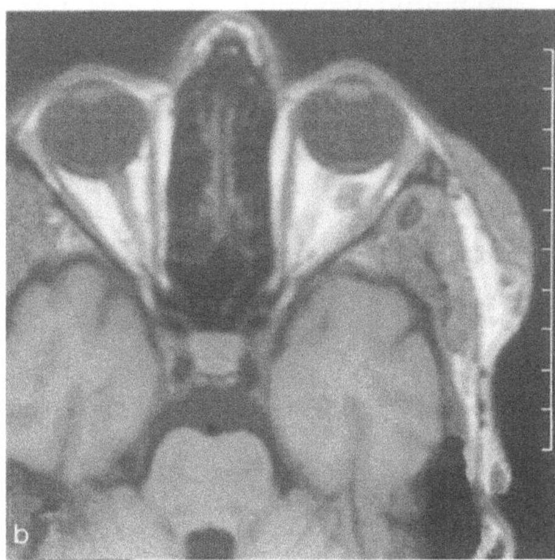

Fig. 5a, b. a Eighteen-year-old boy with diffuse venous malformation of left face. b An additional retroorbital vascular anomaly

Complications

Somatic complications of various types appear within at least 8% of congenital vascular disorders (Fig. 5). The psychosocial stress is not considered. Initial complications are a clear indication for treatment and should lead immediately to a suitable therapy. Some complications occur mainly with hemangiomas, such as ulceration and bleeding, and others with vascular malformations, such as cardial decompensation. Some complications occur in both types of disorders, such as obstruction and compression or hemorrhagic symptoms, which we have seen in giant hemangiomas and in vascular malformations.

Kasabach-Merritt Syndrome

A rare but significant complication is the so-called Kasabach-Merritt syndrome. It describes a thrombocytopenia with possible hemorrhagic symptoms. The real pathomechanism of this serious and life-threatening complication is not known. Besides an increasing consumption of thrombocytes as a result of a capillary injury of the endothelium, microthrombotic changes have been suggested. The syndrome´s dependence on a specific morphologic manifestation is also unclear.

Psychosocial Complications

The psychosocial aspect has to seriously be taken into account. The children are marked by the vascular changes, especially if the sign is in the facial region, which disgusts uninformed nonprofessional onlookers and creates considerable obstacles to normal social integration. In addition the children are hidden by their parents, who feel ashamed, or the mother imagines that it was her own faulty behavior during pregnancy that caused the hemangioma.

Even if the hemangioma is able to regress spontaneously over years, it represents long-term stress for children and parents if in an exposed area. The ensuing problems of fear and worry should not be underestimated. Parents feel that they cannot show their children in their normal social environment. Often the fear is expressed that they would not be able to cope with a possible injury or scratching. Normal social integration is hindered in the kindergarten or nursery school if affected children are teased or excluded from playing with the others. When children grow older, they react with increasing aggressiveness, depression, nervousness, and concentration problems [4].

In the case of a port-wine stain, where somatic complications with tuberous transformation and an increasing hypertrophy of the affected regions has to be taken into acount, the psychosocial stress on patients and relatives should not be underestimated by dismissing it as a problem of cosmetic appearance.

Staged Program for the Treatment of Hemangiomas

Treatment of hemangiomas is still controversial. Until recently, the "wait-and-see" approach was recommended because of the strong tendency for spontaneous regression exhibited by these lesions and the considerable complication rate of former therapeutic modalities. However, one has to consider why this recommendation was made. All other therapeutic procedures have shown a considerable complication rate in comparison with the possibility of a spontaneous regression. In this context it should be remembered there were severe side effects after radiotherapy.

Through the further development of therapeutic modalities, especially of laser technologies, an early and careful therapy has become possible [8], so that hemangiomas can be treated in prodromal or early phases to avoid an expansion.
1. Hemangiomas in the face and anogenital region have to be treated as emergencies and should be treated within a few days.
2. If there is a clear growth increase in the early phase when the hemangioma is located in another part of the body, it should be treated within the following week.
3. Hemangiomas of the orotracheal tract should also be treated as emergencies and make use of a laser in order to avoid the necessity of a tracheotomy.

In the hemangioma treatment protocol the main decision has to be made according to the region where the hemangioma occurs. On the face and in the anogenital region we do not wait for spontaneous regression. Following color-coded duplex ultrasound (CCDS) and sometimes magnetic resonance tomography (MRI), we immediately start laser treatment to prevent further growth and other complications. In the therapy of Kasabach-Merritt syndrome, before con-

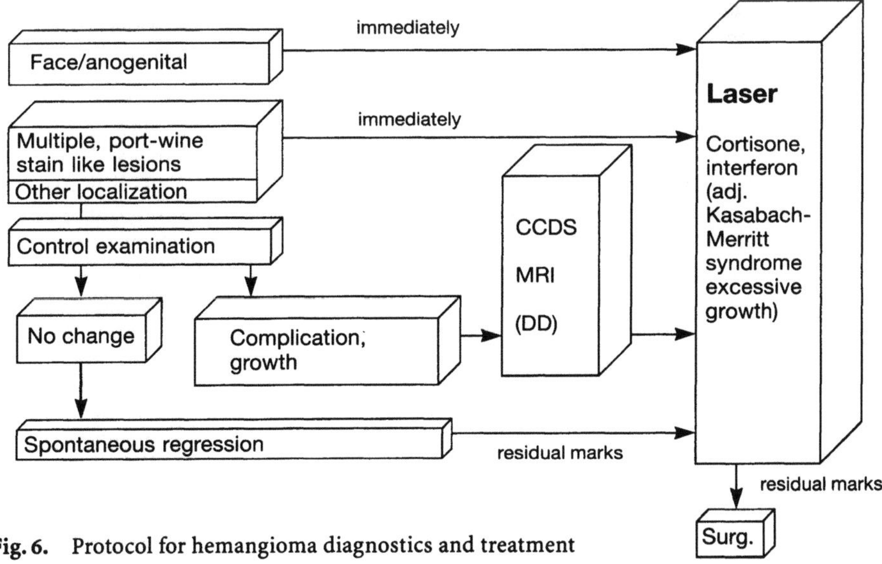

Fig. 6.   Protocol for hemangioma diagnostics and treatment

clusive studies as to the effects of interferon or cortison therapy have been conducted, laser therapy can be initiated (Fig. 6).

In all other locations we generally wait for spontaneous regression. If, instead of regression, growth or other complications are noted, we start treatment. Spontaneous involutional hemangiomas can leave disruptive residuals which require continuous therapy to achieve a favorable cosmetic result [2].

Staged Program for the Treatment of Vascular Malformations

Conversely, it is generally agreed that vascular malformations require treatment since they show no spontaneous regression and can lead to considerable complications.

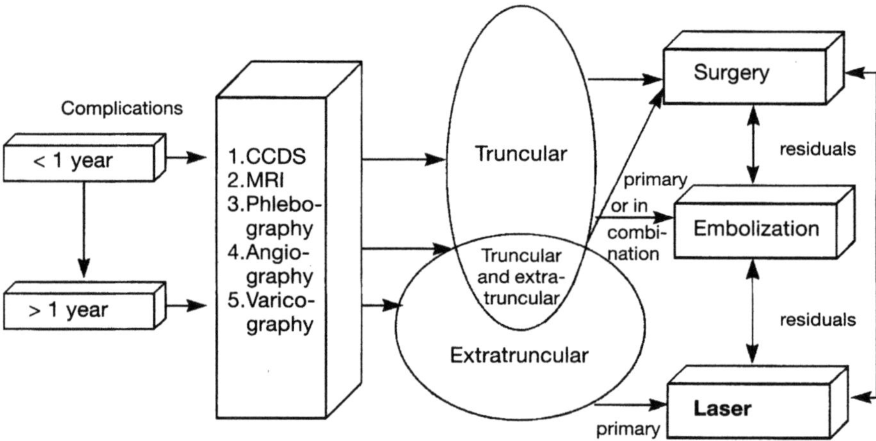

Fig. 7.   Protocol for vascular malformation diagnostics and treatment

In truncular malformations, laser intervention is secondary following vascular surgery, embolization, or sclerotherapy. In venous extratruncular malformations with smaller vessels, laser therapy is the first choice treatment.

The treatment should start early to minimize the secondary symptoms caused by the pathologic blood circulation. If complications arise, such as cardiac decompensation, therapy should be started without delay (Fig. 7). Vascular malformations have to heal completely, in contrast to hemangiomas, unless residuals are acceptable to the patient.

Summary

Distinguishing between CVDs, e.g., hemangiomas and vascular malformations, often presents special problems. The clinical symptoms can be misleading and diagnosis requires complete and careful evaluation of the patient´s history and in some cases further diagnostic measures. A clear histologic classification is limited to cases in which a surgical resection is indicated and the minimally invasive therapy is no longer possible. However, the diagnosis should be made in a very early stage as the different types of congenital vascular disorders require different types of management. While hemangiomas should be treated in their very early stages, the treatment of some vascular malformations can be postponed until the diagnostic and therapeutic measures are of acceptable risk for the patient.

References

1. Belov S, Loose DA, Weber J (1989) Vascular malformations. Einhorn, Reinbeck (Periodica Angiologica 16), pp 19–30
2. Berlien HP, Cremer H, Djawari D, Grantzow R, Gubisch W (1993/1994) Leitlinien zur Behandlung angeborener Gefäßerkrankungen. Paediatr Prax 46: 87–92
3. Finn MC, Glowacki J, Mulliken JB (1983) Congenital vascular lesions: clinical application of a new classification. J Pediatri Surg 18 (6): 894–900
4. Grantzow R, Schmittenbecher PP, Klima-Lange D, Spreng G (1990/1991) Problematik der Therapie von Riesenhämangiomen. Paediatr Prax 41: 311–320
5. Jacobs AH, Walton RG (1976) The incidence of birthmarks in the neonate. Pediatrics 58 (2): 218–222
6. Philipp C, Poetke M, Berlien HP (1993/1994) Klinik und Klassifikation angeborener Gefäßerkrankungen. Paediatr Prax 46: 75–83
7. Poetke M, Philipp C, Mack M, Berlien HP (1997) Hämangiom oder vaskuläre Malformation? Differentialdiagnostische Überlegungen in der Frühtherapie kindlicher Hämangiome und vaskularer Malformationen. Kinderarzt 28 (in press)
8. Poetke M, Philipp C, Berlien HP (1996) Die Laserbehandlung von Hämangiomen und vaskulären Malformationen. Indikationen, Parameter und Applikationstechniken. Zentralbl Kinderchir 5: 138–150

Ten Years of Laser Treatment of Hemangiomas and Vascular Malformations: Techniques and Results

M. Poetke, C. Philipp, and H. P. Berlien

Introduction

Laser treatment of hemangiomas and vascular malformations, collectively referred to as congenital vascular disorders (CVD), is based on a program that seeks to match the type of lesion with the most effective type of therapy. Early treatment of hemangiomas was a point of controversy in earlier publications. Until recently, the "wait-and-see" approach was recommended because of the strong tendency toward spontaneous regression and the complication rate of formerly used therapeutic modalities. Conversely, it is generally accepted that vascular malformations require treatment since they show no spontaneous regression and can lead to considerable complications.

Since 1984, we have employed various types of lasers and application modalities in the management of hemangiomas and vascular malformations. Larger and deep-seated lesions were treated with percutaneous interstitial or intraluminal laser irradiation. For the treatment of subcutaneous lesions to a depth of 2–5 mm, we employ a transcutaneous Nd:YAG laser application with skin protection through local cooling. In combination with the direct Nd:YAG laser coagulation with short pulses, the flashlamp-pumped dye (FDL), and the argon laser treatment of superficial and small vascular disorders, we have a full range of safe and effective tools for the therapy of congenital vascular disorders.

Although the etiopathogenesis of hemangiomas is different from that of vascular malformations, the treatment concept is similar. Depending on the form, localization, and perfusion of vascular disorders, the different irradiation parameters and application procedures are used with the intention of either definite coagulation or the induction of a stasis in vessels with minimum lateral damage and subsequent regression (Table 1).

Table 1. Differential laser therapy of congenital vascular disorders

---

Prodromal phases, capillary, intracutaneous
- Flashlamp-pumped dye laser
- Argon laser
- Nd:YAG laser

Thickness 1–5 mm, intra- and subcutaneous portions
- Nd:YAG laser with continuous surface cooling

Subcutaneous, deep seated
- Nd:YAG laser with interstitial bare fiber technique

Argon Laser Treatment

For the treatment of intracutaneous parts of CVD, the argon laser is used in noncontact with a focussing hand piece. While doing so, single pulses with minor focus (0.05–2.0 mm), 2–3 W, and short exposure times such as 0.1 s are applied. Multiple exposures and overlapping of single irradiation areas have to be avoided. With these parameters, the effective depth is limited to 1 mm with a low risk of damaging the overlaying epidermis, especially if one uses a glass plate. The glass plate has a higher heat conductivity than air. If you put a drop of water between the skin surface and the glass plate you produce an immersion of water, so that the heat is released much faster from the epidermis than from the epidermis to air. A second advantage is the possibility of compressing the vessels in order to simplify coagulation of all vessel parts and to minimize the shielding effect of absorption.

FDL Treatment

Port-wine stains can be treated with the argon laser, but especially with the FDL laser. The high pulse peak power of the FDL disrupts the vessels; furthermore, this laser is characterized by a greater focus, so that a larger area can be treated more easily.

A significant reduction of pain as well as skin protection during laser treatment can be achieved by a cooling chamber with a flexible membrane on the side facing the skin. It allows a smooth contact even on curved surfaces, but also compression of superficial vessels by using valves to build up pressure in the

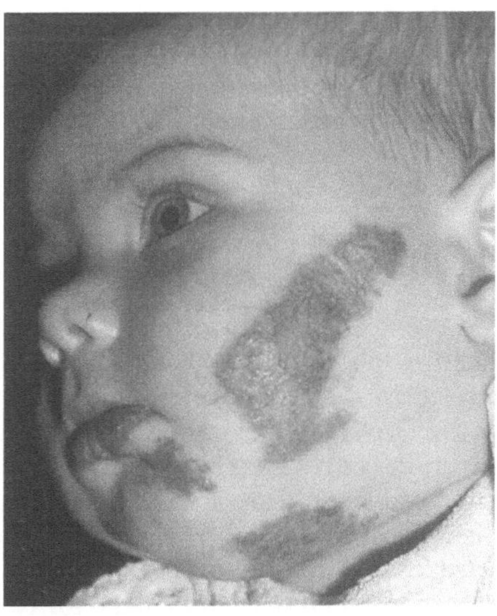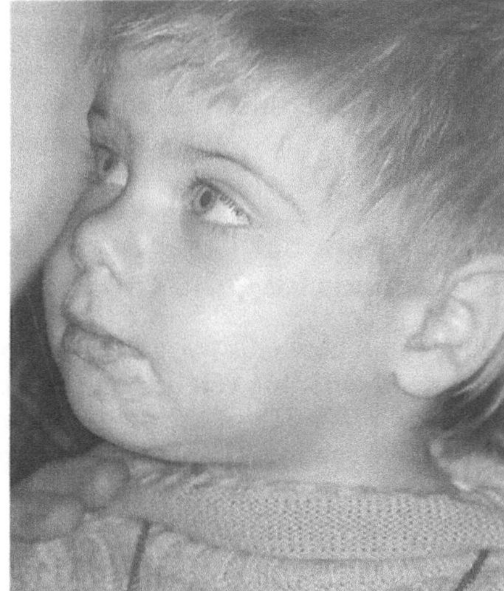

Fig. 1a,b. Cutaneous hemangioma prior to (a) and after (b) laser therapy

chamber. Due to the temperature of the cooling fluid and its flow, the cooling effect can be precisely adjusted to various needs and can be used either for the treatment of port-wine stains or intracutaneous hemangiomas. The anesthetic effect of the cooling is of great advantage, especially in the treatment of children (Fig. 1).

Nd:YAG Laser Treatment

The clinical use of the Nd:YAG laser was proven to be successful in the treatment of hemangiomas and vascular malformations. The Nd:YAG laser emits light in the infrared wavelength range (1064 nm) which will be significantly more strongly absorbed in blood than in the surrounding tissue. As a result of scattering in the tissue the laser irradiation is relatively uniformly distributed. This being the case, it can be observed that the endothelial structures are injured more easily than surrounding connective tissue. With heat conduction an interaction depth can be reached of up to 10 mm.

Transcutaneous Laser Application

For intracutaneous areas of congenital vascular disorders (excepting the special laser therapy of the port-wine stain), the laser beam of the Nd:YAG laser is directly applied in a *repetitive mode*. Multiple exposures of the same area and overlapping of single irradiation areas have to be avoided. An application of the "polka dot technique" is helpful in avoiding confluenced coagulation of the skin. The distance between the single application spots should be as large as the focus diameter. With these parameters the effective depth is limited to 1 mm; furthermore, there is a low risk of damage to the skin. Carbonization or even evaporation of the skin has to be avoided.

To minimize the risk of any destruction of the regenerative skin layers, an additional application procedure was established: transcutaneous laser application with continuous surface cooling.

Transcutaneous Laser Application with Continuous Ice Cube Cooling

With transcutaneous Nd:YAG laser application in *continuous mode* a coagulation depth of 8 mm can be reached. Less selective water absorption and reflection and remission of the emitted laser beam would damage the skin without protective cooling. Highly sufficient protection is provided by clear ice cubes placed directly on the skin [1, 2]. The defocused laser beam should be applied directly through these ice cubes. With the help of an ice cube pressing on the skin surface, the coagulation depth can be increased up to 10 mm (Figs. 2, 3).

Local skin cooling can reduce the risk of thermal epidermal damage for two reasons. First, due to the cooling effect of water of a constant temperature of

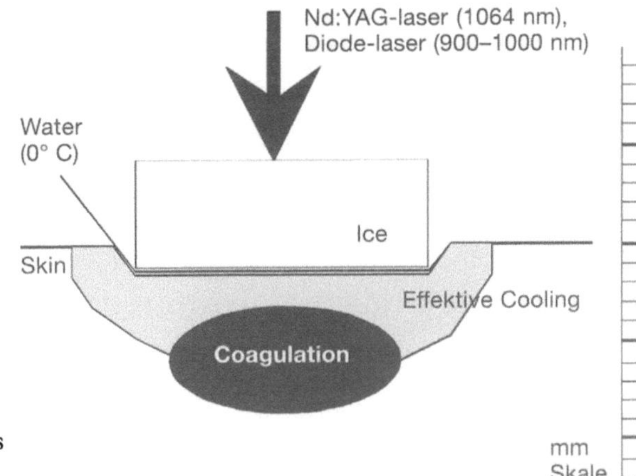

Fig. 2. Principle of continuous ice cube cooled irradiation

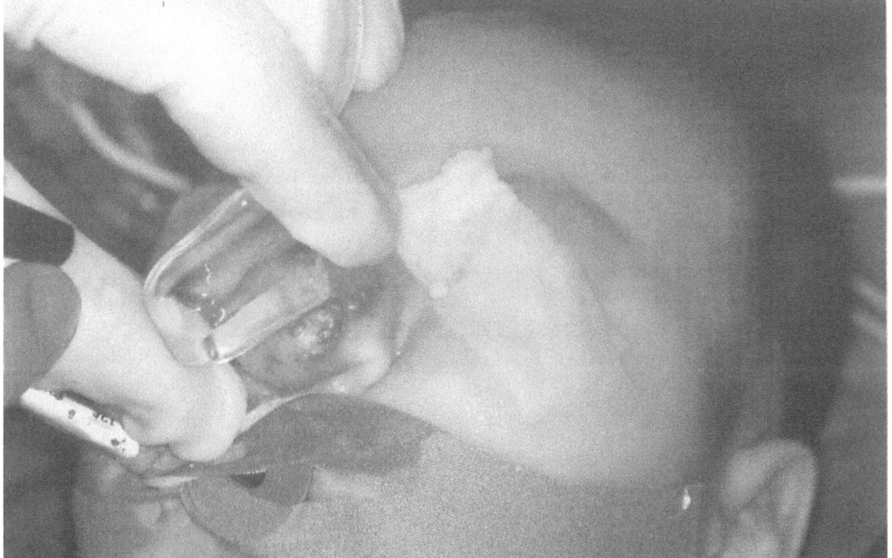

Fig. 3. Continuous ice cube cooling during the transcutaneous irradiation of a growing hemangioma

0°C melting on the contact surface of the ice and skin, the heat transfer from the superficial layers into the water is very effective and the skin can be spared coagulation. At a depth of approximately 1.5 mm where cooling has no effect because of the limited heat conduction of the skin, the temperature rises to more than 60°C with a resulting coagulation zone. Secondly, by pressing the ice cube on the skin surface, the epidermal thickness is reduced so that a lesser amount of laser irradiation is absorbed into this layer.

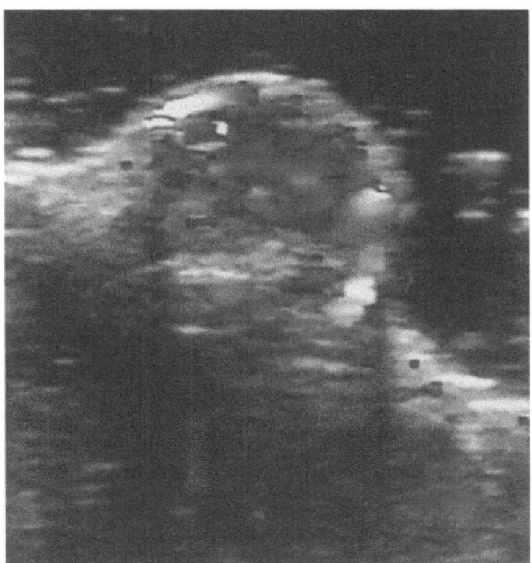

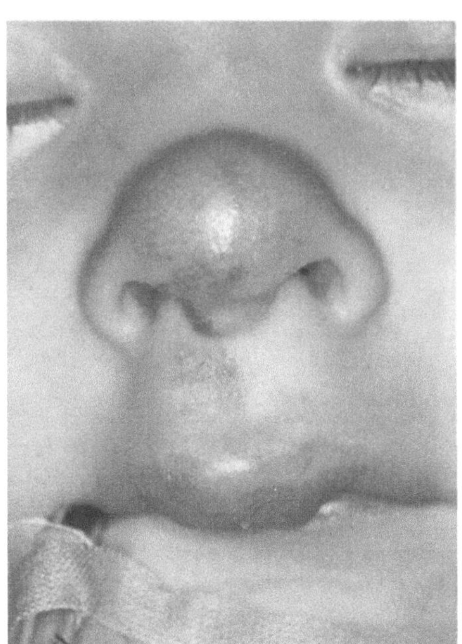

Fig. 4a, b.   A 6-month-old boy with a growing subcutaneous hemangioma (**a**) with high flow characteristics (**b**)

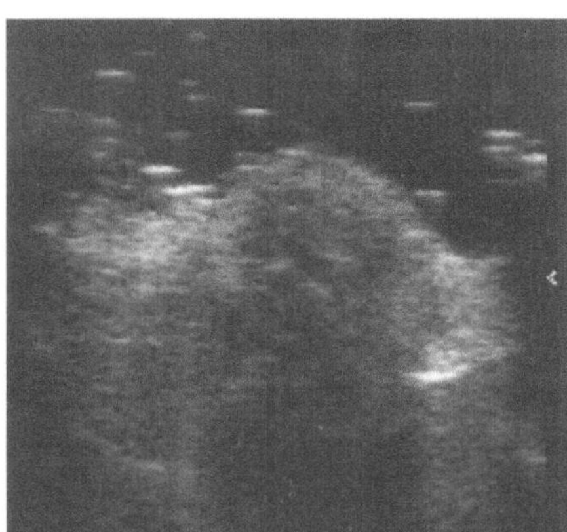

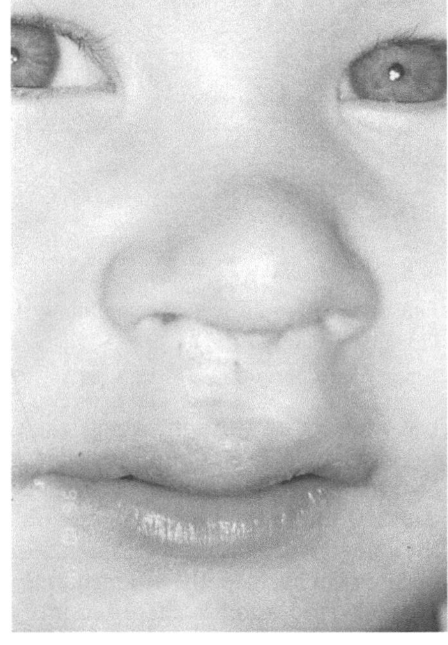

Fig. 5a, b.   After two transcutaneous laser treatments of patient in Fig. 4, we achieved the preservation of the lip and nose with full function and sensibility (**a**). The decrease of coloration by perfusion in the color-coded duplex ultrasound is notable (**b**)

Using this method, one must remember to change the ice cubes regularly since they melt during laser irradiation. Generally, irradiation should be terminated when initial blanching becomes visible or after a 20-s irradiation period of the same region. By doing so, thermal damage to the skin can be avoided (Figs. 4, 5).

Percutaneous Interstitial or Intraluminal Bare Fiber Technique

If a lesion is located deep in the subcutis or if there is a congenital vascular disorder with a high-flow vessel, percutaneous application has proven to be very useful [3, 4]. Using this technique, direct puncturing of the lesion is performed by a teflon cannula (Abocath G16) through which a newly fractured bare fiber is introduced. One has to be aware that there is a distance of about 5 mm between the end of the bare fiber and the end of the teflon cannula, in order to avoid damage to the cannula.

The red helium–neon pilot beam can often be used as a positioning aid. The correct position of the fiber end can be easily and clearly identified in a dimmed room by the pilot light up to a depth of approximately 2 cm or with ultrasound.

Two different kinds of interstitial application are possible:

1. Leaving the bare fiber and the abocath in the same position during the irradiation of an area: the area is changed afterwards.
2. Withdrawing the bare fiber and the abocath simultaneously at a speed of 1 mm/s during laser treatment.

If possible, the first technique should be applied because one adds a specific amount of energy to a definitive area.

A power of 5 W and an irradiation time of 180 s at the maximum should be chosen because longer application time or higher power can cause carbonization of the tissue and the fiber. To avoid a coagulation necrosis of the superficial

Table 2. Laser parameters for the Nd:YAG laser treatment of congenital vascular disorders (except port-wine stain)

Transcutaneous (depth 0–1 mm)
  Nd:YAG laser (1064 nm)
    20 W, 0.1 s
    1 mm spot diameter

Transcutaneous with ice cube cooling (depth 0–8 mm)
  Nd:YAG laser (1064 nm)
    25–30 W, cw
    5–7 mm spot diameter, focussing hand piece
    Irradiation through the ice cube, good contact to skin obligatory

Percutaneous (depth >2 mm)

Interstitially	Intraluminally
Nd:YAG laser (1064 nm)	Nd:YAG laser (1064 nm)
Max. 5 W, continous wave	Max. 10 W, continous wave
bare fiber, newly fractured	Bare fiber with additional rinsing

layers, the temperature of the irradiated skin region has to be controlled using two fingers placed on the skin surface of the treated area. However, one must be careful not to press the skin directly onto the fiber tip because the laser beam could then damage the skin.

Since 1992, color-coded duplex sonography has been used for the online control of this procedure. This technique provides complete information, for example, for determination of the precise puncturing route, control of the fiber position, visualization of tissue changes during the procedure, as well as for depiction of the reduction of tumor perfusion and coagulated volume (Table 2).

Postoperative Care

Postoperatively the irradiated area will swell considerably as a symptom of the induced inflammation reaction. This is not a complication but an intended tissue reaction. After treatment a therapy-free interval of 4 to 6 weeks is necessary to allow complete healing of the induced inflammation and restitution of the skin.

After laser therapy the treated body area should be protected from mechanical stress and excessive sunlight strain. Blisters may appear and should not be opened because restitution should not be endangered. Minor crust formation is possible.

Results

Of a total of about 2798 patients with CVD who were referred to our clinic by colleagues and other centers, we have completed the treatment of 965 patients between 1984 and 1994. In particular, 599 patients presented with hemangiomas with more than 872 lesions; 121 of them were capillary and 751 tuberous. Another 366 patients showed vascular malformations. We saw 165 patients with venous, 42 with lymphatic, and 159 with capillary malformations.

Distribution of Type, Age, Localization, and Multifocal Appearance

Of all of the 599 hemangioma patients, more than 60% received laser treatment in their first year of life. The reason for this is the large amount of proliferating hemangiomas in this initial phase of childhood. In fact, 151 cases were presented at 1–3 years of age. Most of them showed large, often tuberous lesions with continuing growth or complications; 61 patients between 4 and 7 years of age were treated for noninvoluting hemangiomas or the removal of residuals.

The distribution of age is slightly different from that of patients with vascular malformation. The largest group – with 185 cases – was older than 14 years. In the group with the youngest patients, the group of up to 1 year of age had 29 cases and that of 1–3 years 37 cases. The vascular malformations were mostly located in the head and neck region or the thorax and showed rapid enlargement, relevant shunting, or complications. The patients in the other groups who were between 4 and more than 14 years old (mostly venous malformations of various sizes and locations) were presented. Some showed residuals after sclerotherapy or surgical resection. Some were recognized at a later age; often a trauma was remembered by the patients or their parents with a subsequent development of vascular malformation.

In both groups of CVD, we saw a multifocal appearance of lesions. If the lesions were close to each other, they were counted as one. Only if different body regions or structures were involved were the lesions counted separately. Up to 30 hemangiomas were counted in a newborn after 2 weeks, but most of the hemangioma patients showed one or two lesions. In the vascular malformation group a multifocal appearance of lesions was more seldom. In 25 cases of hemangiomas, organs such as the parotid or the trachea were involved and in eight cases vascular malformations as well.

We performed 170 transcutaneous treatments with an argon, FDL, or Nd:YAG laser, 1044 treatments transcutaneously with ice cube cooling, 517 treatments interstitially, and 65 treatments endoscopically with bare fiber (Table 3).

The treatments were performed either on an in- or outpatient basis according to age, localization, and size with good to excellent results in most cases and a complication rate of less than 2%.

Table 3. Side effects of laser treatment of congenital vascular disorders

Side effect	Management
Superficial treatment	
Skin burn second degree	Instant cooling for reduction of thermal effects
Hyperpigmentation	Mostly temporary (1–2 years), Active reduction of pigmentation possible with argon or Q-switched Nd:YAG laser (532 nm)
Hypopigmentation	Only seen in argon laser use with wide spot
Interstitial treatment	
Swelling	Intraoperative corticoid i.v. in patients with orotracheal lesions
Paresthesia	Control examination

Hemangiomas

The mean number of treatments was 1.03 for all cases.

In prodromal stages, a single treatment is sufficient in most cases for complete and scarless removal via argon or FDL laser. Thus, active treatment can be indicated on a broad basis with regard to the previously proven growth tendency. In plane lesions, a single treatment is sufficient for prevention of further growth. Involution is often seen within the next few weeks. Tuberous hemangiomas require repeated treatments (two to three times) with the Nd:YAG laser. Since they often grow extensively, one should treat them as soon as possible. Even if they do not show any change in size, laser treatment can reduce the volume of hemangiomas, initializing the process of regression.

Vascular Malformations

The number of treatments was 3.0 for venous and 2.07 for lymphatic malformations.

Extratruncular venous malformation is a primary indication for laser therapy, while truncular malformations require embolization and/or vascular surgery in most cases. Lymphatic malformation of the head and neck region show prolonged progression and should be continuously followed up. The treatment can prevent complications, such as tracheostomy, by being repeated.

Conclusion

Due to the development of new therapeutic modalities (especially new laser technologies), an early therapy of CVD with low complication rates is possible. Hemangiomas can be treated in the prodromal or early phases to prevent expansion and to induce regression. Furthermore, extratruncular vascular malformations should be treated in time to minimize secondary symptoms caused by the pathological circulation.

Summary

From 1984 to 1994, we treated 965 children with more than 1238 lesions of congenital vascular disorders such as hemangiomas and vascular malformations. Most of the patients ($n = 599$) presented hemangiomas of the face and the anogenital region, and some were located in the trachea or mouth or in the urogenital tract. All of these hemangiomas were growing prior to intervention or showed complications such as bleeding, ulceration, superinfection, or obstruction. Furthermore, 366 patients presented with vascular malformations, either of the singular-vessel type, involvement or mixed-vascular origin (venous, arteriovenous, venolymphatic, lymphatic) with various complications such as tracheal obstruction or recurrent thrombophlebitis.

According to our staged program, the hemangiomas were treated as early as possible, while the vascular malformations were only treated with laser when no other therapeutic technique (embolization, resection) seemed suitable. The lasers used were flashlamp-pumped dye laser, argon laser, and Nd:YAG laser with transcutaneous application with or without surface cooling or interstitial laser application.

References

1. Berlien HP, Müller G, Waldschmidt J (1986) Correct selection of different types of laser treatment of surface and deep located vessel anomalies. 3rd Congress of the European Laser Association (ELA), Amsterdam
2. Berlien HP, Waldschmidt J, Müller 6 (1988) Laser treatment of cutaneous and deep vessel anomalies. In: Waidelich W (ed) Laser optoelectronics in medicine. Springer, Berlin Heidelberg New York, pp 526–528
3. Berlien HP, Müller G, Waldschmidt J (1990) Lasers in pediatric surgery. Prog Pediatr Surg 25: 5–22
4. Poetke M, Philipp C, Berlien HP (1996) Die Laserbehandlung von Hämangiomen und vaskulären Malformationen. Indikationen, Parameter und Applikationstechniken. Zentralbl Kinderchir 5: 138–150

Diagnosis and Therapy of Pediatric Airway Obstructions

J. ENGERT

Introduction

Any stenosis of the tracheal or bronchial lumen can, depending on the degree and nature of the stenosis and on the age and maturity of the afflicted child, by itself or by additional closure of the remaining lumen by swelling, secretion, loose hemorrhagic-suppurative or crusty material, granulation tissue, foreign bodies etc. lead to a life-threatening emergency situation which allows only little time for diagnosis and therapy. The diagnostic and therapeutic procedures depend on the etiology, nature and degree of the obstruction and on its localization and must be individually adapted to the maturity of the anatomy and the age of the child.

Tumors, Stenoses, and Strictures of the Tracheobronchial Tree

When tracheal and bronchial malacias, vascular stenoses and papillomatosis are not considered, probably most tracheal stenoses in childhood are due to traumatic intubation and long-term intubation and suction procedures during long-term artificial respiration [2, 4] and are accordingly found mainly in the upper trachea or, in the case of tracheostomas, just cranial to the stoma. The frequency is 54% in some series [13].

The importance of inflammatory stenoses, including necrotizing tracheobronchitis (NTB), is not reported uniformly and amounts to 25% in some series [11]. Tumors and angiomas account for approximately 14% [11]. Congenital lesions and stenoses are correspondingly much rarer and more frequently involve the lower trachea [2, 4]. When the congenital forms are classified according to the predominant symptoms, 90% of the stenosing malformations are laryngeal anomalies [16]; 75% of these are the prognostically favorable laryngomalacia.

Total congenital atresias of the larynx, the trachea, or the lungs are incompatible with survival; isolated atresias associated with an otherwise intact bronchial system provide a theoretical chance of survival.

Congenital Stenosing Malformations

Supraglottal Stenoses

Supraglottal stenoses due to laryngeal cysts, membrane stenoses, hemangiomas, and papillomas belong to the congenital obstructing malformations. Congenital

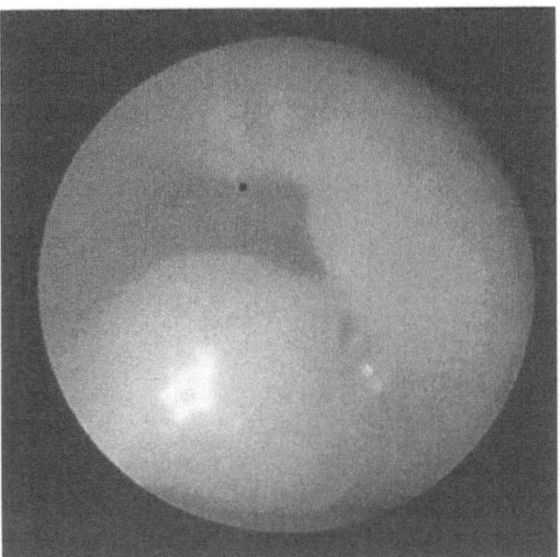 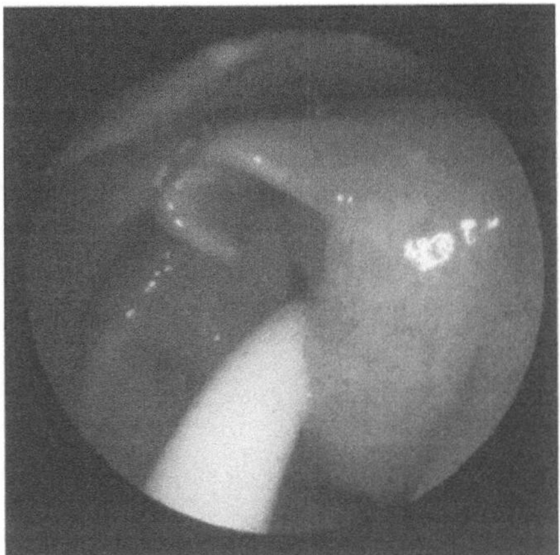

Fig. 1.   Congenital laryngoceles producing typical stridor

laryngoceles (Fig. 1) only seldom cause an intraluminal or intramural obstruction and usually present later in childhood. Simple retention cysts must be distinguished from laryngoceles. Laryngo-esophago-tracheal clefts, hamartomas, and malformations of the larynx itself as well as the extremely rare intralaryngeal struma with typical, slowly worsening stridor require differentiated diagnosis and therapy; in the context of laser treatment their diagnostic and therapeutic importance goes beyond endoscopy.

Anterior Glottal Membranous Stenoses

Anterior glottal membranous stenoses, which may extend into the subglottal space and cause a protruding thickening of the cricoid (hyperplastic cricoid stenosis), or

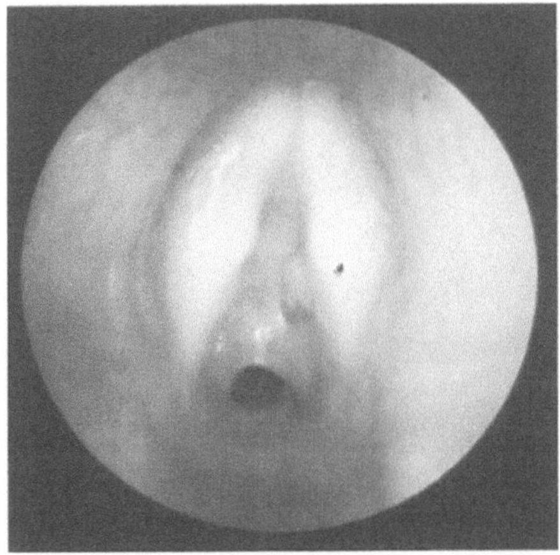 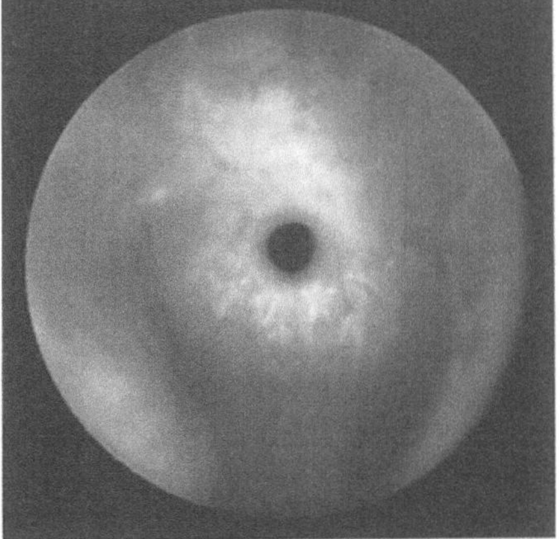

Fig. 2.   Glottal membranes producing high-grade stenosis at the level of the vocal chords

glottal membranes in the form of membranous synechiae at the level of the vocal chords (Fig. 2), possibly in combination with supraglottal membranes, are characterized by "voiceless crying." Some lesions of the recurrent nerve, which cause unilateral or bilateral vocal chord paralysis (stridor, "week cry", respiratory distress syndrome) and which are present in 10% of these malformations, are combined with other central nervous or cardiovascular anomalies. These, as well as ankylosis of the cricoarytenoid joints, which is also characterized by vocal chord immobility, must be diagnosed immediately.

Subglottal Stenosis

The relatively common congenital subglottal stenosis, either circumscribed or extensive, presents as hyperplastic cricoid stenosis (possibly an abortive form of laryngeal atresia) with a lumen diameter of 2–3 mm (Fig. 3) or as connective tissue hyperplasia immediately below the vocal chords and has a relatively good prognosis. In addition, there are membranes, fibrous cicatritial diaphragms, hemangiomas, glandular cystic hyperplasias and also papillomatosis, which will not be discussed here. Moore than 85% of subglottal hemangiomas (Fig. 4) become symptomatic during the first year of life. They are located in the posterior or lateral subglottal space and, aside from hoarseness, dyspnea, and feeding difficulties due to vascular engorgement during crying, may produce only the typical, gradually worsening croupous stridor as the sole symptom. Some subglottal hemangiomas are the partial expression of a hemangiomatosis (Fig. 5) with further localizations in the regions of the head, neck, hypopharynx and larynx. Intralaryngeal and tracheal strumas are extremely rare and present with approximately the same clinical picture. Also to be mentioned, in the other parts of the trachea, are vascular malformations (hemangiomas), cysts, lipomas, lymph nodes, hypoplasia and cartilaginous anomalies such as complete cartilage rings, dystopias and cartilage bridges, fibrovascular hamartomas, mucosal

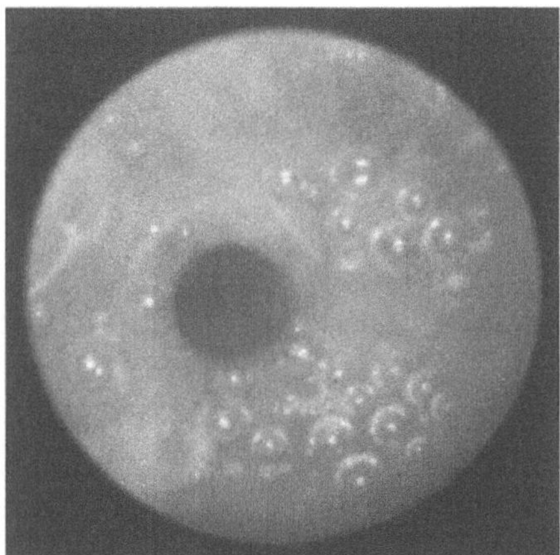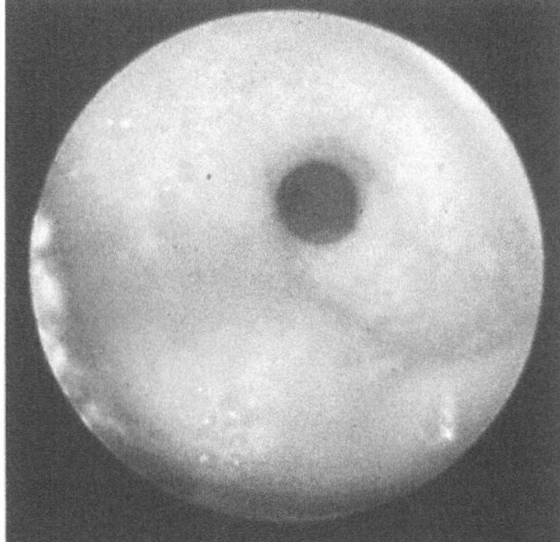

Fig. 3.   Congenital *(right)* and acquired *(left)* subglottal stenosis

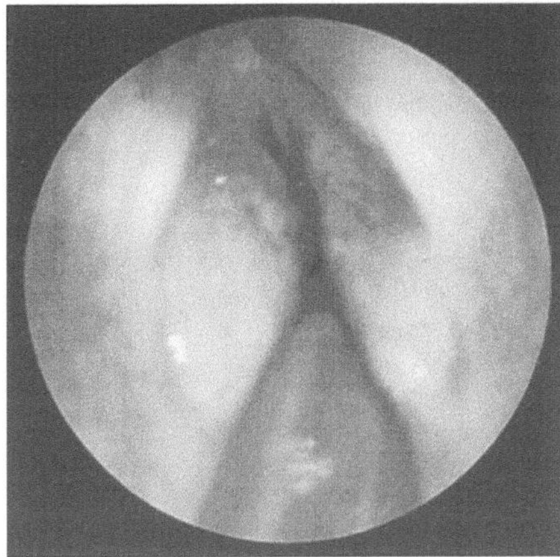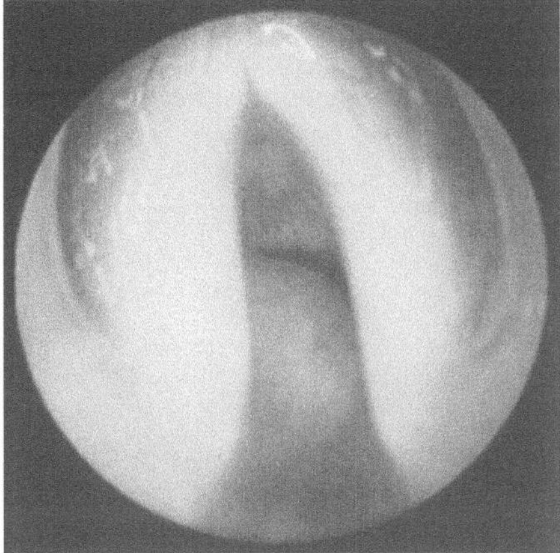

Fig. 4. Glottal and subglottal hemangioma. (Acknowledgements to K. Mantel, Munich)

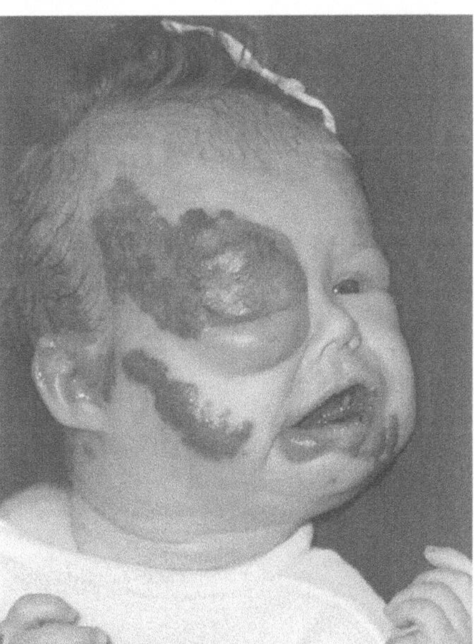

Fig. 5. Hemangiomatosis (vascular malformation) of the head and neck associated with subglottal hemangioma

folds with and without cul-de-sac (Fig. 6) after correction of esophageal atresia as well as rare tumors and trifurcated or T-shaped tracheas.

Acquired Stenoses

Postintubational Lesions

Among the secondary, acquired stenoses of the tracheobronchial tree the postintubational lesions are, besides the lesions of the vocal chords (Fig. 7a, b),

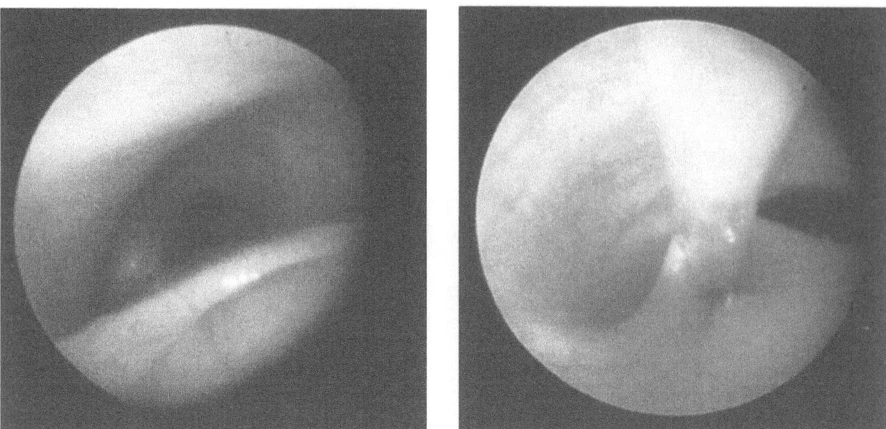

Fig. 6. Mucosal fold and cul-de-sac after correction of esophageal atresia

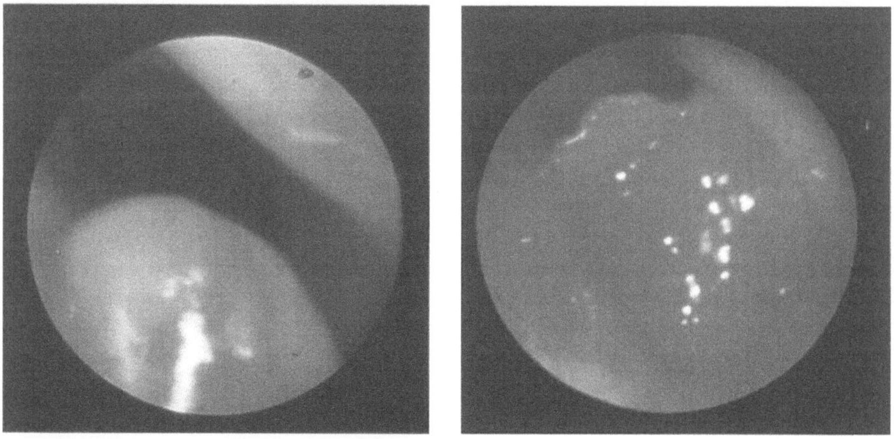

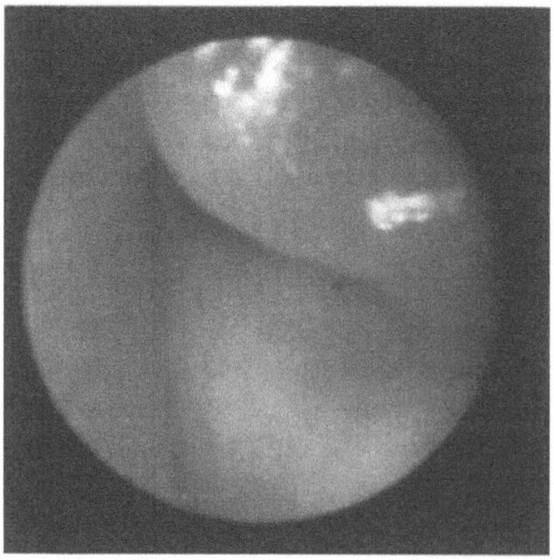

Fig. 7a

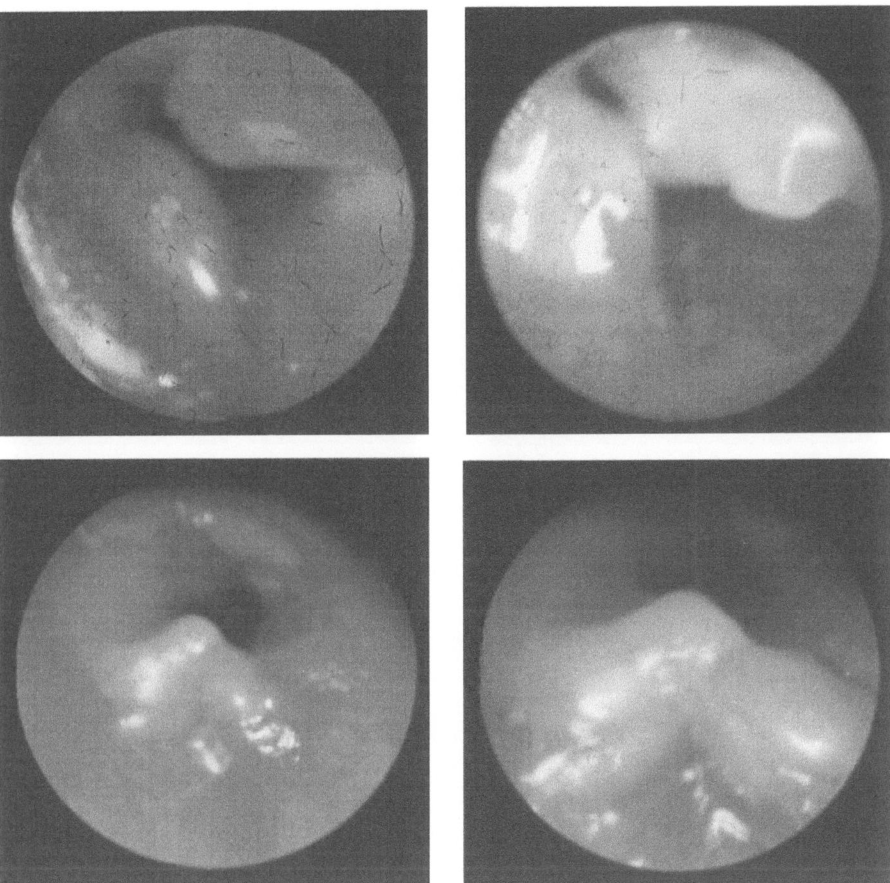

Fig. 7a, b.   Postintubational lesions of the vocal chords and the subglottal trachea

the most important entity: a traumatic intubation typically injures the subglottal trachea by tangentially separating the mucosa from its understructure and sometimes also by destroying its continuity. Furthermore, the endotracheal tube has extensive contact at the level of the cricoid, the only anularly closed cartilaginous ring, which also has the smallest diameter in the infant trachea, so that here, even when there has been no direct injury, compression lesions with subsequent cicatritial stenosis can result [4].

Although a rate of 1.6%–6.7% of postintubation stenosis was reported by Parkin et al. (1976 as quoted in [11]) the actual frequency in dependence on the maturity of the child and other underlying disturbances is below 1%. Adequate dimension of the tube, acceptance of a slight air leakage, better fixation, control of infections, and limitation of the duration of intubation can reduce postintubational lesions (Fig. 8a, b) but, because of the increasing numbers of especially small premature infants requiring long-term artificial ventilation, cannot eliminate them entirely.

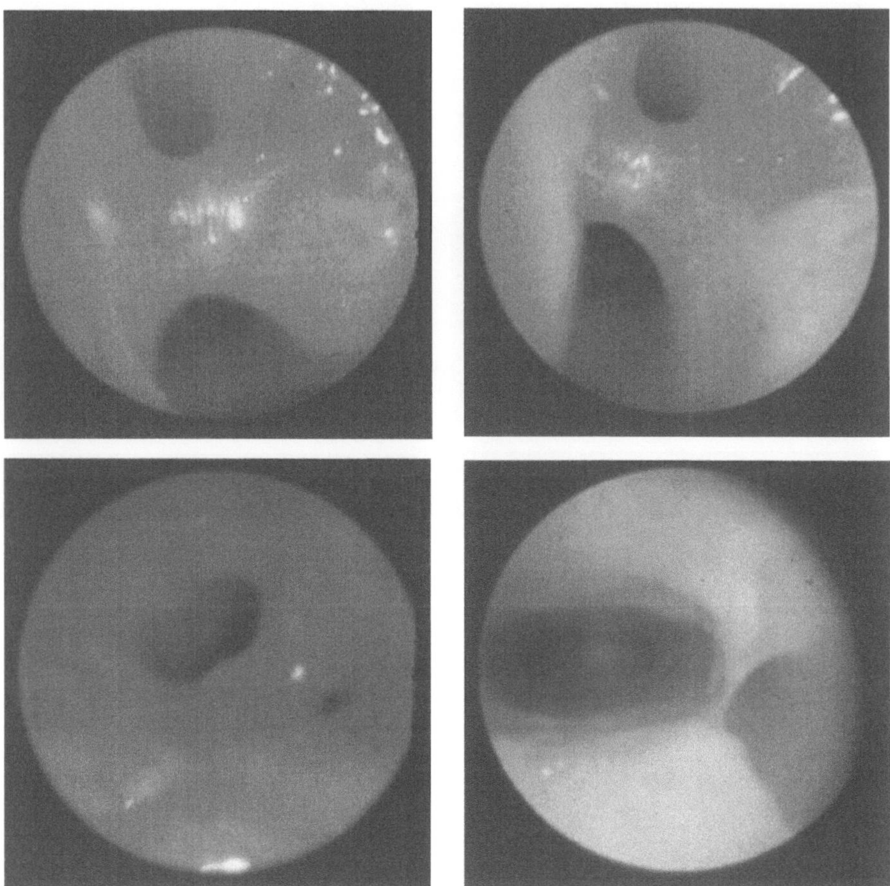

Fig. 8a

Postinfections Granulomas and Cicatritial Stenoses

Postinfectious granulomas and cicatritial stenoses result from necrotizing tracheobronchitis (NTB) not exclusively, but most severely, in premature infants
with a pronounced deficiency in immune competence. Sometimes multiple,
short, or extensive tracheal stenoses develop from deep ulcerations; serosal
sequestrations with persisting excessive granulation, obstructing crusts, and
constricting scars may even close the lumen completely (Fig. 9a, b).

Tracheostomas

Tracheostomas, which should be avoided if possible because of the danger of
infection of potential operation sites, are almost regularly accompanied by the

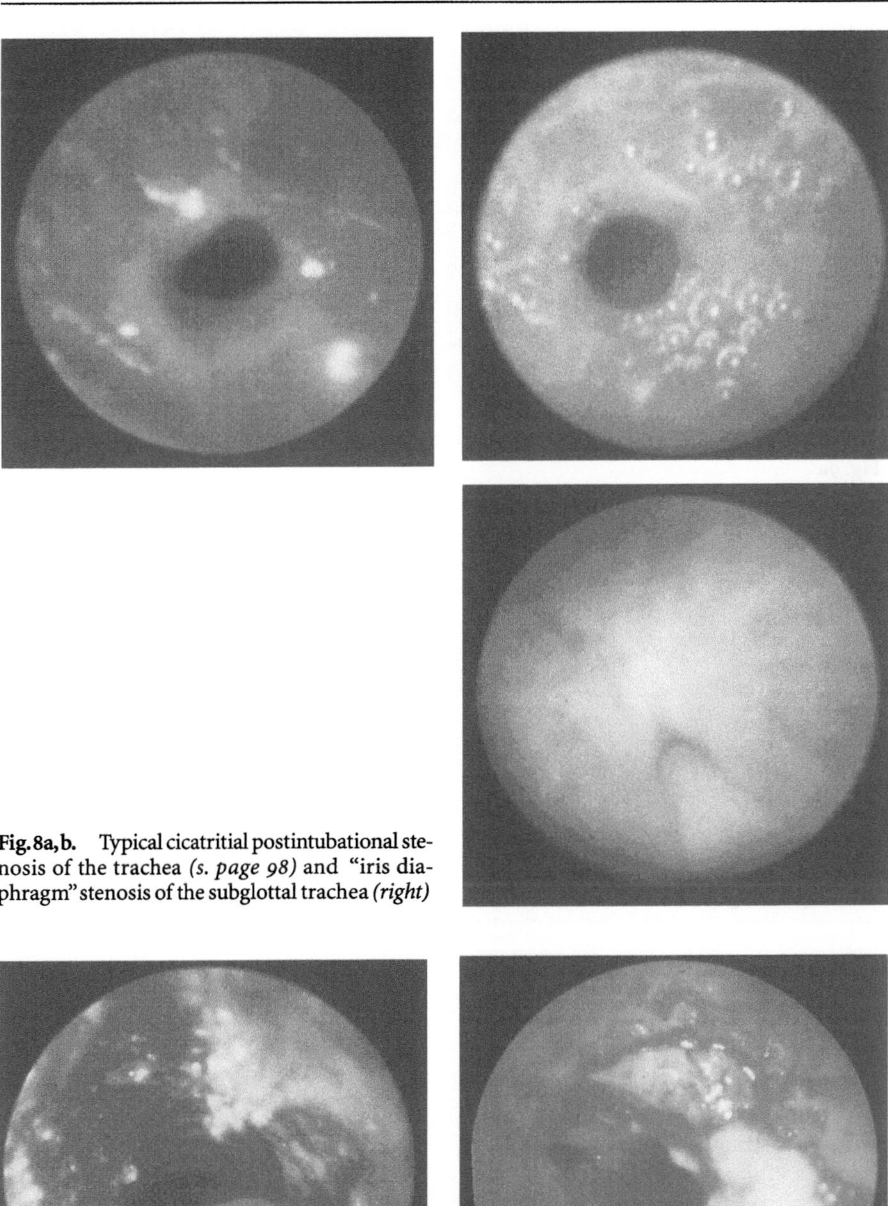

Fig. 8a, b. Typical cicatritial postintubational stenosis of the trachea *(s. page 98)* and "iris diaphragm" stenosis of the subglottal trachea *(right)*

Fig. 9a

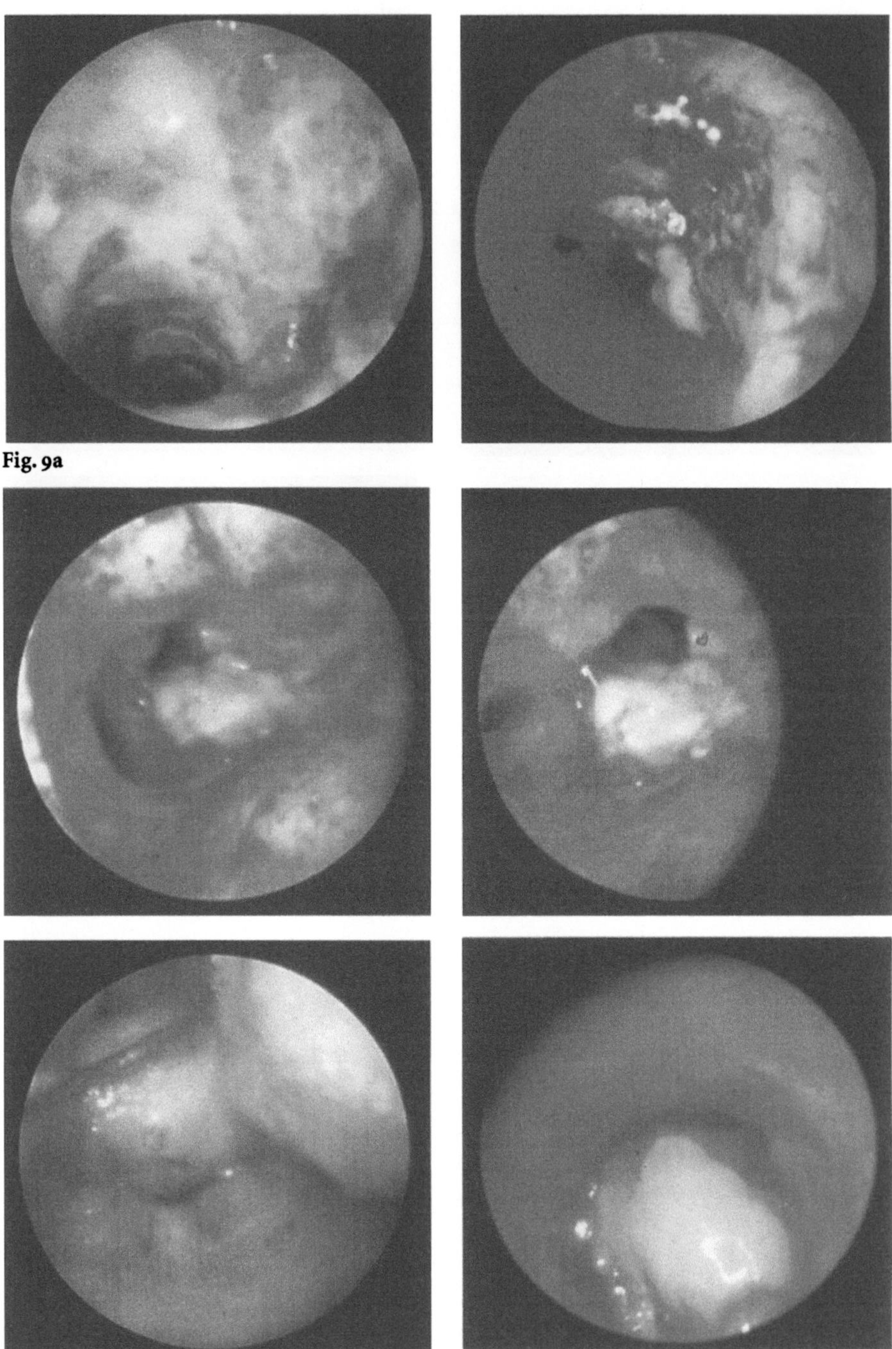

Fig. 9a, b. Necrotizing tracheobronchitis (NTB) with persisting excessive granulation and almost complete closure of the trachea

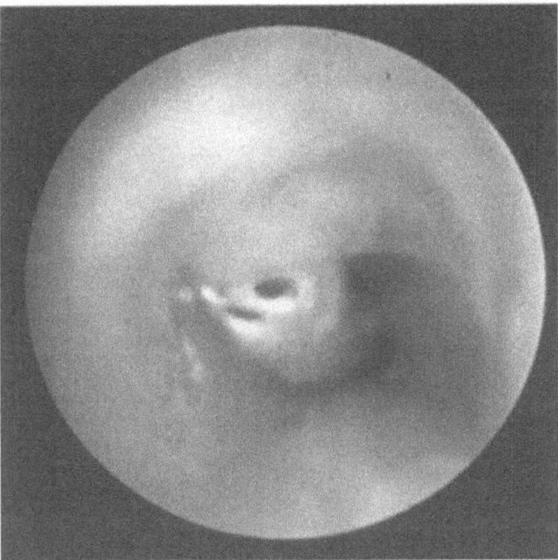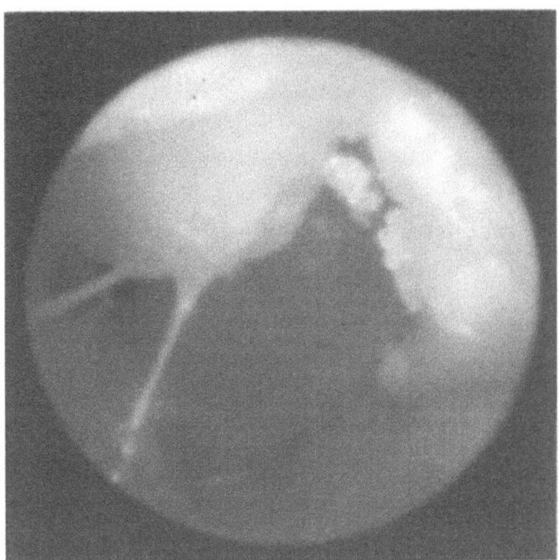

Fig. 10.   Granuloma formation surrounding a plastic cannula (silver cannula on the *left*)

formation of granulomas for which neither inadequate surgical technique nor dwelling time nor material alone are responsible. Frontocranial to the stoma considerable thickening of the wall, excessive granulation, and granulomas may develop which must be diagnosed and removed before decannulation at the latest (Fig. 10).

Injuries

Direct accidental injuries to the trachea and bronchi are relatively rare but, especially in connection with certain sports, tearing, crushing, or penetration can lead to defects including isolated malacias, cicatrices, cicatritial contraction, and stenosis.

Aspiration of Foreign Bodies

The aspiration of foreign bodies is being increasingly treated immediately as an emergency so that secondary alterations with mucosal and bronchial wall lesions have become infrequent. However, typical neoplastic granulations, scars, contractions, and stenoses are still seen, primarily at the intermediary, lobal, and segmental bronchial levels (Fig. 11a, b).

Inhalational (Caustic) Injuries

Inhalational (caustic) injuries in older children are complex traumas with orally commencing extensive damage to the laryngeal, tracheal, and bronchial mucosa (and walls) similar to necrotizing tracheobronchitis and have overall – not only locally – poor prospects.

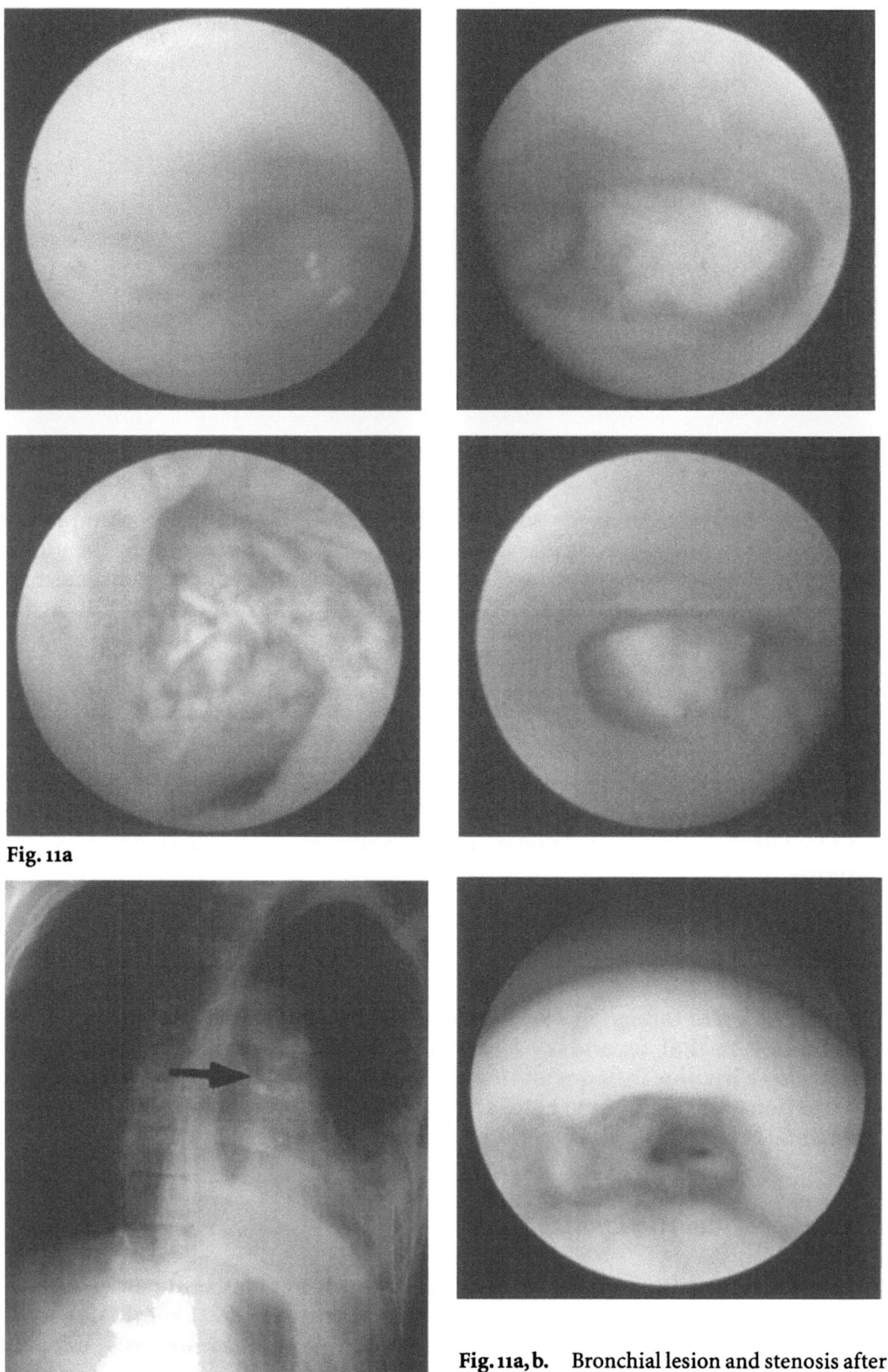

Fig. 11a

Fig. 11a, b. Bronchial lesion and stenosis after neglected foreign body aspiration

Clinical Picture and Diagnosis

Anamnesis

A history of frequent bronchopulmonary infections or intubations is of particular significance when organic airways obstruction is suspected, but acute dyspnea in mature or immature neonates post partum, after intubation or during the first year of life can also present without anamnesis even in cases of severe stenosis. Depending more on the degree of the stenosis than on its location, the children develop signs of dyspnea, croupous and strained breathing, and intercostal, jugular, and subcostal drawing in of breath, in- and expiratory stridor and cyanosis which can culminate in manifest respiratory distress. In both congenital and acquired (usually postintubational) stenoses the symptoms can be either delayed or develop so acutely that only diagnostic measures that also restore ventilation are possible.

Diagnostic Methods

The primary diagnostic methods are radiological: conventional X-ray imaging in the sagittal and lateral planes, possibly additional application of contrast medium in dynamic studies as well as tomography. Only when these methods are inefficient is computer tomography with fast-scan technology, digital subtraction angiography (DAS) or magnetic resonance imaging (MRI) or MR echography indicated.

Depending on the age of the child and on how urgent, the conventional techniques of' fluoroscopy, seriography, and transtubal contrast imaging with corresponding documentation – both planes – may be applied in premature and full-term neonates. Except in cases of practically certain postinflammatory stenoses, examination with these methods should be performed before tracheobronchoscopy or tracheobronchography. Orientational endoscopy can be performed with the flexible bronchoscope under general anesthesia (mask) in spontaneous respiration. Considering the anatomical dimensions and in order to avoid further mucosal lesions, the exclusive use of rigid optics is advisable. The use of sedation alone seems risky and focal anesthesia in small children is justifiable only when the examination is limited to the larynx or in malacias [6]. In urgent cases the rigid bronchoscope is mandatory in order to maintain ventilation. For diagnosis at the bronchial level, combinations of bronchoscopy, bronchography (extent of the stenosing process), and angiography may be helpful. In older children, when there is enough time and especially for diagnosis of extratracheal conditions or accompanying malformations, axial and sagittal and sometimes frontal MR tomography, partially in conjunction with angiography or esophagography, are most productive, especially in the presence of anomalies of the aortal arc or "pulmonary-artery-sling" syndrome. This applies also to middle and distal tracheal stenoses to show vascular calibers and the location, extent, and degree of the stenoses, MRI and bronchoscopy are a useful combination both pre- and postoperatively since they can be performed during the same anesthesia.

In acute respiratory distress, when diagnostic procedures can be performed only with rigid bronchoscopes and with tracheotomy and jet ventilation in readiness, additional invasive operative intervention must be immediately available. The aim of all endoscopic diagnosis is the definite determination of the localization and extent of the lesion.

Therapy

Since adequate therapy of all malformations and diseases obstructing the airways is dependent on the condition, age, maturity, and weight of the child, on the etiology of the stenosing process with intra- or extraluminal obstruction, on occlusion (synechiae, membrane, tumor, edema, secretion, foreign body, granulation tissue, cicatrix) or constriction, localization (supraglottal, glottal, infraglottal, intrathoracic-tracheal or bronchial), on the degree of obturation (Cotton I–IV), on the progression of the stenosing process, and, finally, on concomitant malformations and disorders [12], the therapeutic procedure must be subordinate to the possibilities and necessities and not to a single therapeutic principle. Besides surgical resection, augmentation, stabilization, and transection of extrinsic obstructions, laser therapy has, for more than 10 years, been a proven adjunct in the therapy of intrinsic obstructions [8]. Independent of whether adjuvant or complementary techniques or combined treatments are employed, all endoscopic methods, including laser, are in principle limited to intrinsic stenoses. General indications for the application of laser are, in our opinion, all stenoses with more than 70% obstruction (Cotton II) or with definite signs of progression. Before laser therapy of short peripheral stenoses, preliminary dilation with a Fogarty or angioplasty catheter can be useful to visualize the anatomy (perhaps with contrast medium) in order to optimize the use of the laser, or, in long stenoses, to reduce them quantitatively by removing granulomatous and cicatritial alterations with the Volmar ring knife.

Laser Techniques

Amoung the numerous types of laser available, the KTP-, the Nd:YAG- and the CO_2 laser have proven suitable for tracheal and bronchial application:
1. The KTP laser (532 nm) can be inserted through rigid and flexible bronchoscopes into the trachea and into the branches of the bronchial tree, i.e., into the segmental bronchi. With poor absorption by water but good absorption by hemoglobin, coagulation of mucosal hemorrhages and vessels smaller than 0.5 mm is possible. With a spot size of 0.5 mm, the laser is equally suitable for cutting and vaporizing.
2. The Nd:YAG laser with a wavelength of 1064 nm can be used with flexible as well as with rigid bronchoscopes. Poor absorption by water and good absorption by hemoglobin provide good hemostasis (vessels larger than 0.5 mm) and vaporization with good visibility of the operative field but poorer cutting qualities than the CO_2 laser. Because of its high scattering rate, the depth of

penetration is relatively difficult to control so that there is, in principle, the danger of injury to the tracheal and bronchial wall (clinical complications are approximately 2%) [1], which through necrobiosis and cell necrosis, collagen coagulation, and homogenization of the vascular walls can lead, by way of new granulation, to renewed cicatrization. In practice, however, exact application is the rule and the necrotic zone is small, the edema slight, the sealing of the resection zone good, and epithelization rapidly concluded when, for the reasons named, the instrument is guided exclusively tangentially to the wall structures. Here, as in the use of rigid and flexible bronchoscopes, the "learning curve" is significant for success. More recent techniques, for example, with a "fiber tome" laser (Medi Las 40 N), use a special feedback mechanism which protects the tip of the "bare fiber" by energy control from thermic destruction, improves the cutting characteristics [14], and permits intentional resection in immediate proximity to the bronchial wall.

3. The CO_2 laser (10.6 μ) has a high absorption coefficient in water and a low scattering rate. This results in a laser effect that can be focused on the target with an accuracy of 0.5 mm. Good cutting qualities are combined with minimal edema formation and good tissue sealing. The hemostatic effect is relatively poor; only vessels smaller than 0.6 mm can be coagulated. The danger of deeper wall lesions is less than with the Nd:YAG laser [7]. The CO2 laser cannot be used with flexible bronchoscopes and its use is limited caudally at the carina.

The possibilities and limitations of the various types of laser are determined by the site of operation and the type of bronchoscope that can be used there. Rigid bronchoscopes, which allow direct ventilation or endoscopically controlled jet ventilation in the distal portions of the trachea, good suctioning of burning products [15], and scavenging of various materials, "palpation" of tumor contours, and temporary hemostasis by compression as well as a broad application of instruments, but which always require general anesthesia, do not reach all distal bronchial lesions. In principle, however, it is possible to operate further distally with rigid optics and "bare fiber." Comparing instruments, the Wolff bronchoscope (diameter 4 mm, length 15 cm), because it has no Hopkins optics in the center, affords better visibility and escape for the combustion-supporting anesthetic gases. Flexible bronchoscopes, aside from their undisputed value in orientational diagnosis in local anesthesia in very small and in older children, especially in the upper airways, can only be used otherwise with a tube size of 6 mm or more, which generally means not in emergencies, not for foreign bodies and hemorrhages, and not with instruments.

Use of Laser

General Indications

Laser treatment is generally indicated for all intrinsic stenoses, with which 75% of the patients are afflicted, i.e., for the congenital anomalies of the tracheobronchial tree such as synechiae, membrane stenoses, mucosal folds, fibrous plaques, cartilage and tissue heterotopias, cartilage bridges, cysts, angiomas and tumors as well as for acquired stenoses in the form of overlays of granulation tissue, granulomas and cicatritial (or membranous) stenoses, inasmuch as these do not involve the cartilaginous skeleton of the trachea or the bronchi. Intramural, stenosing alterations caused by cartilage hypoplasia, complete cartilage rings, submucosal fibrous pads and posttraumatic cartilage (i.e., wall) distortions and constrictions are only occasionally accessible to laser techniques, when, after interposition grafting procedures, augmenting and stabilizing operative plastic methods, one or more of the above complications result. When intrinsic obstructions treatable by laser are accompanied by additional malformations of the tracheobronchial tree, the esophagus or the vessels such as the laryngo-tracheo-esophageal cleft, atresia or stenoses of the esophagus, tracheo-esophageal fistula, vascular rings, sequestration, accessory lungs, anomalies of the bronchial tree or lobar emphysema [12, 9], sequential or combined endoscopic and open surgical therapy can be advantageous. Together with auxiliary instruments such as balloon catheters (Fogarty and angioplasty catheters) and the Volmar ring knife, the Nd:YAG laser has proven successful in our experience and, applied without exception through rigid bronchoscopes, can be adapted individually to the lesions to be treated.

Granulations

Granulations are removed with the "bare fiber" (diameter 400 µm) with the contact technique with 15-W power, 200-ms pulse duration and intervals of 200–300 ms. Alterations over a short length of the trachea (Type A; Fig. 12a, b), extensive stenosis of the intrathoracic trachea (Type B; Fig. 13a, b) and even involvement of the entire inspectable tracheobronchial tree (Type C) can, in principle, be treated with laser. However, long segmental and multiple A- and B-Type stenoses mean not only a quantitative difference in treatment and laser application but also

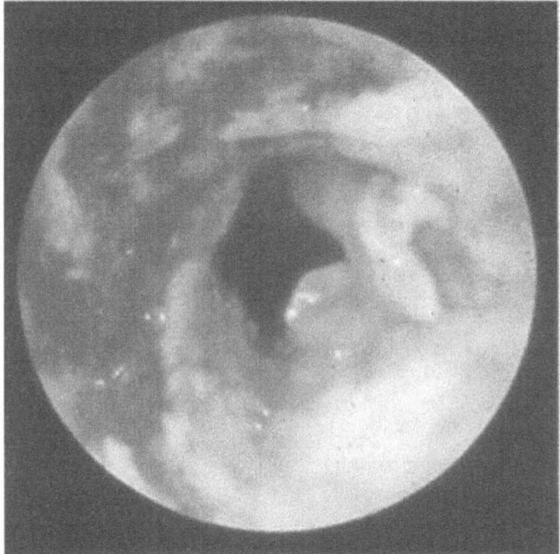
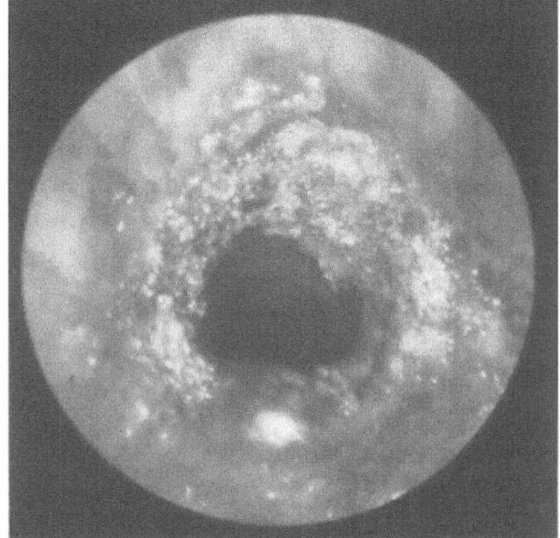

Fig. 12a

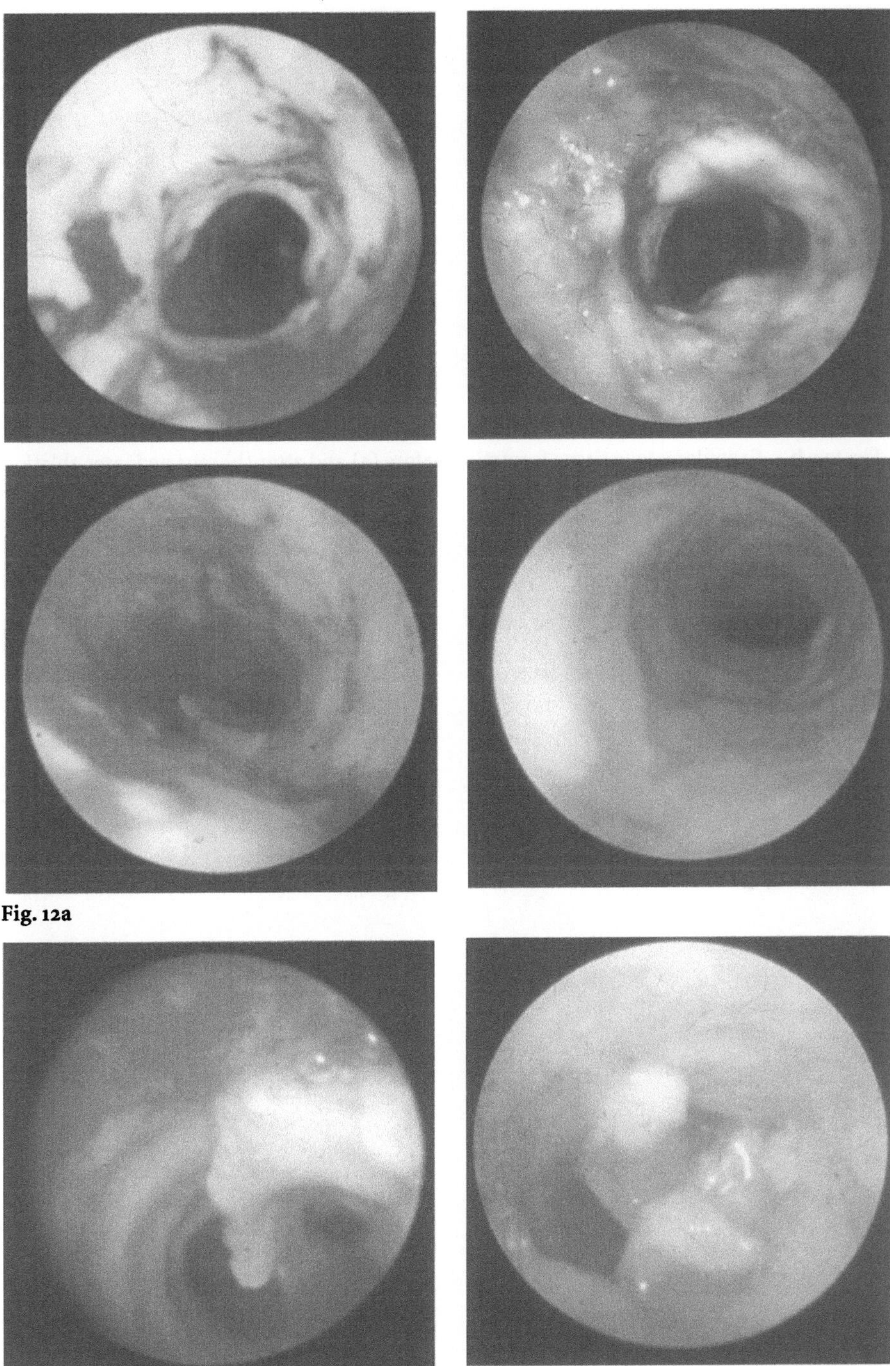

Fig. 12a

Fig. 12b

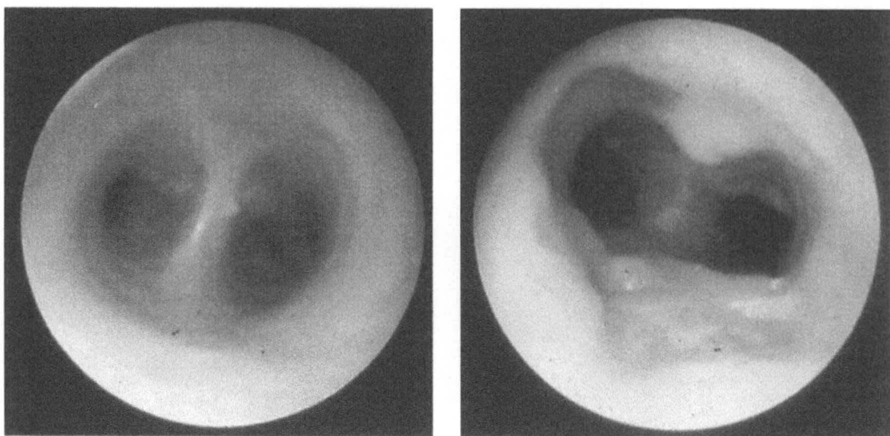

Fig. 12a, b.   Granulomatous tissue formation before (**a**) and after (**b**) repeated laser ablation

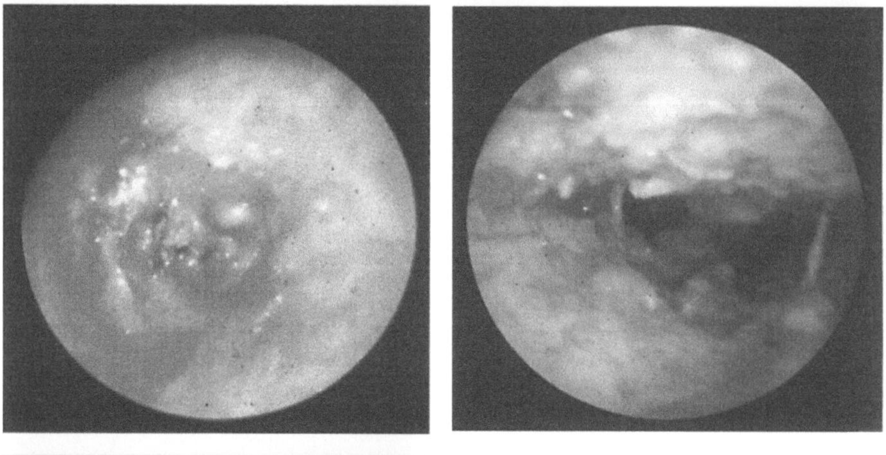

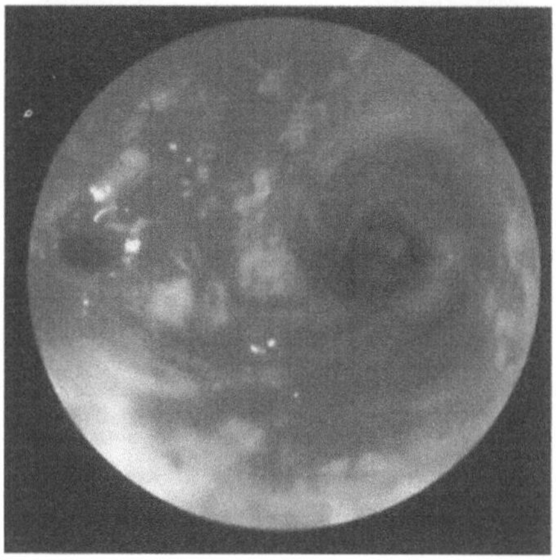

Fig. 13a

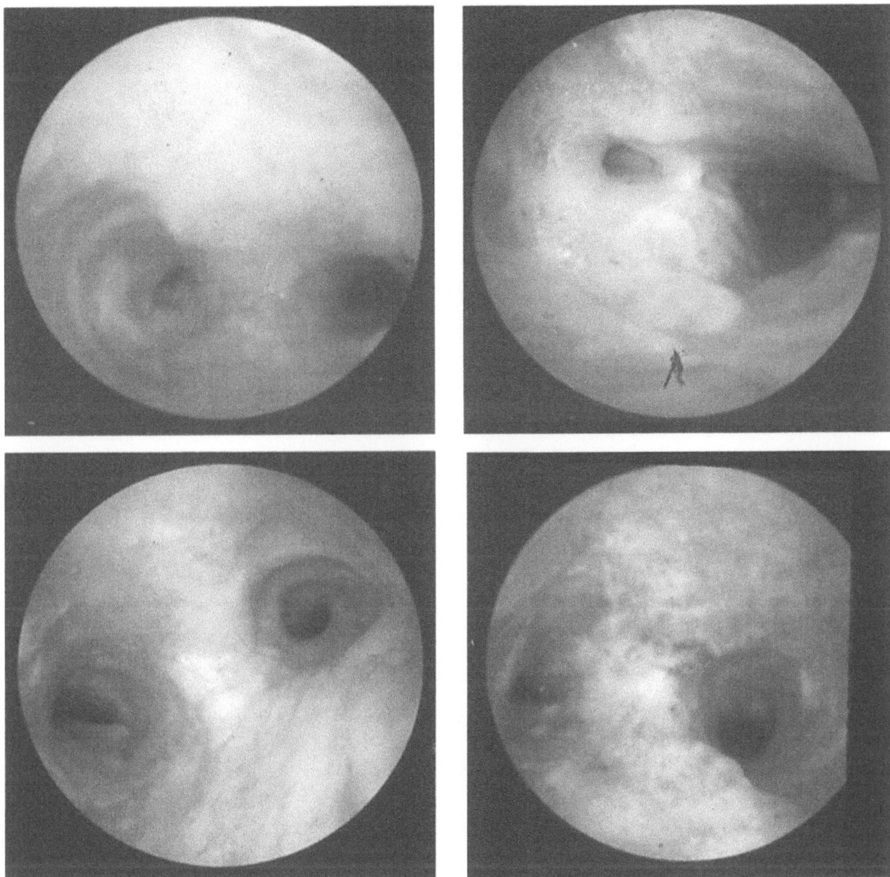

Fig. 13a, b.   Extensive granulomatous and fibrous stenosis of the intrathoracic trachea and left primary bronchus before (**a**) and after (**b**) repeated laser resection

show such a disparate prognosis that the complementary insertion of silicone-incubated tubes and stents in increasing size (Lichtenberger´s technique), to gently dilate the lumen, must be considered, despite the known side effects, as well as the general time plan (intervals) and quantitative limitation of laser application.

Scar Tissue

Scar tissue requires for resection higher power of 25 (to 30) W with an impulse duration of 200–300 ms and intervals of 200 ms. Vascularized scars and diaphragms (membranes) or "active scars" (Fig. 14) relapse more frequently than "old scars," which have a better prognosis and may require only one laser treatment [10].

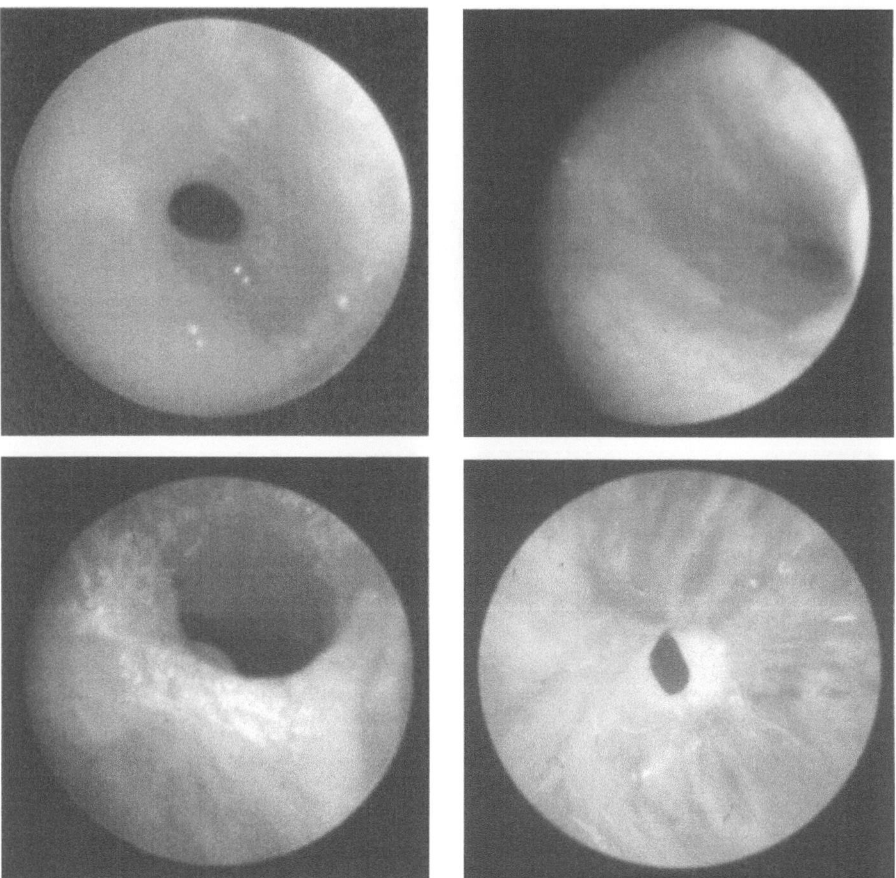

Fig. 14.   Different vascularized membrane stenoses

Angiomas

Angiomas are treated with the noncontact technique at 20 W, with an impulse
duration of 300 (to 500) ms, and with the same interval. Hemorrhages are
definitively controlled with 20 W, 400-ms impulses, and intervals of 500 ms.

Special Indications and Limitations

Larynged and Tracheal Cysts

Laryngeal and trachea cysts are opened by laser, biopsied, and then extirpated.
Except in the case of hemangiomas, tumors (lipomas, fibrovascular hamartomas, fibrohistiocytomas, and papillomas) [cf. 9] are histologically diagnosed
and then ablated by laser with the noncontact technique in one or more ses-

sions. Subglottal hemangiomas, which can reach a considerable size, do not necessarily have a poor prognosis. If spontaneous regression does not occur (capillary hemangiomas), they are treated with the non-contact technique. When they are an expression of a hemangiomatosis (see above), tracheostomy, otherwise to be strictly avoided, may be recommended. Since this is not possible in the case of distal tracheal and bronchial hemangiomas, laser treatment is only permissible with immediately available thoracic surgical intervention. Intralaryngeal strumas require surgical extirpation. Laryngo-tracheoesophageal clefts and malformations of the larynx itself can only be treated by laser excision when subsequent bonding with fibrin is possible [11].

Glottal Membranes as Membranous Synechiae

Glottal membranes as membranous synechiae at the level of the vocal chords, possibly combined with supraglottal membranes, must be exactly laser-ablated (alternatively surgically excised), sparing the vocal chords.

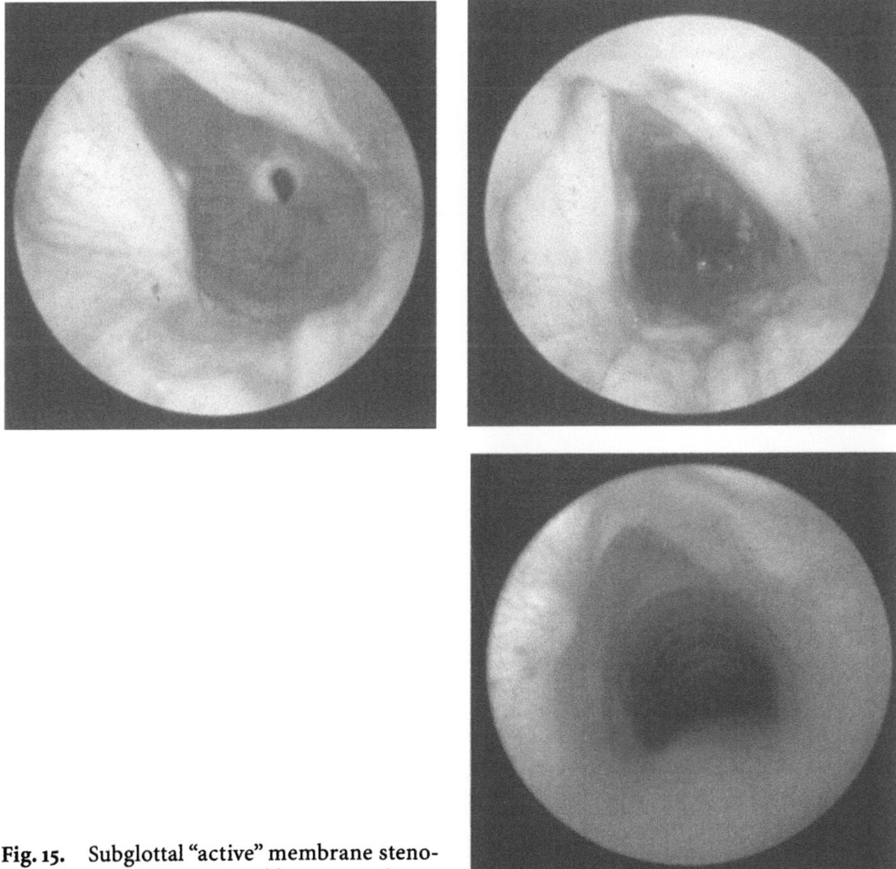

Fig. 15. Subglottal "active" membrane stenosis before and after repeated laser resection

Glottal Stenoses

Glottal stenoses (Fig. 15) and obstructions at the level of the cricoid may require more than one session in order to avoid laser-induced local cicatritial contractions. If cartilage injuries occur, plastic surgical dilation is indicated after interim silicone stent treatment. Bougienage at this localization is useless.

Granulation Tissue or Granulomas

Persisting granulation tissue or granulomas of often considerable size can be expected after tracheostomy; they must be resected before decannulation at the latest and the wound worked over and sealed by laser (Fig. 16). Since there is no more irritation by the cannula, this therapy is usually unproblematic.

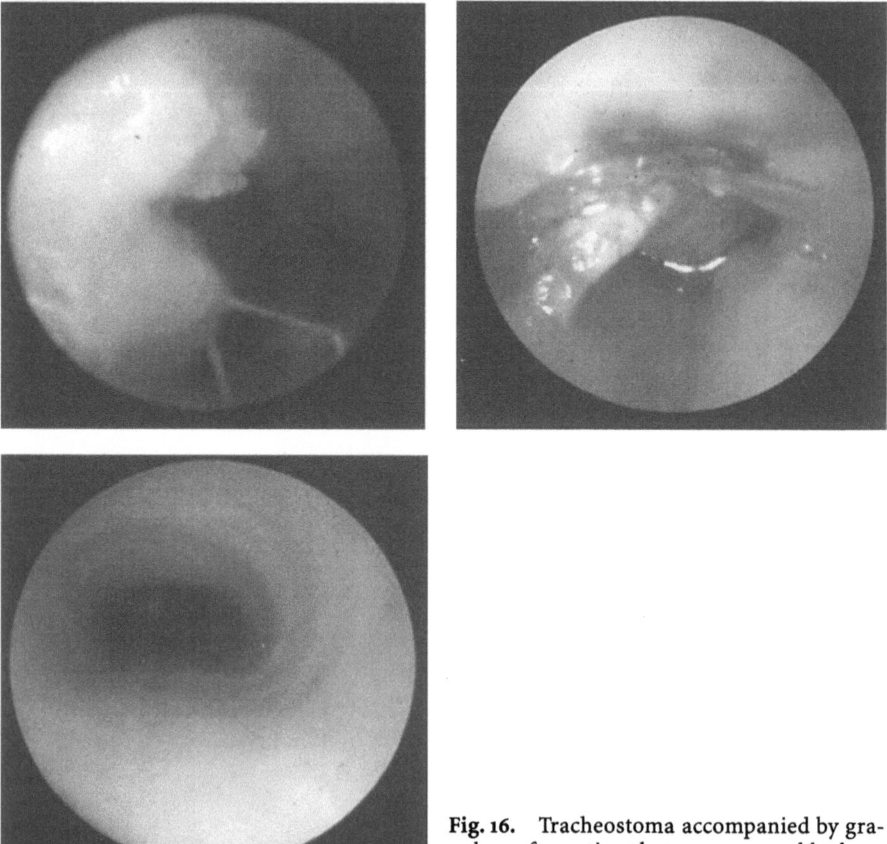

Fig. 16. Tracheostoma accompanied by granuloma formation that was removed by laser ablation

Cicatritial Stenoses

Disobliteration or laser ablation of extensive intraluminal cicatritial stenoses of the trachea and the bronchi, which in addition to contraction and distortion of the entire wall of the trachea or bronchi have led to stricture, can be attempted (Fig. 17a, b), but plastic surgical dilation is often unavoidable. The precise differentiation between purely intrinsic, intramural, and combined stenoses is particularly important but difficult. The combination of laser treatment with bougienage with silicone-intubated tubes or stents is justified in individual cases. An exception is localization at the cricoid (see above); this technique is also problematic in the distal trachea and at the carina. As yet, there is no extensive experience.

Circular cicatritial stenoses are not a general contraindication for laser therapy. When involvement of the cartilaginous tracheal or bronchial wall cannot be definitely excluded, partial, i.e., one-sided laser ablation has been satis-

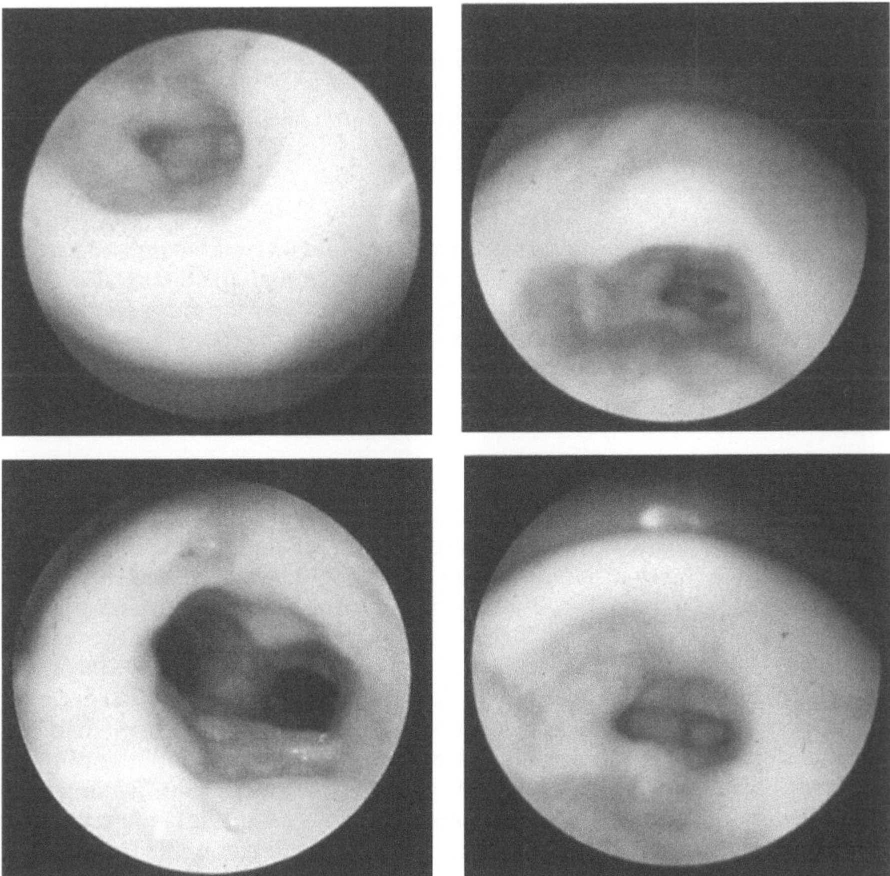

Fig. 17a

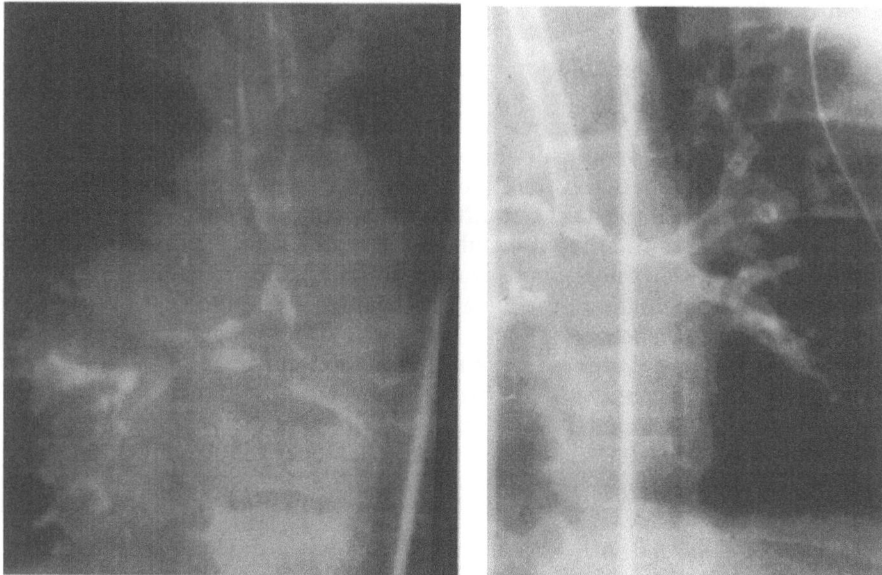

Fig. 17a, b.   Cicatritial stenosis of the distal trachea before (**a**) and after (**b**) repeated stenting and laser ablation

factory, not only for us [5]. When the cartilaginous skeleton is undamaged and remains so, circular stenoses can be corrected at a single sitting. However, stenoses that are limited to only one tracheal cartilage are more favorable. In the case of extensive stenoses it must be taken into account that a dynamic laser effect by one-time application may contract the wall with new scars.

Necrotizing Tracheobronchitis

In the usually fulminant necrotizing tracheobronchitis (NTB) (Metlay 1983 as quoted in [13]), deep extensive ulcerations (Fig. 18), mucosal-submucosal sequestrations, and the formation of crusts and granulation tissue can result in life-threatening, more or less complete closure of the trachea and the bronchi which cannot be overcome by suctioning and mechanical pressure ventilation. Only immediate disobliteration through a rigid bronchoscope can restore ventilation within seconds. The primary use of laser is prevented by poor visibility and difficult orientation; it can only be used, if at all, for hemostasis. Whereas an interim, proxy therapy with silicone-incubated tubes is initially effective in the trachea, it is problematic at the bronchial level, where repeated disobliteration with adjuvant laser application may have to be performed. In our opinion, it is important that all inflammatory reactions have subsided completely prior to the actual laser therapy of cicatritial stenoses. The silicone-incubated tubes or stents left in situ mitigate inflammation by preventing excessive granulation and by restituting the mucosa (at the same time preventing contraction) and subsequently allow laser

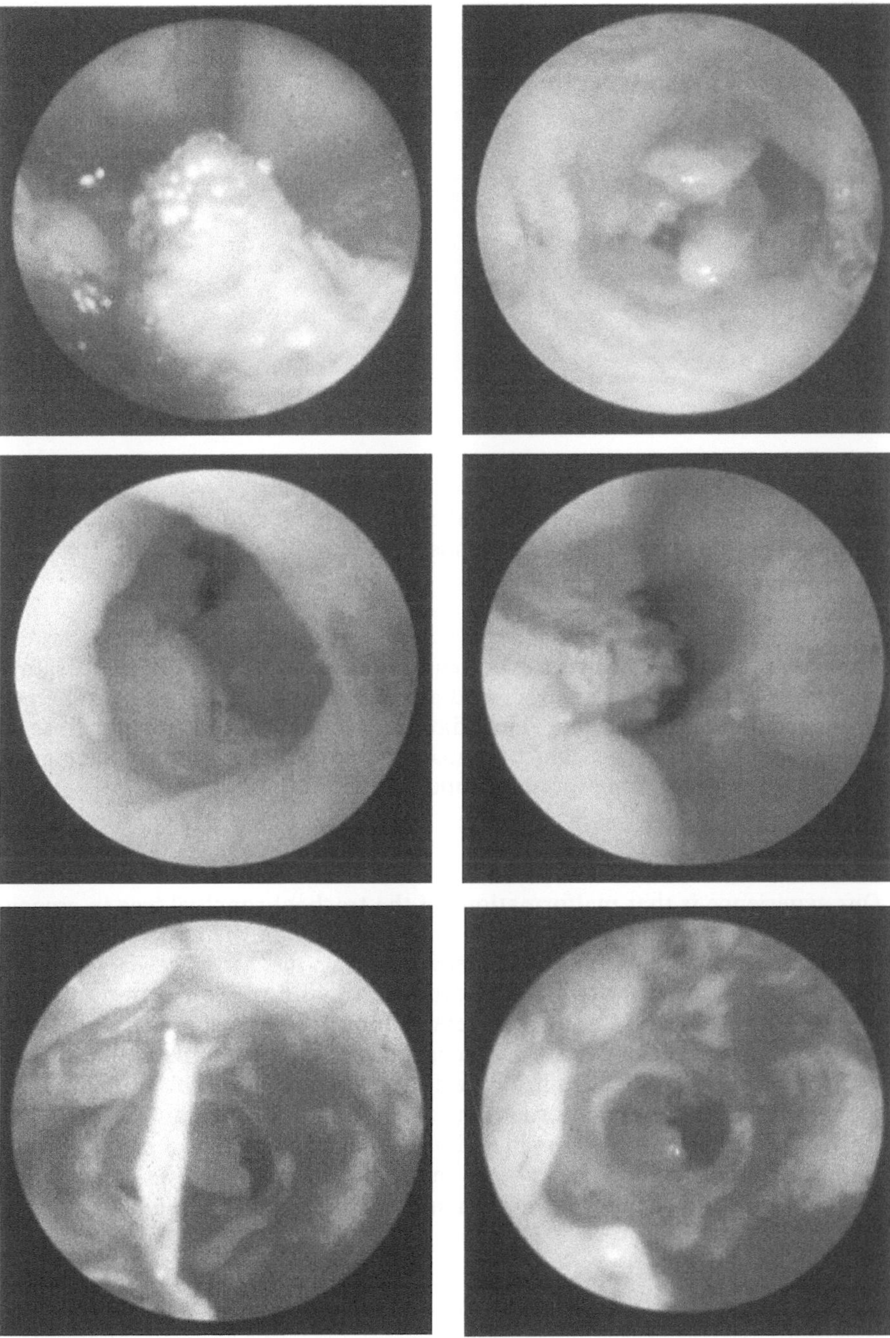

Fig. 18

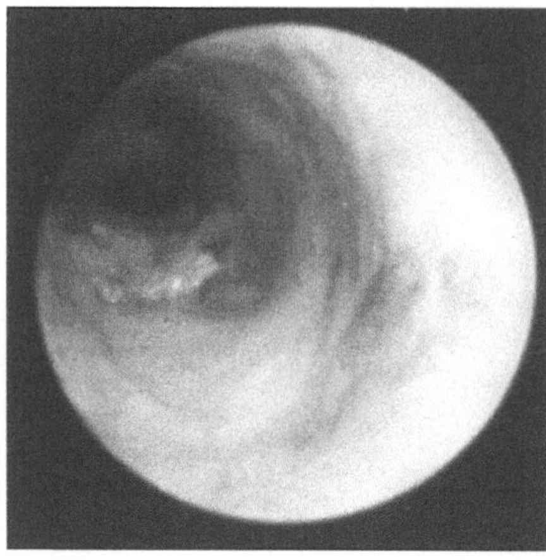

Fig. 18. Fulminant necrotizing tracheobronchitis (NTB) with ulceration, mucosal-submucosal sequestration and lesion of the cartilage

ablation of the stenosing portions of the bronchi. These sequelae of NTB, as
also those of inhalational traumas, take very difficult and tedious courses and
still have the most unfavorable prognosis.

Peripheral Stenoses

Peripheral stenoses (down to the segmental bronchi) may be successfully
treated with the technique described above when the resections can be performed without injuring important adjoining anatomical structures such as the
bifurcations of further bronchi. Diagnosis and possibly preliminary bougienage
(anatomy, see above) are especially important in this context.

Malformations

Our experience is that malformations of the tracheobronchial tree in association with esophageal atresia, such as mucosal folds in the upper, middle, and
distal trachea and cul-de-sac fistula remnants (Fig. 19a, b), especially when they
are near the carina or are of large caliber but with narrow communication
with the trachea, cause a more or less pronounced mechanical handicap in
about a quarter of the patients with esophageal atresia Vogt III B and III C,
which typically leads to chronically recidivating infections. The situation is ag-
gravated by additional malformations of the tracheobronchial tree, especially
by tracheal superior lobe bronchi and bronchial stenoses. The airways obstruction can be relieved and the patients made symptomless by laser coagulation,
by equalizing and removal of mucosa and by fibrin bonding (Fig. 20).

Author´s Results

During a period of 10 years, 1986–1995 (5 of which with laser) we treated a total
of 79 tracheal and bronchial stenoses with various localization (Table 1) and

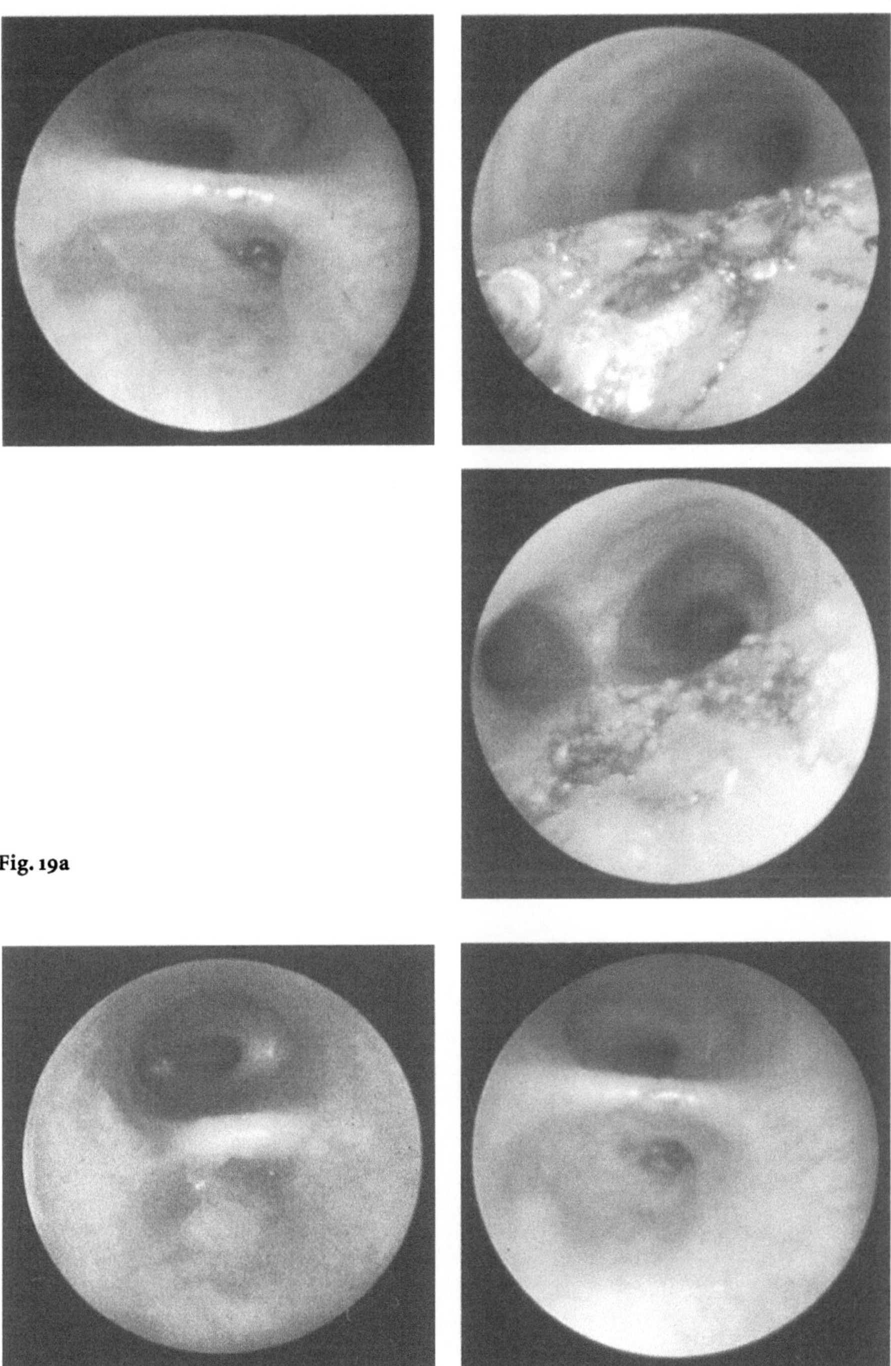

Fig. 19a

Fig. 19b

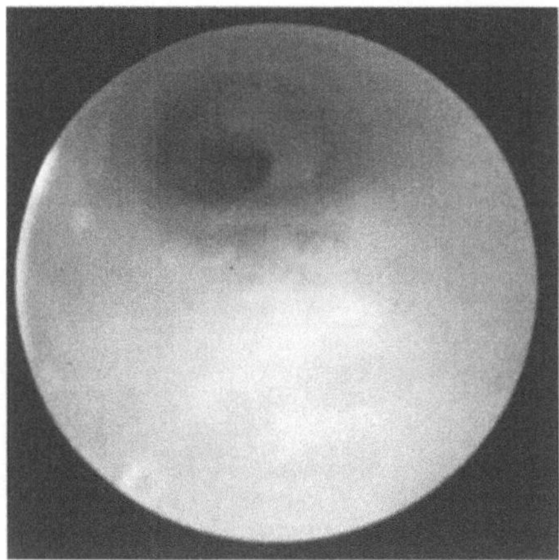

Fig. 19a, b. Mucosal folds and cul-de-sac fistula remnants of the distal trachea after laser ablation

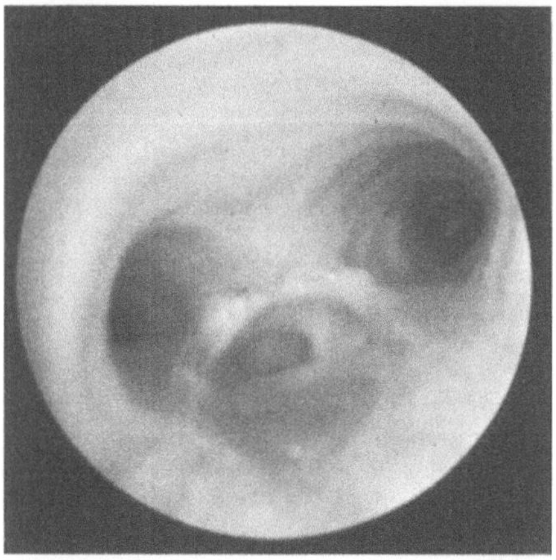

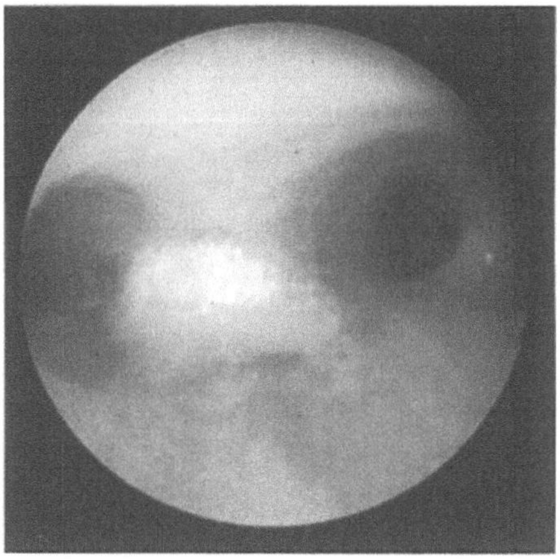

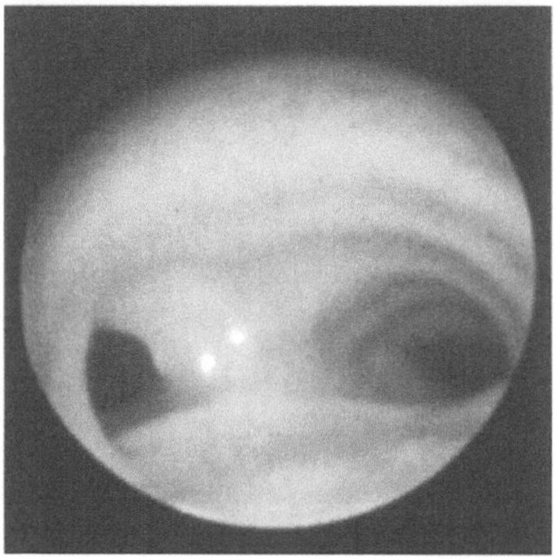

Fig. 20. Cul-de-sac fistula remnants at the level of the carina. Removal of mucosa and fibrin bonding

Table 1. Intraluminal and bronchial stenoses, 1986–1995 ($n = 79$)

	Treated	No success as yet	Still stoma	Still Deaths tube
1. Supraglottal	2			
2. Glottal/supraglottal	25	3		
3. Upper trachea	4	–		
4. Middle trachea	5	1		
5. Tracheostoma	11	–		
6. Distal trachea/carina	13	1		
7. Extensive (>1 cm)	(4)	1		
8. Principal/lobar bronchus (R)	10	2		
9. Principal/lobar bronchus (L)	9	1		

Table 2. Etiology of intraluminal tracheal and bronchial stenoses, 1986–1995 (n = 79)

1. Postintubational	34	
2. NTB/inflammation	13	
3. Tracheostoma	11	
4. Unknown	4	
5. Congenital	3	
6. Trauma	3	
7. Foreign body	3	
8. Tumor/cystic	3	
9. Caustic	3	
10. Tuberculosis	2	

NTB, necrotizing tracheobronchitis

genesis (Table 2). In ten cases we were either unsuccessful or the treatment has not yet been concluded. Five patients still have tracheostomas, four of which were executed elsewhere. One child is still intubated with a silicone-incubated stent. Three children died from the sequelae of obliterating panalveolitis before the laser period. In 25 children with corrected esophageal atresia, cul-de-sac remnants, which represent a more pronounced mechanical handicap because of recidivating bronchitis, were ablated and the tracheal wall smoothed (in some cases prophylactically) or, alternatively, closed with fibrin after removing the mucosa.

Possibilities and Limitations of Laser Therapy

The introduction of laser techniques into the treatment of stenosing processes of the tracheobronchial tree has markedly improved therapeutic prospects. Until then, the final states of cicatri and also of intraluminal obstructions had to be treated surgically, mainly resective and dilative surgery, usually involved a stoma, or required electro- or cryosurgical procedures and was attended by

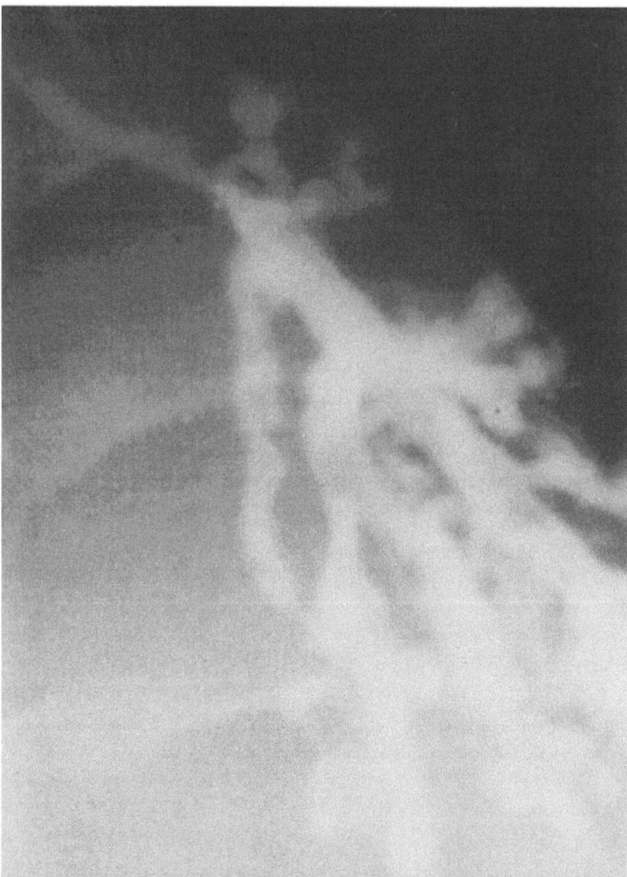

Fig. 21. Bronchiectasis due to stenosis of the left primary bronchus. Laser treatment is not indicated because resective therapy is necessary

frequent and serious complications. Now, with individually selectable lasers as described above, most intraluminal stenosing processes can be efficiently eliminated and 90% of stomas can be avoided [11]. The success of laser therapy depends not only on its quality but also very essentially on the indication.

Contraindications are cartilaginous stenoses, tracheal malacias at the level or the vicinity of stenoses, and total occlusions.

Natural limits to the method, not all universally accepted, are:

1. Congenital anterior webs, some of which occupy the subglottal space and cause tissue thickening and protrusion of the cricoid; they are not suitable for laser treatment because of frequent scar formation [7, 10].
2. Irreversible lesions of the tracheobronchial tree and the lungs distal to the obstruction which are accessible only to resective methods (e.g., bronchiectases; Fig. 21) or global irreversible lesions subsequent to NTB or thermic inhalational traumas.

3. Additional or combined, i.e., intraluminal and extraluminal, stenoses which require plastic surgical dilation or resection.
4. Unknown anatomy of distal stenoses despite bougienage and disobliteration; operative dilative and resective methods must be chosen here.
5. Lack of tangible progress in tedious endoscopic or laser treatment when operative methods would be more efficient; this decision is espcecially difficult after NTB and thermic inhalational traumas.

Prerequisites for successful laser use are considerable experience and a command of the additional open-surgical techniques possibly necessary. Success is essentially determined by a restrictive indication for laser use and by the quality of diagnostic and therapeutic teamwork.

Summary

The application of laser during the past 10 years in the treatment of intraluminal stenosing processes in the tracheobronchial tree has meant progress with respect to effectivity, length of treatment and early and late complications, which is not attainable with electrosurgical, cryosurgical, or mechanical techniques. Indications are all tracheal and bronchial, congenital and acquired intraluminal tumorous processes which do not involve the cartilage, i.e., all supraglottal, glottal and subglottal cysts, tumors, vascular and hamartomatous malformations, membranes, fibrous scarry diaphragms, cartilaginous dystopias and bridges, postintubational and postinfectious granulomas, and cicatritial stenoses, granulomas following tracheostomas, scarry stenoses following injuries and inhalational lesions and foreign body aspiration which reduce the lumen by more than 70% or are progressive.

Essential for successful, age-dependent treatment are careful anamnesis and diagnostic methods that allow reliable evaluation of the localization, nature, and extent of the stenosis and permit immediate restoration of ventilation, possibly with the aid of operative measures. Combination of individually applicable laser types with mechanical and operative techniques, either in one session or sequentially, may be indicated on the findings, especially in the presence of accompanying malformations. Laser treatment reaches natural limits in congenital stenoses with tissue accretion at the cricoid because of frequent cicatrization after laser application and irreversible lesions of the tracheobronchial tree and the lungs distal to an obstruction which allow only resective methods, in the presence of accompanying or combined intraluminal, intramural and extraluminal stenoses. Further limits are set by the anatomical impossibility of laser resection of distal stenoses, or when a lengthy course of laser treatment is expected and insufficient progress is made, and when operative methods would be more efficient.

Adequate experience, expertise in open-operative techniques possibly also necessary and the restriction of laser application to suitable cases are requisite for success.

References

1. Becker HD (1993) Bronchoscopic diagnosis and options of treatment of laryngo-tracheal lesions in children: Oral presentation at the 3rd International Wullstein Symposium on "Diagnosis and Treatment of Laryngo-Tracheal Lesions in Children," 22–23 April 1993, Würzburg, Germany
2. Bronscheid D, Krysa S, Vogt-Moykopf J (1991) Tracheal stenosis. In: Fallis JC, Filler RM, Lemoine C (eds) Pediatric thoracic surgery. Elsevier, Amsterdam, pp 161–162
3. Engert J (1991) Bedeutung und Behandlung oesophago-trachealer Fistelgangreste und Schleimhautfalten nach Korrektur von Ösophagusatresien, In: Hasse W (ed) Funktionsgerechte Chirurgie der Oesophagusatresie. Fischer, Stuttgart, pp 285–288
4. Johnson DG (1991) Tracheal stenosis. In: Fallis JC, Filler RM, Lemoine G (eds) Pediatric thoracic surgery, Elsevier, Amsterdam, pp 151–160
5. Kaufmann R (1992) Mid-infrared lasers. Oral presentation at Laser 1992, 19–21 November 1992, Münster, Germany
6. Mantel K (1993) Laryngo-tracheal lesions in children: indications and use of rigid endoscopes for diagnosis and treatment. Oral presentation at the 3rd International Wullstein Symposium on "Diagnosis and Treatment of Laryngo-Tracheal Lesions in Children," 22–23 April 1993, Würzburg, Germany
7. Monnier P (1993) Partial cricoid resection with primary tracheal reanastomosis in children: technique and results. Oral presentation at the 3rd International Wullstein Symposium on "Diagnosis and Treatment of Laryngo-Tracheal Lesions in Children," 22–23 April 1993, Würzburg, Germany
8. Nowak W (1992) Indikationen, Erfolg und Grenzen der endobronchialen Laserbehandlung. Oral presentation at Laser 1992, 19–21 November 1992, Münster, Germany
9. Schmittenbecher PP (1992) Laserapplication in airways obstruction in childhood, Laser 1992, 19–21 November 1992, Münster, Germany
10. Strunk CL (1991) Laser treatment of congenital lesions of the tracheobronchial tree, In: Gans SL (ed) The principles and practice of the pediatric surgical specialities; tracheal reconstruction in infancy. Saunders, Philadelphia, pp 111–124
11. Waldschmidt J (1992) Endoscopic laser surgery of the airways, oral presentation 8. Steglitzer Kinderchirurgisches Symposium, Endoscopic Surgery in Children, 4./5.12.1992, Berlin
12. Waldschmidt J (1993) Pediatric tracheal stenosis: therapeutical aspects of the pediatric surgeon. Oral presentation at the 3rd International Wullstein Symposium on "Diagnosis and Treatment of Laryngo-Tracheal Lesions in Children," 22–23 April 1993, Würzburg, Germany
13. Waldschmidt J (1994) Endoscopic treatment of stenosis of the larynx, trachea and in the bronchial system. III. International Congress for Children-Endosurgery 31 Januar–2 Februar, 1994, Münster, Germany
14. Wittmann M (1992) Endobronchiale Lasertherapie im Kontaktverfahren (Nd:YAG-Fibertom-Laser) Laser 1992, 19–21 November 1992, Münster, Germany
15. Wöllner W (1992)
16. Zimmermann T (1993) Congenital malformations of larynx and trachea. Oral presentation at the 3rd International Wullstein Symposium on "Diagnosis and Treatment of Laryngo-Tracheal Lesions in Children," 22–23 April 1993, Würzburg, Germany

Laser Treatment of Recurrent Respiratory Papillomatosis

C. DESLOOVERE and C. VON ILBERG

Introduction

Laryngeal papillomatosis was first described in the seventeenth century by Marcellus Donalus as warts in the larynx [13]. In the past 15 years a lot of research data indicate that recurrent respiratory papillomatosis is probably caused by a viral infection [5, 21, 41]. Human papilloma virus (HPV) types, mostly HPV 6 and 11 [1], could be isolated in 50%–100% of papillomata [6, 8, 13, 36].

According to Matt et al. [22], the incidence amounts to about seven per million per year with 1500 individuals per year requiring treatment in the United States. The disease most frequently starts in early childhood with a peak incidence between 2 and 4 years [13, 27]. According to the literature [5, 8, 15, 27] the disease was initially observed in 37%–83% of patients before the age of 5 years. The pathway of infection is still unclear. Recent data [13, 29] indicate that it could take place intrauterinely through the placenta. First symptoms are a hoarse voice, stridor and/or airways obstruction [5, 13].

The most frequent localization of recurrent respiratory papillomatosis (RRP) is the larynx in about 90% [13] of cases. The papillomata can finally spread along the entire respiratory tract. Tracheobronchial papillomata are rarely observed in patients without laryngeal lesions and uncommon where a tracheotomy has not been performed [5]. In patients with tracheostomy an incidence of tracheal spread of papillomatosis between 7% and 76% has been cited in several studies [6, 8, 12, 39, 45]. Cole et al. [6] have noted tracheal papillomata as soon as 7 weeks after tracheostomy. Risk factors include the presence of subglottic disease at the time of tracheostomy and prolonged cannulation [6, 7]. Mucosal disruption due to the incision and the cannula manipulation could promote distal spread [7]. Most authors agree that tracheostomy should be avoided in patients with RRP whenever possible and if necessary to decannulate them early [5–8, 35, 39].

Other localizations of papillomatosis such as the oral cavity, nasopharynx and nose and ear canal are seldom [13, 41].

Generally, laryngeal papillomata appear as solitary, multiple or sometimes superficially spreading red, soft, cauliflower-like lesions [27]. As yet the natural course of papillomatosis is unpredictable; some papillomata grow very slowly and others take a fulminant course with early respiratory obstruction. The importance of the host-virus immune interaction is still unclear [8, 13].

Many different therapy modalities have been developed for treatment of recurrent laryngeal papillomatosis so far. Basically four approaches have been used [5, 8]:

1. Chemical inhibition of papilloma growth: antimetabolites, hormones or podophyllum
2. Physical removal: cup forceps removal, cryosurgery, ultrasound or laser
3. Enhancement of the immune response: vaccines, transfer factor or interferon
4. Antiviral agents

During the past decade laser surgery has become the standard method for primary treatment of RRP [13, 14]. We combine laser surgery with interferon therapy. For severe RRP it recently proved possible to achieve some promising results with newly developed antiviral drugs

Anesthesia for Laser Surgery of RRP

Laser surgery of RRP is generally carried out under general anesthesia. The use of the carbon dioxide laser for treatment of RRP has necessitated changes in anesthetic techniques. There are three major problems to be dealt with: the risk of combustion in the upper airways, the risk of spreading papillomata in the lower airway, and the need for good exposure of the larynx and trachea. Up to the present, three types of anesthesia are used to manage these problems: jet ventilation, endotracheal intubation, and intermittent apneic anesthesia [16, 38].

Among the jet-ventilation techniques one has to distinguish between proximal (supraglottic) and distal (subglottic) ventilation. In the latter technique a catheter is placed in the subglottis or trachea, combined with high pressure oxygen ventilation [20]. If the glottis is (for the most part) obstructed – a frequent situation in RRP – this method can be dangerous. Complications arise from the high pressure in the lower airways caused by the proximal obstruction: pneumomediastinum, pneumothorax, or trapdoor obstruction with barotrauma to the airways [20, 43]. An advantage of this technique is the unlikelihood, that a papilloma would be blown into the tracheobronchial tree [20]. In cases where a major glottic obstruction is suspected, some authors [20, 31] start with a regular endotracheal intubation with a small tube. After debulking of the glottis using laser, anesthesia is continued with distal jet ventilation. Under this precaution, in a survey of the literature of 423 patients, Koufman et al. [20] described an incidence of severe barotrauma of 1.7%.

With proximal (supraglottic) jet ventilation, the risk of barotrauma is nearly nonexistent [20]. Koufman et al. [20] did not encounter such problems in 668 procedures. The catheter is placed in one of the light carrier lumina of the laryngoscope [20, 31]. According to Koufman et al. [20], infants can usually be ventilated at pressures of 6–12 psi, most children at pressures of 10–16 psi, and most adults at pressures of 12–18 psi. The authors recommend a 1- to 1.5-s insufflation time and a ventilation rate of 20/min [20, 31]. To control ventilation, thorax movements and oxygen saturation are checked.

The advantages of this method are a clear view into the larynx and the absence of any combustible material in the larynx. Several disadvantages are described [31]:

1. Difficulty of placing the laryngoscope with the catheter for jet ventilation.
2. Supraglottic jet ventilation possibly displacing papillomata and blood into the trachea. Until today, however, no case of seeding of papillomata caused by jet ventilation has been reported [7, 20, 31, 43].
3. The glottis must be patent
4. Dry gas insufflation causing unnecessary desiccation of the laryngeal tissue. Therefore constant moisturizing is necessary [38].
5. Due to displacement of the ventilation catheter, gastric distension may occur. Therefore most authors recommend stomach suction routinely after jet ventilation [20, 31].

For the above reasons we abandoned this technique in favor of an endotracheal intubation technique with intermittent apneic anesthesia. Continuous measurement of the blood O_2 level is mandatory with this technique.

Recommended for laser surgery are tubes wrapped with aluminumfoil as well as metal tubes [16, 29, 43]. Romeo et al. [29] recommend using silicone tubes because of their high resistance to ignition and burn which makes them burnless intensively than polyvinyltubes. Polyvinyltubes also release hydrogen chloride, a potent pulmonary toxin. The entire tube should be covered with aluminumfoil, particulary the distal end and the cuff [24]. The cuff has to be filled with saline solution and possibly tinted with methylene blue, which serves as a built-in sprinkler and indicates whether the cuff has been inadvertently penetrated by the laser beam [29]. As cited in the literature [18], ignition not only occurred through direct contact with the laser beam, but also indirectly through heat accumulation. Wet cotton patches or wet Merocel should be used to protect the distal end of the cuffed endotracheal tube and also the non-target area of the larynx [29, 38]. Constant suction promotes an adequate evacuation of laser beam smoke and heat during the procedure [29].

Further attention should be given to the gas mixtura applied to the patient. Experimentally, Hirschman et al. [18] found that vinyl plastic, red rubber, and latex tubes ignited in the presence of 100% O_2, 100% NO_2 and any combination of the two. Tubes did not burn in air; 25% O_2 weakly supported combustion. Therefore it is recommended [18, 24, 29, 43] that the inhaled oxygen concentration be reduced to the lowest safe level (preferably below 40%) before laser use begins. We personally use room air or air with oxygen below 40% for ventilation during laser procedures flammable anesthetic agents should be reduced [43].

In the past years new flexible, smooth metal tubes have been made available with and without cuff [43]. They are now easy to handle and safe because they are not inflammable, although they can become hot through repeated laser interference. The cuff, however, is not isolated, so the precautions discussed above have to be taken. At present we prefer the use of metal tubes.

Our technique consists of primary endotracheal intubation either with a metal tube (Mallinckrodt) or less frequently with an aluminum-coated silicone tube (Xomed Laser Shield). In older children and adults we use a Kleinsasser laryngoscope, in small children we prefer a Riecker laryngoscope. The largest laryngoscope that can be safely inserted should be chosen. After insertion and photodocumentation of the sita with a 0° Wolff optic, all visible papillomata in the supraglottic region and anterior part of the vocal cords are carefully removed with the CO_2 laser. Then the patient is hyperventilated with 100% oxygen and 1.5%–2% isoflurane for 1–2 min until oxygen saturation reaches 99%–100% on the pulse oximeter. The endotracheal tube is then removed and the remaining papillomata are ablated during apnea. As soon as oxygen saturation falls below 97%, the patient is reintubated through the laryngoscope under direct view. In younger children the apneic period is limited to 1.5–2.0 g min, in children over 5 years to 3.5–4.0 min [38]. This procedure can be repeated until all papillomata are removed. Afterwords the child is reintubated through the laryngoscope under direct view and it can be removed without disturbing the tube, due to the lateral slit in the Riecker laryngoscope.

We definitely feel that this method is advantageous over the jet ventilation technique because of its low rate of complications, the mucosa not being desiccated by the anesthetic gases, and the low risk of dissemination of papillomata due to the gentle reintubation through the laryngoscope under direct view.

CO_2 Laser Technique for RRP

Before discussing operation techniques one has to keep in mind that RRP is caused by the human papilloma virus and that virus material has been found in normal-appearing mucosa adjacent to the papillomata [13, 36]. Thus, even with radical operation methods, it is not possible to eradicate the disease. Therefore the primary goal of laser surgery should be to establish an airway and to reduce the mass of the papillomata as much as possible, minimizing secondary destruction and functional impairment of the larynx [23, 36]. The insertion of the laryngoscope is carried out in a patient in extended position for optimal visualization. Fixation is achieved by a Kleinsasser suspension arm, which is not supposed to be in contact with the patient´s chest to avoid movements due to respiration. The laryngoscope should have a rough surface to minimize laser beam reflection (no black laryngoscopes because of heating up). Most types are armed with two light carrier channels. On one side we insert the light carrier; on the other side a suction catheter is placed. We use the Sharplan 1075 laser in combination with a Zeiss microscope. An objective lens of 400 mm is inserted. The usual magnification setting on the microscope is 16x, for smaller lesions a 25 × magnification might be necessary. A Sony video camera is attached to one side of the microscope. The laser is fitted with an acuspot laser micromanipulator. The diameter of the CO_2 laser acuspot is 120 µm.

Before starting the laser procedure, the nontarget areas of the face, including the external parts of the anesthetic tubes, are covered with a wet towel. The cuff of the anesthetic tube and the nontarget areas of the larynx are covered with moist Merocel. Most authors advocate moist cotton swabs armed with surgical wire [3, 18, 24, 29]. We abandoned this because the cotton can be desiccated due to laser beam interference and heat. Dry cotton ignites very easily and has to be kept constantly moist. Merocel proved to be more resistant; even dried out it does not burn when hit by the laser beam.

We generally use the laser on pulse or superpulse mode with single pulse duration of 0.05 or 0.1 s for small lesions. For larger lesions the laser is set in repetition mode. The intensity should be as low as possible; our usual settings are between 3 and 10 W. Similar settings are cited in the literature [3, 4, 7, 33]. Due to the small spot size, energy density is high enough to vaporize papillomata. The use of the laser on continuous burn is not as safe as pulsed application because tissue temperatures rise to a higher level and may produce a second or third degree burn with resultant edema and pain. Larger papillomata on the vocal cords can be grasped with a fine pair of cupped forceps, a plane of cleavage produced in Reinke´s space by laser burning, and laser dissection carried out along the plane of cleavage [3]. Since papillomata are localized in the epithelium, great care has to be taken not to damage the vocal muscle [33]. The free margin of the vocal cords should be preserved as much as possible, especially at the anterior commissure. Care should be taken not to denude both free edges of the anterior 3 mm of the true or false vocal cords in order to prevent anterior webbing [3, 8, 23]. In the case of bilateral anterior papillomata, a second laser treatment for the contralateral side has to be planned after healing has been accomplished. To obtain access to ventricular papillomata, Dedo and Jackler [8] propose cutting the false cord back until its raw inferior edge rests upon intact mucosa of the ventricle floor. We usally treat papillomata in this area by keeping free the false cord with the suction catheter.

After removal of papillomata in the supraglottic region and the anterior part of the vocal cords, we generally use the intermittent apneic anesthesia technique to continue the operation. After extubation an optimal view on the posterior portion of the vocal cords, the posterior commissure and the subglottic region is achieved, so papillomata can easily be removed from these areas. As described earlier, apneic episodes are repeated until all papillomata are removed. Matt et al. [21] developed a subglottoscope, 5.7 mm (minimal inside diameter) by 18.6 mm (maximum outside diameter) and 158.57 mm long. After induction of general anesthesia by mask, they introduce the subglottoscope through the larynx as distally into the trachea as necessary to visualize the most distal lesion and then suspend it Anesthetic gases are insufflated down the subglottoscope through a catheter introduced into a lateral channel. Spontaneous breathing is required [22]. Distal disease is treated first and the airway is firmly maintained. The advantage of this technique for subglottic and tracheal disease is the possibility of using the microscope with a micromanipulator [22], as opposed to the laser bronchoscope.

CO_2 laser bronchoscopes are still the standard equipment for treatment of tracheal papillomatosis. Because they are bulk and difficult to use simultaneous for suction and tissue manipulation, the procedure is rather difficult especially in small children [7, 8, 22]. However, appropriate flexible carriers for the CO_2 laser beam are going to be developed in the near future. Alternatively, Nd:YAG lasers are used in this area. The Nd:YAG laser light can be transmitted through a flexible fiberoptic carrier and can therefore be easily applied to the trachea. In a regular flexible bronchoscope, the laser fiber can be passed through the operation channel. As a major disadvantage, its large and deep coagulation zone even with the contact method compared to that of a CO_2 laser lesion has to be mentioned. Especially in small children, Nd:YAG laser energy can pass through the tracheal cartilage and be absorbed outside the trachea [9, 42]. This could produce undesired effects, e.g., on the tracheal cartilage.

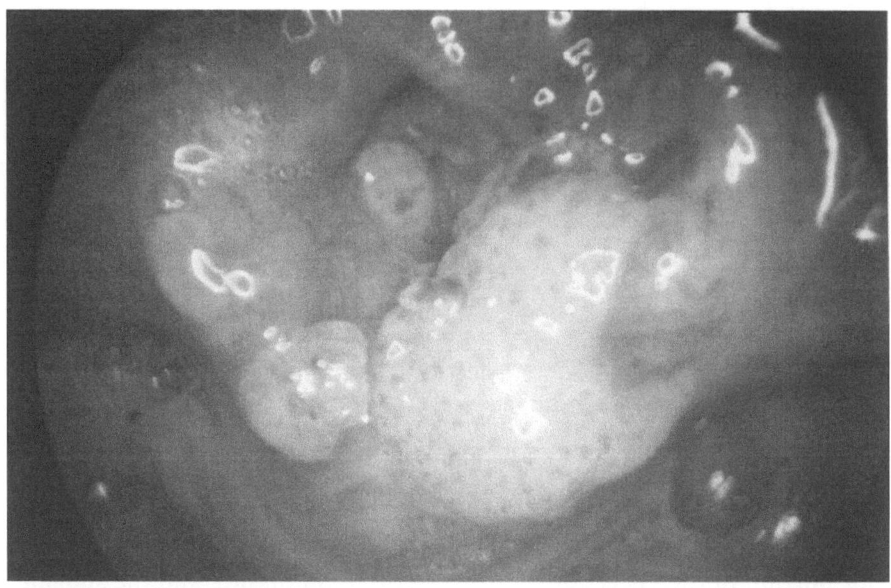

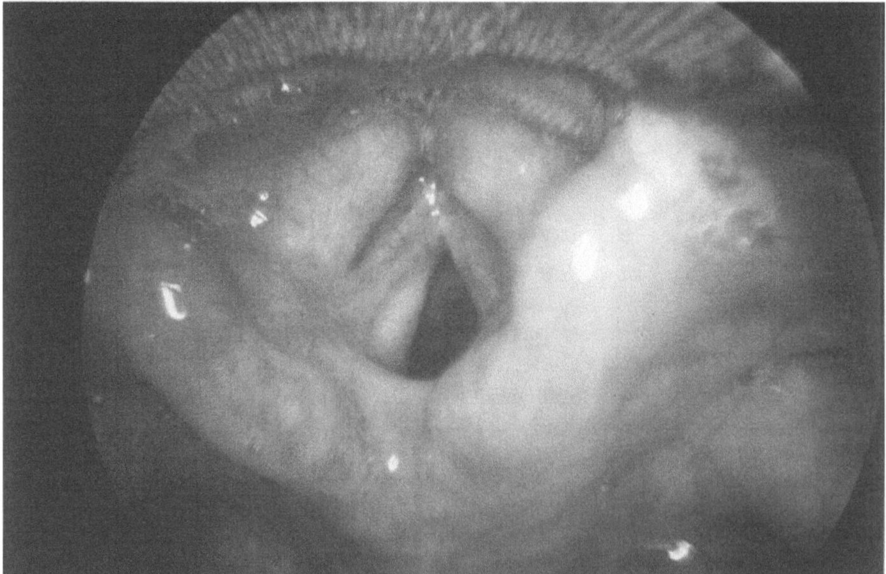

Fig. 1a, b.　**a** Laryngeal papillomatosis in a 4-year-old child before treatment. **b** The same child during clinical remisssion after combined treatmant with laser surgery and interferon

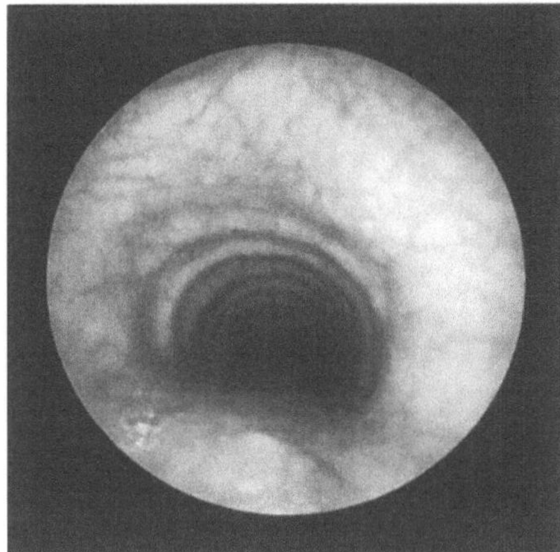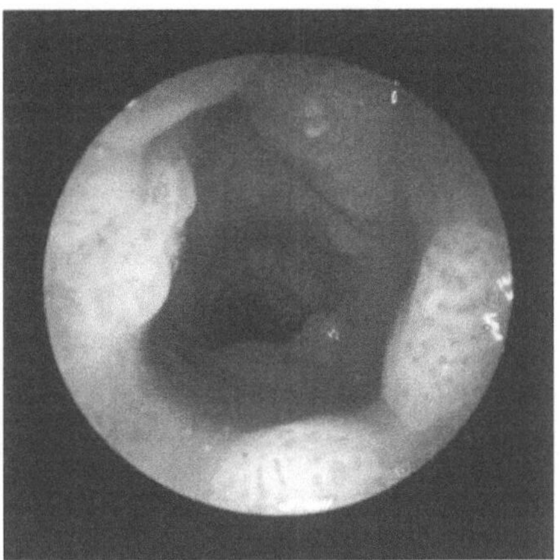

Fig. 2a, b.   a Tracheal papillomatosis in a 3–year-old child before treatment. **b** The same child during clinical remission after combined treatment with laser surgery and interferon

One of the advantages of CO_2 laser surgery for RRP is the opportunity to perform precise microsurgery with minimal or no bleeding, thus minimizing the risk of spread of papillomata [3, 17]. In addition, it produces little adjacent tissue reaction (edema) [3, 23] in comparison to cup forceps removal. We therefore only apply cortisone intravenously at the beginning of the operation in cases of severe papillomatosis to prevent subsequent edema.

Durkin et al. [10] experimentally demonstrated a delayed healing of surface epithelium with increased formation of fibrous tissue in the subepithalium following removal of normal epithelium of the vocal cords in dogs with the CO_2 laser versus removal with forceps. Macroscopically, no difference could be found after 3 weeks. Other authors only found a small delay in the healing process of laser-induced wounds of the vocal cords with rather little scar tissue [15, 25, 30, 33].

Figures 1 and 2 show an example of laryngeal and tracheal papillomatosis before and after full remission of the RRP. Even after several laser procedures, scar tissue is minimal.

Complications

Complications following laser surgery can be differentiated into immediate and delayed sequelae. The incidence of immediate complications is estimated to be between 0.2% and 3% [3, 7, 12, 44].

Complications of anesthesia include hypoxia, pneumothorax, and pneumomediastinum with jet ventilation. Complications following surgery include burns of nontarget areas (tongue, eye, lip), air-way fires, laryngeal edema, postoperative hemorrhage, cottonoid ignition, endotracheal cuff lesion and pharyngeal burn [7, 11, 33, 42]. Because of laryngeal edema about 8% of our patients had to be reintubated for 2–4 h postoperatively. All patients could be successfully extubated.

Highly significant seem to be the delayed complications of tissue injury. Crockett et al. [7] described a linear relationship between frequency of laser microlaryngoscopy and delayed complications. They observed a complication incidence of 36%, yet mostly minor ones. The most important delayed complications are: anterior web, posterior web, interarytenoid scar bands, glottic stenosis, and voice disorders. The most frequent complication seems to be the webbing of the anterior commissure [7, 35, 36]. For smaller webs we prefer CO_2 laser surgery with postoperative covering of the surface with fibrin glue. For larger webs an intracheal keel is used [6, 44]. Any kind of functional surgery should not be carried out before final remission of RRP.

Further Lasers in RRP Therapy

Some experience in the treatment of RRP with the argon laser on two patients has been reported by Brophy et al. [24]. During their animal experiments the authors detected vital virus particles in the vapor created during the laser procedure, thus bearing the danger of infection by inhalation [4, 32]. The argon laser therefore seems to be too dangerous for treatment of RRP.

Abramson et al. [1] described first results after treatment of RRP with hematoporphyrin combined with argon laser to induce photodynamic activation of hematoporphyrin. The results in two patients are promising. According to Feyh and Kastenbauer [11], who treated 12 patients with this photodynamic laser therapy, papilloma showed a whitish livid color 24 h after treatment. During the following 3–5 days the papilloma tissue was sloughed and the true and false vocal cords were covered by fibrin. Some 3–4 weeks later, the endolaryngeal mucosa was reepithelialized in all patients with no signs of residual disease. They observed recurrence in four cases within a maximal observation time of 1.5 years. A major disadvantage of this method is the necessity of avoiding day light exposure for 14 days because of the risk of photosensibilization of the skin. This is difficult to impose on children [11]. Further research is necessary.

Results

Due to numerous publications on small patient collectives, numbers, multiple combinations of therapy modalities, and the unpredictability of the disease, the results of laser treatment are difficult to evaluate. Most authors consider RRP to be cured if no relapse occurs within 5 years [8, 45], although even beyond 5 years relapses have been described [5]. There is some evidence, that solitary lesions can be cured by laser surgery alone [5, 45]. Motta et al. [26] state that laser surgery promotes definitive remission of disease.

For those children who show severe papillomatosis or rapid progression of RRP necessitating a tracheotomy, we combine laser surgery with al alpha-interferon therapy to improve results. Interferons are potent, antiviral, antiproliferative and immunmodulating proteins produced by many cells in the human organism. Alpha-interferon has been widely used as a purified human substance or a product of recombinant bacteria. This treatment is carried out in collaboration with the children´s ward of the university clinic and will not be discussed here [13].

References

1. Abramson AL, Waner M, Brandsma J (1988) The clinical treatment of laryngeal papillomas with hematoporphyrin therapy. Arch Otolaryngol 114: 795–800
2. Bomholt A (1983) Interferon therapy for laryngeal papillomatosis in Adults. Arch Otolaryngol 109: 550–552
3. Brondbo K, Alberti PW, Crowson N (1983) Adult recurrent multiple laryngeal papilloma: laser management and socioeconomic effects. Acta Otolaryngol (Stockh) 95: 431–439
4. Brophy JW, Scully PA, Stratton CJ (1982) Argon laser use in papillomas of the larynx. Laryngoscope 92: 1164–1167
5. Cohen SR, Geller KAA, Seltzer S, Thompson JW (1980) Papilloma of the larynx and the tracheo-bronchial tree in children: a retrospective study. Ann Otol 89: 497–503
6. Cole RR, Myer C, Cotton RT (1989) Tracheotomy in children with recurrent respiratory papilloma-tosis. Head Neck 11: 220–230
7. Crockett DM, McCabe BF, Shive CJ (1987) Complications of laser surgery for recurrent respiratory papillomatosis. Ann Otol Rhinol Laryngol 96: 639–644
8. Dedo HH, Jackler RK (1982) Laryngeal papilloma: results of treatment with the CO_2 laser and podophyllum. Ann Otol Rhinol Laryngol 91: 425–430
9. Duncavanage JA, Ossof RH (1990) Laser application in the tracheobronchial tree. Otolaryng Clin North Am 23: 67–76
10. Durkin G, Duncavanage JA, Toohill RJ, Tien TM, Caya JG (1986) Wound healing of true vocal cord squamous epithelium after CO_2 laser ablation and cup forceps stripping. Otolaryngol Head Neck Surg 95: 273–277
11. Feyh J, Kastenbauer E (1992) Die Behandlung der Larynxpapillomatose mit Hilfe der photodynamischen Lasertherapie. Laryngorhinotologie 71: 190–192
12. Fried MP (1984) A survey of complication of laser laryngoscopy. Arch Otolaryngol 110: 31–34
13. Gerein V (1992) Molekularbiologische und klinisch-biochemische Untersuchungen zur Ätiologie, Pathogenese und Therapie bei rezidivierender Papillomatose der Atemwege. Habilitationsschrift, University of Frankfurt/Main
14. Goepfert H, Guterman JU, Dichtel WJ, Sessions RB, Cangir A, Sulek M (1982) Leucocyte interferon in patients with juvenile laryngeal papillomatosis. Ann Otol Rhinol Laryngol 91: 431–436
15. Haglund S, Lundquist PG, Strander H (1981) Interferon therapy in juvenile laryngeal papillomato-sis. Arch Otolaryngol 107: 327–332
16. Hawkins DB, Joseph M (1990) Avoiding a wrapped endotracheal tube in laser laryngeal surgery: experi-ences with apneic anesthesia and metal laser-flex endotracheal tubes. Laryngoscope 100: 1283–1287
17. Heipcke TH, Pascher W, Röhrs M (19S7) Stimmfunktion nach Lasertherapie. HNO 35: 234–241
18. Hirschman CA, Smith J (1980) Indirect ignition of the endotracheal tube during carbon dioxide la-ser surgery. Arch Otolaryngol 106: 639–641
19. Irwin BC, Hendrickse WA, Pincott JR, Bailey CM, Evans JN (1986) Juvenile laryngeal papillomatose. J Laryngol Otol 100: 435–445
20. Koufman JA, Little FB, Weeks DK (1987) Proximal large-bore jet ventilation for laryngeal laser sur-gery. Arch Otolaryngol 113: 314–320
21. Lusk RP, McCabe BF, Mixon JH (1987) Three-year experience of treating recurrent respiratory papillomata with interferon. Ann Otol Rhinol Laryngol 96: 158–162
22. Matt BH, McCall JE, Cotton RT (1990) Modified subglottoscope in the treatment of recurrent respi-ratory papillomatosis. Laryngoscope 100: 1022–1024

23. McCabe BF, Clark KF (1983) Interferon and laryngeal papillomatosis. Ann Otol Rhinol Laryngol 92: 2–7
24. Meyers A (1981) Complications of CO_2 laser surgery of the larynx. Ann Otol 90: 132–134
25. Mihashi S, Jako GJ, Incze J, Strong MS (1988) Laser surgery in otolaryngology: interaction of CO_2 laser and soft tissue. Ann N Y Acad Sci 40: 263–294
26. Motta G, Villari G, Pucci V, De Clemente M (1987) The CO_2 laser in the laryngeal microsurgery. Int Surg 72: 175–178
27. Neumann OG, Klopp L (1980) Klinische und histologische Klassifizierung der Larynxpapillome und Papillomatosen. Laryngol Rhinol 59: 57–65
28. Rampil IJ (1992) Anesthetic considerations for laser surgery. Anasth Analg 74: 424–435
29. Romeo YL, Kenney CL (1986) Precaution and safety in carbon dioxide laser surgery. Otolaryngol Head Neck Surg 95: 239–241
30. Rudert H (1988) Laser-Chirurgie in der HNO-Heilkunde. Laryngol Rhinol Otol 67: 261–268
31. Scamman FJ, McCabe BF (1986) Supraglottic jet ventilation for laser surgery of the larynx in children. Ann Otol Rhinol Laryngol 95: 142–145
32. Scully PA, Stratton CJ, Brophy JW (1983) Stereoscanning electron microscopy of argon laser excised laryngeal papilloma. Laryngoscope 93: 188–195
33. Shapshay SM, Rebeiz EE, Bohigian RK, Hybels RL (1990) Benign lesions of the larynx: should the laser be used? Laryngoscope 100: 953–957
34. Shikowitz MJ, Steinberg BM, Abramson AL (1986) Hematoporphyrin derivative therapy of papillomas. Arch Otolaryngol 112: 42–46
35. Shikowitz MJ, Steinberg BM, Winkler B, Abramson AL (1986) Squamous metaplasia in the trachea: the tracheotomized rabbit as an experimental model and implications in recurrent papillomatosis. Otolaryngol Head Neck Surg 95: 31–36
36. Steinberg BM, Topp WC, Schneider PS, Abramson AL (1983) Laryngeal papillomavirus infection during clinical remission. N Engl J Med 308: 1261–1264
37. Trucker HM (1980) Double-barreled (diversionary) tracheotomy in the management of juvenile laryngeal papillomatosis. Ann Otol 89: 504–507
38. Weisberger EC, Miner JD (1988) Apneic anesthesia for improved endoscopic removal of laryngeal papillomata. Laryngoscope 98: 693–697
39. Weiss MD, Kashima HK (1983) Tracheal involvement in laryngeal papillomatosis. Laryngoscope 93: 45–48
40. Wellens W, Snoeck R, Desloovere C, Van Ranst M, Naesens L, De Clerq E, Feenstra L (1997) Treatment of severe laryngeal papillomatosis with intralesional injection of Cidofovir [(S)-1-(3-hydroxy-phosphonylmethoxypropyl)cyostine, HPMPC, Vistide]. Proceedings of XVI World Congress of Otorhinolaryngology. Head and Neck Surgery, Sydney, pp 455–459
41. Welsh RL, Gluckman Jl (1984) Dissemination of squamous papilloma by surgical manipulation: a case report. Laryngoscope 94: 1568–1570
42. Werner JA, Rudert H (1992) Der Einsatz des Nd:Yag-Lasers in der Hals-, Nasen-, Ohrenheilkunde. HNO 40: 248–258
43. Werner JA, Schade W, Jeckstrom W, Lippert BM, Godbersen GS, Helbig V, Rudert H (1990) Comparison of endotracheal tube safety during carbon dioxide laser surgery: an experimental study. Laser Med Surg 6: 184–189
44. Wetmore SJ, Key JM, Suen JY (1985) Complications of laser surgery for laryngeal papillomatosis. Laryngoscope 95: 798–801
45. Wolters B, Eichhorn TH, Kleinsasser O (1984) Kritische Betrachtungen zur Therapie der juvenilen Kehlpapillome. Laryngol Rhinol Otol 63: 396–400

The Treatment of Laryngeal Papillomas
with the Aid of Photodynamic Laser Therapy

J. Feyh and P. P. Schmittenbecher

Introduction

Humanpapilloma virus (HPV) associated papillomas are the most common benign laryngeal tumors in children and show a similar distribution in both sexes. Papillomas and condylomas are caused by HPV which belongs to the family of papovaviruses [2]. Numerous studies have shown that there are at least 16 HPV subspecies apparent in man, causing different diseases [13]. In children larynx papillomas are histologically benign whereas in adults papillomatosis turns into cancer in 10%–20% of cases [4, 15, 16]. Conventional therapy is based on surgical removal of the papillomas by means of CO_2 laser systems. Because of the recurrent character of this disorder, the increasing number of surgical interventions leaves scars in the mucous membranes of the vocal cords of the larynx. This results in an increasing malfunction of the larynx.

All other treatment agents that have been added to surgery such as steroids [3], aureomycine [11], idoxoridine [5], podophyllin [6], vaccine [12], and interferon [14] showed no significant effect in prolonging the treatment interval for recurrent larynx papillomatosis.

As new treatment modality, photodynamic therapy (PDT) has been performed in children with frequently recurring papillomatosis of the larynx. PDT is based on an intravenous administration of a photosensitizing drug (hematoporphyrin derivative) which is selectively retained in neoplastic tissue [9]. Laser light illumination of the photosensitized tissue of a wavelength of 630 nm leads to destruction of the neoplastic tissue by means of a phototoxic process. The phototoxic reaction is based on the excitation of the photosensitizer, and an energy transfer to oxygen leads to the production of singlet oxygen. The neoplastic cell itself is destroyed by this mechanism as is the microcirculatory network of the tumors [10]. In a study of the treatment of malignant tumors in the head and neck area, the impact of PDT has been demonstrated with success [7, 8]. These results justified the introduction of PDT into the treatment of frequently recurring laryngeal papillomas.

Method

Seven children (4 male; 3 female) with recurrent larynx papillomas have been included in the study. Three to 70 surgical interventions had been done before the first PDT; three children had a tracheostomy. A hematoporphyrin-

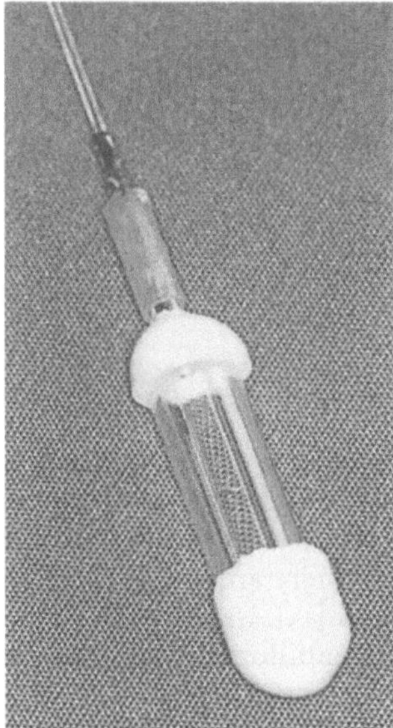

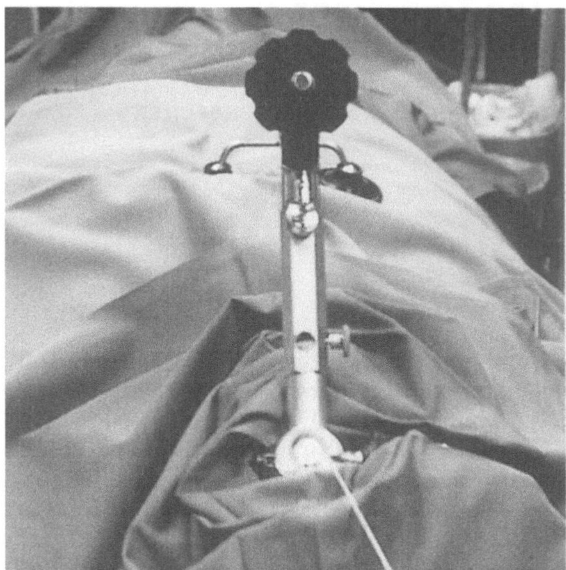

Fig. 1.   Laser light applicator for photodynamic therapy of the larynx

Fig. 2.   Intraoperative situs during direct laryngoscopy. The laser light applicator is inserted into the endolarynx

derivative (Photoscan-3) was administered of a dose of 2.0 mg/kg body weight intravenously. Following the injection, the patients were kept in darkened rooms in the hospital. Forty-eight hours after the injection an integral laser illumination of the endolarynx was performed by means of a cylindrical laser light diffuser (Fig. 1) during direct laryngoscopy and under general anesthesia (Fig. 2). The light applicator system provided a laser light homogeneity of about 5%. An argon dye laser system (coherent, 630 nm) was used as light source. All patients received a light power density of 100 mW/cm^2 and a total energy amount of 100 J/cm^2. The duration of the laser light application was 16.6 min. After PDT the patients spent the first postoperative night on the intensive care unit.

Results

None of the patients showed laryngeal edema causing dyspnea following PDT. Twenty-four hours after PDT, the papilloma tissue was livid and avital. Three to 5 days after PDT, fibrin layers could be observed in the former area of the papillomas. After 3–4 weeks, the endolarynx of all patients reepithelialized without any signs of residual papillomas (Figs. 3, 4). In none of the cases treated could a synechia be observed. Over a follow-up period of 12–17 months, four out of seven patients showed a recurrence of their disease within a relapse time of 4–6 months. All other patients are still free of disease.

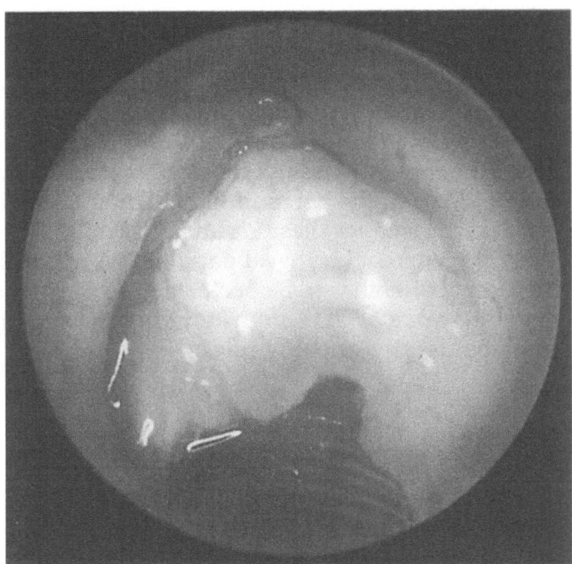

Fig. 3. Endoscopic view on the papillomatosis of the larynx of a 12-year-old boy prior to photodynamic therapy

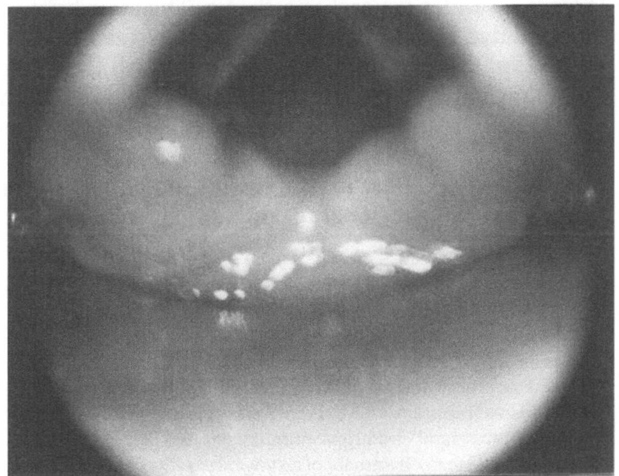

Fig. 4. Fourteen days after photodynamic therapy the vocal and false cords can be identified without residual papilloma tissue

Discussion

Adult and juvenile recurrent laryngeal papillomas show macroscopic complete remission following PDT. As a side effect no damage or scarring to the normal laryngeal tissue could be observed. The mechanism of the selective photosensitization of papilloma tissue still remains obscure. Although all patients included in this study showed recurrence of their disease in their medical history following surgical removal after 3–4 months, only four of seven showed a recurrence following PDT. A selective impact of PDT on HPV-associated papillomas has been shown in animal experiments [1]. At present nothing more is known about the mode of action of PDT on papillomas. Probably this tissue retains hematophorphyrin derivatives in a greater amount than in the surrounding normal tissue because of its increased proliferation. Based on these results, PDT might be a hopeful tool for the treatment of recurrent laryngeal papillomas expecially in children in whom a tracheostomy often has to be performed to prevent dyspnea. Clinical studies will show the value of PDT in prolonging the time interval for the treatment of recurrent laryngeal papillomas.

Summary

Laryngeal papillomas represent a disease of head and neck that can be treated only symptomatically by surgical means. Seven patients with recurrent laryngeal papillomas were admitted to a pilot study for PDT (Fig. 3). Forty-eight hours after intravenous administration of a hematoporphyrin derivative, PDT was performed by means of a specially developed laser light applicator (Figs. 1, 2) under general anesthesia. The laser light was generated by an argon-pumped dye laser system operating at a wavelength of 630 nm. On endoscopic evaluation the papilloma showed a whitish livid color 24 h after PDT. During the following 3–5 days the papilloma tissue was sloughed, and the true and false vocal cords were covered by fibrin. Three to 4 weeks after PDT the endolaryngeal mucosa had reepithelialized in all patients with no signs of residual disease (Fig. 4). Despite the initial multifocal nature of the papilloma, even beyond the anterior commissure, no synechia developed.

References

1. Abramson AL, Waner M, Brandsma J (1988) The clinical treatment of laryngeal papillomas with hematoporphyrin therapy. Arch Otolaryngol Head Neck Surg ??: 114
2. Brandsma JL, Abramson AL (1989) Association of papillomavirus with cancers of the head and neck. Arch Otolaryngol Head Neck Surg 115: 621–625
3. Broyles EM (1940) Treatment of laryngeal papilloma in children with estrogenic hormones. Bull John Hopkins Hosp 66: 318–322
4. Cohen SR, Geller KA, Seltzer S, Thompson JW (1973) Papillomas of the larynx and tracheobronchal tree in children. Ann Otolaryngol Rhinol Laryngol 82: 649–655
5. Cook TA, Cohn AM, Brunschwig JP, Goepfert JS, Butel W, Rawls E (1973) Laryngeal papilloma: etiologic and therapeutic considerations. Ann Otolaryngol Rhinol Laryngol 82: 649–655
6. Dedo H, Jackler RK (1982) Laryngeal papilloma: results of treatment with the CO_2 laser and podophyllum. Ann Otol Rhinol Laryngol 91: 435–430
7. Feyh J, Goetz A, Martin F, Lumper W, Müller W, Brendel W, Kastenbauer E (1989) Photodynamische Lasertumortherapie mit Hämatoporpyrin.Derivat (HpD) eines Spinozellulären Karzinoms der Ohrmuschel. Laryngol Rhinol Otol 68: 563–565
8. Feyh J, Goetz A, Müller W, Königsberger R, Kastenbauer E (1990) Photodynamic therapy in head and neck surgery. J Photochem Photobiol 7: 353–358

9. Feyh J, Goetz A, Schneckenburger H, Müller W, Kastenbauer E (1991) Zeitaufgelöste Laserfluoreszenzmikroskopie von Hämatoporphyrin-Derivat in vivo. Laryngol Rhinol Otol 1: 41–44
10. Feyh J, Goetz A, Heimann A, Königsberger R, Kastenbauer E (1991) Mikrozirkulatorische Effekte der photodynamischen Therapie mit Hämatoporphyrin-Derivat. Laryngol Rhinol Otol 2: 99–101
11. Holinger PH, Johnson KC, Anison GC (1950) Papilloma of the larynx: a review of 109 cases with a preliminary report of aureomycin therapy. Ann Otolaryngol 59: 547–564
12. Holinger PH, Schild JA, Mazurizi D (1968) Laryngeal papilloma: review of etiology and therapy. St Louis 78, 1462–1474
13. Mounts P, Shah KV (1984) Respiratory papillomatosis: etiological relation to genital tract papillomavirus. Prog Med Virol 29: 90–114
14. Schouten TJ, Weimar W, Bos JH, Bos CE, Cremers CWRJ, Schellekens H (1982) Treatment of juvenile laryngeal papillomatosis with two types of interferon. Laryngoscope 92: 686–688
15. Toso G (1971) Epithelial papillomas. Laryngoscope 78: 1524–1531
16. Yoder MG, Batsakis JG (1980) Squamous cell carcinoma in solitary laryngeal papilloma. Otolaryngol Head Neck Surg 88: 745–748

Laser Treatment of Tracheoesophageal Fistulae

P. P. Schmittenbecher and K. Mantel

Introduction

The value of endoscopic techniques in surgery has changed. For several years only a diagnostic procedure, endoscopy is now being used in surgical therapy, especially in the esophagus and the trachea. In general surgery, for example, the recanalization of tumorous obstructions in trachea or esophagus or in the treatment of malignant tracheoesophageal fistula are carried out by surgical endoscopists [14, 16, 24].

In pediatric surgery the importance of interventional endoscopy is also growing. Percutaneous endoscopic gastrostomy represents an example of a procedure in the upper gastrointestinal tract [12].

Correction of tracheoesophageal fistulae in children is usually done via a cervical or thoracic surgical approach [18, 19]. Since 1975 endoscopic closure of such fistulae by the use of fibrin glue, cyanoacrylate glue, diathermia or laser application has been a topic of discussion [6, 21, 23, 26]. This idea aims at the advantage of combining a diagnostic endoscopic procedure directly with therapeutic intervention.

Basic Information

In newborns with tracheoesophageal fistulae with or without esophageal atresia about 1.8%–8.3% of fistulae are of the isolated "H"- or "N"-type [19]. Furthermore, in 3.6%–5% recurrence of a fistula develops after the correction of esophageal atresia [26]. In childhood, acquired fistulae are extremely rare and most often caused by ingestion of alkaline batteries or other foreign bodies [25].

Fistulae are noticed clinically by coughing, choking, aspiration, and cyanosis during feeding, atypic respiratory infection, recurrent pneumonia and gas bloating of the stomach [2–4, 19]. The diagnosis is confirmed either by a tube esophagogram or by tracheoscopy. Sometimes multiple X-ray examinations are necessary to show the fistula (Fig. 1). In tracheoscopy, certain clues such as mucosal retraction can be identified (Fig. 2), and the fistula is established by selective catheterization [2, 4, 10, 15].

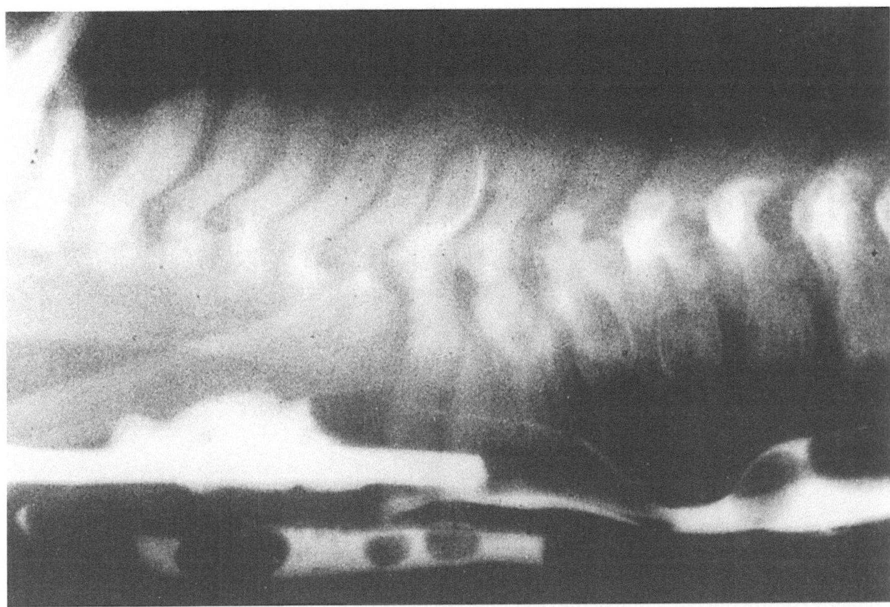

Fig. 1. Tube esophagogram in a 51-day-old boy, carried out with the abdomen hanging downwards. The contrast medium is passing over to the trachea

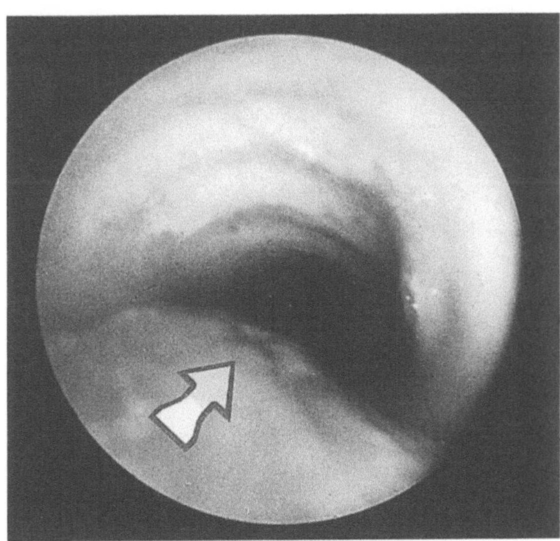

Fig. 2. Tracheoscopy of the same patient showing a small mucosal hill with a central retraction equivalent to the entrance of the fistula

Laser Instruments and Operation Procedure

As described elsewhere [23], we use a Nd:YAG laser mediLas 2 (Dornier Medizintechnik GmbH, Germering, Germany), a wavelength of 1.06 µm, and a

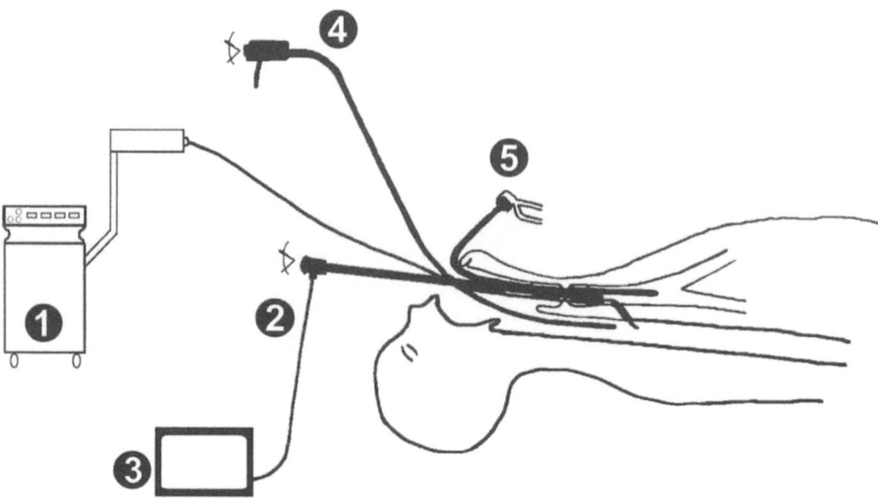

Fig. 3. Diagram of the interventional procedure showing *(1.)* the laser (Nd:YAG, 1.06 µm, bare fiber, 600 µm), *(2.)* the rigid bronchoscope (3.5 mm) inserted in the trachea to position and subsequently control the retraction of the laser fiber (tracheoscopy), *(3.)* video illustration and documentation, *(4.)* the flexible bronchoscope (4 mm) for control of the esophageal end of the fistula (esophagoscopy), and *(5.)* the ventilation tube (3.0 mm)

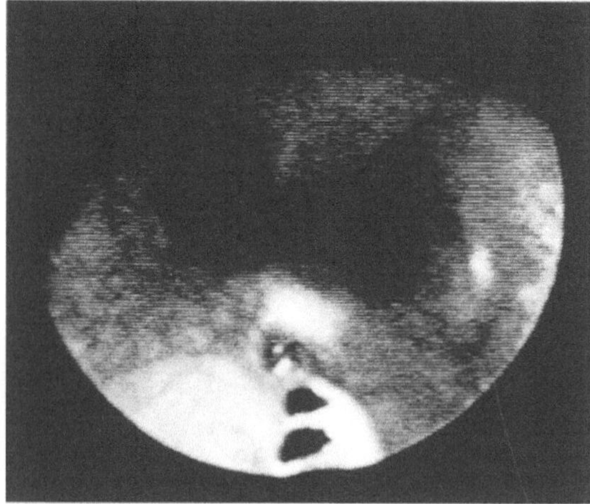

Fig. 4. The laser fiber is inserted into the fistula. Fiber retraction and laser pulse application are oriented on the scale marking every 0.5 mm

connected flexible quartz fiber (600 µm outer diameter). The latter is a so-called bare fiber without covering and gas cooling, but it is supplied with a scale marking every 0.5 mm (see Fig. 4). In suspension laryngoscopy, a rigid 3.5-mm bronchoscope is positioned near the tracheal end of the fistula and a 12-gauge central venous catheter is placed into the fistula. The laser fiber is pushed through this catheter up to the esophagus and the catheter is removed. Under visible control of a simultaneously inserted 4-mm flexible bronchoscope placed in the esophagus, the laser fiber is retracted straight to the esophageal end of the fistula to prevent esophageal mucosa from being damaged (Fig. 3). By retracting the laser fiber, step-by-step laser pulses (10–15 W; 0.5–1.0-s pulse duration) are delivered to the tissue every 0.5 mm with tracheoscopic guidance (Fig. 4).

At the end of the intervention it is most favorable to achieve spontaneous breathing as early as possible. Feedings are given by tube for 1 week. A control examination is performed by tube esophagogram or tracheoscopy after a minimum of 4 weeks.

Clinical Application

Since 1987 we have treated eight newborns (four boys and four girls) with a congenital tracheoesophageal fistula. In seven cases an isolated "N"-type fistula was diagnosed; in one case of esophageal atresia type IIIc, the proximal fistula was overlooked during the first endoscopic investigation and during operation. Seven times only a single laser procedure was carried out; in one girl intervention was carried out twice. In two cases fibrin glue was applied finally. Endoscopic intervention was performed between the third and 54th day of life. Table 1 shows patient data and the laser parameters. One child was extubated immediately after endoscopy, five on the first postoperative day, but one boy was reintubated somewhat later. In three cases ventilation lasted for 5 days. In all patients feedings were given by tube for 1 to 3 weeks.

Table 1. Data on patients and laser parameters

No.	1	2	3	4	5	6	7	8
m/f	m	m	f	f	m	f	f	m
Birth weight [g]	2240	2780	2100	2800	3950	2330	3200	2960
Age at intervention [d]	33	47	3	53	12	25/54	51	51
Number of impulses	9	13	7	13	12	16/22	30	26
Duration of impulses [s]	1	1	1	1	1	1/1	0.5	0.5–1.0
Power [W]	19–24	12–15	15–20	18–20	18–20	20/20	15–18	15
Energy [J]	68	159	121	177	205	241/372	213	269
Fibrin glue	–	–	–	–	–	–/+	+	–
Course	OP	+	+[a]	+	OP	OP	OP	+

OP, operated upon
[a] Died

Three to 5 weeks later and after an uneventful course, esophagogram and/or endoscopy demonstrated normal conditions in three children (Fig. 5). One girl, more over, was clinically inconspicuous when she died of trisomy 18 and a complex heart defect. Ten days to 3 weeks after intervention four children pre-

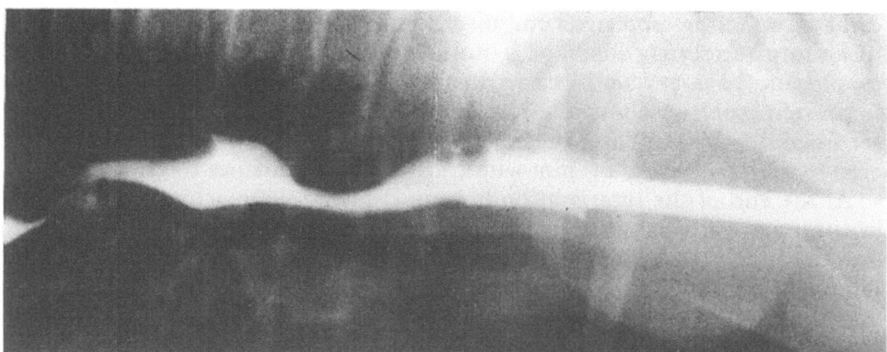

Fig. 5.   Control examination by tube esophagogram 4 weeks after intervention (same patient as in Figs. 1, 2). No flow of contrast medium into the trachea can be identified

sented the clinical signs of recurrence proved by tube esophagogram and endoscopy. In one case the laser energy was much lower than in all the other cases so that technical failing can be considered. Intraoperatively, the fistula was much smaller than before, with a pinlike lumen. In another case, the postinterventional course was uneventful for 2 weeks, but then the fistula recurred. A second laser procedure combined with fibrin glue application yielded the same unsatisfactory result. Surgical correction showed a defect of 1.5 cm between the trachea and the esophagus in connection with a very steep fistula. Two further negative courses including the second case of fibrin glue addition led to operative correction without a second endoscopic intervention. Operative revision showed fistulae with a 2-mm diameter. Postoperative courses were uneventful.

Discussion

In cervical and thoracic operative correction of tracheoesophageal fistulae, complications consist in recurrent laryngeal nerve palsy, secondary vocal cord palsy, longer tracheal intubation, recurrent fistulae, leaks and, though seldom, phrenic palsy, tracheal obstruction, pneumothorax, and mediastinitis [3, 19]. Although these problems are seldom seen, one has also to mention that newborns with an isolated fistula are often small with a birth weight of around 2.5 kg, and thoracotomy is a major intervention in such babies. In a recurrent fistula, after correction of esophageal atresia, operative circumstances are more difficult due to the consequences of the first operation. These considerations led to the search for an endoscopic method.

The first attempts to close a tracheoesophageal fistula by endoscopic intervention were made by Waag et al. [26, 27], Gdanietz et al. [13], Pompino [20] and Daniel et al. [9] in seven cases altogether. Six times a recurrent fistula following the correction of esophageal atresia was treated, once an isolated "N" fistula.

Multiple applications of cyanoacrylat (Histoacryl) have been necessary in every case, in one case finally without success. Only the combination of cyanoacrylate and polidocanol (Aethoxysklerol) was followed by primary occlusion in another case report [1].

Brands et al. [6] supposed that closure of a fistula by cyanoacrylate can function only by chemical-induced inflammation or foreign body reaction. Therefore he used fibrin glue as a more physiologic substance combined with epithelial destruction by diathermia, achieving better success [6,7]. Consequently, the most experience was reported by the Mannheim group in 1992, presenting 17 patients with recurrent ($n = 13$) or "N" fistulae ($n = 4$). In 13 cases the closure was achieved endoscopically using different materials such as cyanoacrylate, fibrin glue, and collagen. In 50% only one endoscopic procedure was performed. Two patients were corrected surgically because of recurrence, and two died [8].

Rangecroft et al. [21] reported two cases of recurrent fistulae closed by diathermic interventions alone although numerous sessions were required.

The idea to close such fistulae by endoscopic laser therapy was prompted by Meier [17], who carried out animal experiments showing that the rat esophagus was comparable in diameter to a human tracheoesophageal fistula. He either primarily welded the rat esophagus, or it was secondarily closed by granulation tissue following laser destruction of the surface epithelium. Laser power between 16 an 22 W for less than 2 s was used. Using these parameters, he protected the nearby trachea from perforation or heat destruction. However, in children, especially in cases with a steep run of the tracheoesophageal fistula, trachea and esophagus are very close to the laser-treated area, implying the risk of heat damage or inflammatory destruction of the respective walls.

Kuntz [16] used the laser to roughen the surface of an acquired malignant tracheoesophageal fistula in an adult patient before closure was attempted by a rapidly hardening amino acid solution (Ethibloc). First clinical laser interventions in children with tracheoesophageal fistulae were performed by Waldschmidt et al. [28] treating five patients with recurrent fistulae after esophageal atresia. Using a bare fiber or a hemispheric sapphire tip the epithelium was destroyed to induce granulation and thus obliteration of the fistula. Additional fibrin glue was administered. In some cases more than one intervention was necessary to close the fistula; in two cases no definite closure was achieved.

Our own experience relates only to primary fistulae. In four cases closure was achieved, although in four cases they recurred. In one negative case only a very small amount of energy was administered to the fistula, perhaps not enough to induce sufficient inflammatory reaction. X-ray control was performed as early as 3 weeks later twice by administration of contrast medium via the tube directly to the known esophageal end of the fistula. At the operative correction, the lumen of the fistula was much smaller than before, so that the early radiologic manipulation may have disturbed the thin adhesions between the fistula walls and terminated an advantageous course. In the other three cases the width and length of the lumen, the steepness of the fistula determining the amount of soft tissue being localized between trachea, fistula and esophagus, the ventilation parameters and questions of feeding are still under discussion. We do not know the reasons for these unfortunate courses and could not find a convincing explanation in the analysis of technical and anatomic circumstances. Surprisingly, even fibrin glue, successful when used in some other reports, was applied without positive effects.

Perhaps the geometry of the laser beam from the bare fiber tip with a beam divergence of 15° is disadvantageous for achieving circular radiation of the fistula wall. Indeed, the wall of the fistula normally collapses during retraction of the laser fiber, followed by laser irradiation of the whole circumference even with small beam divergence. Again this presumes that the fistula is not very extensive in lumen and not rigid or scarred in the wall as is possible in recurrent fistulae. Laser application with a more lateral radiation may ensure circumferential application. Schaarschmidt et al. [33] reported animal experiments with a 115° radial beam. Hemispheric or pyramidal sapphire tips represent an alternative in a fistula of adequate width to accommodate these large applicators. Further investigations have to determine the best application mode.

No method of endoscopic fistula occlusion is well enough established for one to say that this is the procedure of choice. Therefore we have to consider whether the endoscopic laser procedure really presents a lower risk than a surgical approach. In recurrent fistulae, thoracotomy is more or less a very difficult and troublesome procedure, so that perhaps one or more endoscopic interventions are justifiable. In primary "N" fistulae, complications of surgical correction are much more seldom, and repeated laser applications have to be discussed critically. Today we prefer in such cases a single attempt of endoscopic laser coagulation directly with the diagnostic tracheoscopy. In accordance with Gans and Johnson [11], we think that tracheoscopy is the most successful diagnostic method and every child suspected of having a fistula is investigated by tracheoscopy. Recurrence is always corrected surgically.

If newborns with esophageal atresia and tracheoesophageal fistula are in critical condition and a thoracotomy is impossible, endoscopic closure of the fistula could be of great advantage. However, up to now endoscopic techniques also including laser techniques are still not safe and easy enough to recommend them for critically ill premature newborns. In such cases Bloch and Filston [5] use a Fogarty balloon catheter for temporary occlusion of the fistula to allow recovery from respiratory insufficiency before surgical correction is undertaken.

Further experiments already done by groups in Münster, Germany, and Berlin, Germany, may lead to a more advantageous laser occlusion of fistula malformations. This may also be of interest in the treatment of primary and secondary urogenital, anogenital, or urorectal fistulae.

Summary

Since 1975 pediatric surgeons have been searching for methods to close a tracheoesophageal fistula by endoscopic intervention. Laser application is one possibility of destroying the epithelium of the fistula wall and inducing inflammation, granulation, and obliteration. Using a Nd:YAG laser and a bare fiber of

600-μm diameter, we treated eight children between the third and 54th day of life. Four uneventful courses contrast with four unfortunate cases showing recurrence of the fistula. Technical and anatomic aspects as well as postoperative ventilation and feeding procedures should be discussed in these patients. Further investigations have to determine the best application mode, and more clinical experience will elucidate the right postinterventional management.

References

1. Al-Samarrai YAI, Jessen K, Haque K (1987) Endoscopic obliteration of a recurrent tracheoesophageal fistula. J Pediatr Surg 22: 993
2. Beasley SW, Myers NA (1988) The diagnosis of congenital tracheoesophageal fistula. J Pediatr Surg 23: 415–417
3. Bedard P, Girvan DP, Shandling B (1974) Congenital H-type tracheoesophageal fistula. J Pediatr Surg 9: 663–668
4. Benjamin B, Pham T (1991) Diagnosis of H-type tracheoesophageal fistula. J Pediatr Surg 26: 667–671
5. Bloch EC, Filston HC (1988) A thin fiberoptic bronchoscope as an aid to occlusion of the fistula in infants with tracheoesophageal fistula. Anesth Analg 67: 791–793
6. Brands W, Joppich I, Lochbühler H (1982) Use of highly concentrated human fibrinogen in paediatric surgery – a new therapeutic principle. Z Kinderchir 35: 159–162
7. Brands W, Lochbühler H, Raute-Kreinsen U, Joppich I, Schaupp W, Menges H-W, Manegold BC (1983) Die Fibrinklebung angeborener Ösophagusmißbildungen. Zentralbl Chir 108: 803–807
8. Buschulte J, Brands W, Manegold BC (1992) Endoskopischer Verschluß oesophago-trachealer Fisteln. 6th Dreiländerkongreß, Lausanne
9. Daniel P, Martin S, Grahl K-O (1980) Zur Problematik der endoskopischen Verklebung der ösophago-trachealen Rezidivfistel nach Ösophagusatresieoperationen mit Gewebekleber. Zentralbl Chir 105: 1522–1524
10. Filston HC, Rankin JS, Kirks DR (1982) The diagnosis of primary and recurrent tracheoesophageal fistulas: value of selective catheterization. J Pediatr Surg 17: 144–148
11. Gans SL, Johnson RO (1977) Diagnosis and surgical management of "H-type" tracheoesophageal fistula in infants and children. J Pediatr Surg 12: 233–235
12. Gauderer MWL, Ponsky JL, Izant RI Jr (1980) Gastrostomy without laparotomy: a percutaneous endoscopic technique. J Pediatr Surg 15: 872–875
13. Gdanietz K, Krause I (1975) Plastic adhesives for closing oesophago-tracheal fistulae in children. Z Kinderchir 17 Suppl: 137–138
14. Joffe SN, Schröder T (1987) Lasers in general surgery. Adv Surg 20: 125–154
15. Kirk JME, Dicks-Mireaux C (1989) Difficulties in diagnosis of congenital H-type tracheo-oesophageal fistulae. Clin Radiol 40: 150–153
16. Kuntz H-D (1987) "Pulmonale Kachexie" und Hautfistel. MMW 129: 68–73
17. Meier H (1986) Klinische Bedeutung des Neodym-YAG-Lasers in der Kinderchirurgie. Laser 2: 10–16
18. Morita T, Ishida K, Satomi A, Takahashi S (1991) Die Behandlung der angeborenen ösophago-trachealen Fisteln ohne begleitende Ösophagusatresie. In: Hasse W (ed) Funktionsgerechte Chirurgie der Ösophagusatresie. Fischer, Stuttgart, pp 267–270
19. Myers MA, Egami (1987) Congenital tracheo-oesophageal fistula. Pediatr Surg Int 2: 198–211
20. Pompino H-J (1985) Endoskopischer Verschluß ösophago-trachealer Fisteln. Z Kinderchir 27 Suppl: 90–93
21. Rangecroft L, Bush GH, Lister J, Irving IM (1984) Endoscopic diathermy obliteration of recurrent tracheoesophageal fistulae. J Pediatr Surg 19: 41–43
22. Schaarschmidt K, Stratmann U, Lehmann RR, Heinze H, Willital GH, Unsöld E (1992) The rat esophagus: ultrastructure and radiological aspects of tissue response after 1320 nm Nd:YAG laser irradiation. Exp Toxicol Pathol 44: 239–244

23. Schmittenbecher PP, Mantel K, Hofmann U, Berlien H-P (1992) Treatment of congenital tracheo-esophageal fistula by endoscopic laser coagulation: preliminary report of three cases. J Pediatr Surg 27: 26–28
24. Soehendra N (1992) Endoskopie in der Chirurgie. Mitt Dtsch Ges Chir 3 Suppl: G 53
25. Szold A, Udassin R, Seror D, Mogle P, Godfrey S (1991) Acquired tracheoesophageal fistula in infancy and childhood. J Pediatr Surg 26: 672–675
26. Waag K-L, Joppich I, Manegold BC (1975) Endoscopic closure with histoacryl of the recurrent oesophago-tracheal fistula following oesophageal atresia. Z Kinderchir 17: 24–28
27. Waag K-L, Joppich I, Manegold BC, del Solar E (1985) Endoskopischer Verschluß ösophago-trachealer Fisteln. Z Kinderchir 27 Suppl: 93–96
28. Waldschmidt J, Schier F, Charissis G (1992) Laserchirurgie an Larynx, Trachea und Bronchien im Kindesalter. In: Berlien H-P, Müller G (eds) Angewandte Lasermedizin. ecomed, Landsberg, pp VI-3, 8, 6; 1–5

Endoscopic Laser Therapy in Pediatric Gastrointestinal Disorders

P. Spinelli, M. Dal Fante, A. Mancini, and G. Casella

Introduction

The most frequent gastrointestinal diseases in childhood which require endoscopic laser treatment are vascular lesions and familial adenomatous polyposis (FAP). The most frequent vascular disease in pediatric age is blue rubber bleb nevus (BRBN) syndrome with hemangiomas of skin and gastrointestinal tract. FAP is a hereditary disease with autosomal-dominant inheritance characterized by disseminated multiple polyps in the entire colon. FAP is the prototype of a hereditary precancerous syndrome [1].

Material and Methods

Two girls, 6 and 9 years old, were affected by BRBN syndrome with skin lesions distributed all over the body, particularly on the labia, neck, back, arm and forearm, abdominal wall, buttocks, and feet. The principal symptom was melena with secondary anemia. In the clinical history of these patients there were repeated hospitalizations and multiple blood transfusions. Distribution, number, configuration, size, and localization of the bleeding lesions were determined before treatment. A complete study of the gastrointestinal tract with upper and lower endoscopy, X-ray barium swallow of the small intestine, and, in one case, enteroscopy was performed. Complete blood examination was necessary to check hemoglobin and hematocrit levels. Arteriography was not performed in these two cases. Upper gastrointestinal endoscopy and colonoscopy were performed under general anesthesia and maximum care was taken during endoscopic examination so as to avoid repeated suction. A total of 32 vascular lesions were found; 21 lesions with a diameter between 4 and 12 mm were located in the stomach, one with an 8-mm diameter in the duodenum, and ten with a diameter between 6 and 10 mm in the colon. In the stomach, seven vascular lesions were located in the subcardial region, seven on the great curvature, six in the gastric body, and one on the angulus. The duodenal lesion was localized in upper flexure (superior knee) and was treated by Nd:YAG laser (10–15 W). Ten gastric lesions were treated by argon laser (4–5 W) and 11 by Nd:YAG laser (10–15 W). In the colon one lesion was located in transverse, three at the left flexure, three in the left colon, two in the sigmoid colon, and one at rectosigmoid junction. Argon laser was used in three vascular lesions and Nd:YAG laser in the other cases.

In patients affected by FAP (one male and two female 16-year-olds), endoscopic laser therapy (ELT) of rectal polyps was performed at intervals of 3 to 6 months and was always preceded by multiple biopsies of the greatest lesions with histology of tubular adenomas. In one patient, seven sessions were performed to photocoagulate 88 polyps in the rectum by Nd:YAG laser (power output 25–45 W); the size of the lesions was between 3 and 7 mm. At the end of this course of laser treatments, the patient underwent total colectomy with ileorectal anastomosis. After surgery this patient continued the endoscopic follow-up and laser treatment of polyps in the rectal stump. A total of 58 new polyps, 2–5 mm in diameter, were treated by Nd:YAG laser during nine sessions. The other two patients were observed 2 and 3 years after colectomy with ileorectal anastomosis, respectively. A total of 253 polyps were treated with Nd:YAG laser (power output 6.5–40 W) during 19 laser sessions; the dimensions were between 2 and 6 mm. Histology revealed tubular adenoma.

Results

In one patient with BRBN syndrome, the low level of hemoglobin persisted after ELT and five blood tranfusions were needed; a surgical resection of multiple vascular lesions localized in jejunum and ileum was performed. At present, this patient is asymptomatic with a normal level of hemoglobin (follow-up 3 years). No transfusions and no hospitalization were required during the follow-up period.

The other patient remained asymptomatic for 6 years after treatment. Then she was put under our observation with melena and secondary anemia; three blood transfusions were required. A second ELT of ten new vascular lesions in the stomach and three in the sigmoid colon was performed using Nd:YAG laser. At present, the patient is asymptomatic (total follow-up 7 years). No complications were observed in BRBN patients.

The follow-up of patients with FAP is 5 years in one case and 9 years in two cases. The mean number of polyps treated at each laser session was four, nine and 13 at the beginning of endoscopic laser therapy. After treatment of the new polyps at intervals of 4–6 months, the number of polyps is, at present, one, two, and seven, respectively. A major complication consisting of a delayed hemorrhage was observed after treatment of five small polyps in the rectal stump; the endoscopic control revealed the presence of a bleeding ulcer at the site of previous laser treatment. This patient required a transanal suture and blood transfusion (11 blood units).

Discussion

Vascular lesions of the gastrointestinal tract in pediatric patients can be associated with:
a) cutaneous lesions (BRBN syndrome and Osler-Weber-Rendu syndrome),
b) enchondromas (Maffucci´s syndrome), and
c) leg varices and bone hypertrophy (Klippel-Trenaunay syndrome) (Table 1).

Table 1. Syndromes associated with vascular lesion of the gastrointestinal tract in pediatric patient

Blue rubber bleb nevus syndrome
- Inheritance: autosomal-dominant mode?
- Sites of vascular lesions: skin
- Morphology: cavernous hemangiomas, rubber nipple easily compressed
- Sites of gastrointestinal vascular lesions: small intestine, stomach, duodenum, large intestine

Osler-Weber-Rendu syndrome
- Inheritance: familial occurrence (tumors increase in number, variety, and size with age)
- Sites of vascular lesions: mucous membrane, skin, face, lips, nail bed
- Morphology: flat vascular lesions, nodular or stellate angiomata, solid tumors, red or blue color, 1–3 mm in diameter, not obliterated by pressure
- Associated symptoms: epistaxis
- Sites of gastrointestinal vascular lesions: stomach, small intestine, rectum

Maffucci´s syndrome
- Inheritance: unknown
- Sites of vascular lesions: skin
- Associated lesions: enchondromas
- Morphology: large diffuse hemangiomas

Klippel-Trenaunay syndrome
- Inheritance: unknown
- Sites of vascular lesions: leg with varices in soft tissues
- Associated lesions: bone hypertrophy
- Morphology: diffusely infiltrating cavernous hemangioma
- Sites of gastrointestinal vascular lesions: distal colon, sigmoid colon, rectum

In all four syndromes it is possible to have a coagulopathy due to platelet consumption with secondary hemorrhagic diathesis (Kasabach-Merrit Syndrome).

BRBN consists of cavernous hemangiomas involving the skin and the gastrointestinal tract; the term describes cutaneous bluish lesions that feel like rubber nipples. They are easily compressed and return to their original shape with cessation of pressure. The skin lesions are distributed over the entire skin, but they have a higher incidence in the trunk and upper extremities [2]. Visceral localizations include oropharynx, nasopharynx, peritoneal cavity, mesentery, liver, lung, heart [3], eye, urogenital tract [4], and central nervous system [5]. Number, size of skin lesions, and incidence and severity of gastrointestinal bleeding increase with age [6]. Histologically, these lesions are classified as cavernous hemangiomas with a cluster of dilated irregular capillary spaces with a varied amount of fibrous connective tissue [7]. A discrete mucosal nodule with an overlying central bluish red cap is observed at endoscopic study. Bleeding from the gastrointestinal tract and secondary anemia are the clinical features of BRBN; in some cases, a triad of symptoms – thrombocytopenia, hemangiomas, and hemorrhagic diathesis – identifies a Kasabach-Merritt syndrome [1]. The association with coagulopathy and Von Willebrand disease is not frequent. Other symptoms of BRBN include: hematuria, ileal intussusception [6], asphyxia due to hemangioma of the parotid gland [8], ataxia [9], decreased range of mobility and pain or deformity of joints [10], and difficulty in walking due to hemangioma localized on the sole of the foot [10]. Osler-Weber-Rendu or hereditary telangiectasia of skin and mucous membranes has an autosomal-dominant inheritance, and in this disorder, vascular lesions increase in number and variety with age, but the bleeding in these patients is rare before 50 years of age [11]. Osler-Weber-Rendu syndrome is diagnosed when vascular lesions are present on mucous membranes, tongue and nail bed with minute bright red "pinpoints" which are typical endoscopic features of this syndrome and permit a differential diagnosis with BRBN.

Endoscopically vascular lesions should be distinguished from clots, suction artifacts, or erosions [12]. Clinical history is important for suspecting other gastrointestinal hemorrhages related to vomiting, aspirin ingestion, thrombocytopenia, sepsis, severe coagulopathy, or renal failure. Distribution, number, configuration, size, and localization of the bleeding lesions should be determined before treatment. A complete study of the gastrointestinal tract with upper and lower endoscopy, X-ray barium swallow of the small intestine, and, possibly, enteroscopy is fundamental. The hematocrit level should be in the normal range at the time of endoscopy because a low hematocrit level secondary to bleeding does not permit endoscopic detection of the flat vascular lesions [13]. Maximum care must be applied during endoscopic examination to avoid repeated endoscopic suctions because endoscope-induced abrasion may be mistaken for vascular lesions. Vascular lesions may be hidden in folds or in other "blind areas" such as just below the cardioesophageal junction or the rectosigmoid junction and the hepatic and splenic flexures. Arteriography in some cases is not able to detect angiomas because thrombs are present in vascular lesions, and they do not permit the flow of contrast medium. Selective abdominal angiography is useful during bleeding because it demonstrates the nature, location, and extent of hemangiomas [2]. Small (less than 5 mm), flat, discrete angiomata are easier to treat than moderate (5–10 mm) or large (more than 10 mm) angiomata. Large, elevated, or umbilicated angiomata may have extensive submucosal or transmural vascular anastomoses; in these cases, angiography and surgical evaluation should be considered before endoscopic photocoagulation [12]. If the angiomata occupies a large surface area on the entire circumference of the gastrointestinal segment, it is better to consider surgical resection instead of endoscopic photocoagulation because when the vascular lesion grows, the wall becomes thinner. In the treatment of vascular lesions it is important to avoid the use of diazepam and meperidine because these drugs lower blood pressure and blanch the telangiectasia [14]. If meperidine has to be given to allow the endoscope to pass, early administration of naloxone is better for reversing the effect of the drug. The use of glucagon – to distend the stomach and to diminish peristalsis – and mild insufflation of air are recommended [14]. Endoscopic treatment can be performed in emergencies during active bleeding, or it can be carried out as an elective procedure when vascular lesions do not bleed. For emergency cases, it is preferable to use an endoscope with a large single suction channel (3.7 mm or more) or with two channels (3.7 and 2.8 mm). In some cases, side or semilateral viewing endoscopes are useful for photocoagulation of gastric and duodenal angiomata. For patients affected by gastrointestinal bleeding of obscure origin, the source of bleeding is often localized in the small bowel, and

enteroscopy is the most important procedure in these cases. In push-enteroscopy a particular overtube localized in the stomach permits the enteroscope to advance 50–60 cm beyond the ligament of Treitz. An internal channel of a diameter of 2 mm allows the intestinal contents to aspirate, biopsy forceps and cytology brushes to pass, and possibly a laser fiber to be inserted [15]. Pushenteroscopy is diagnostic in 17%–38% of cases [15, 16].
ELT can be performed using argon or Nd:YAG lasers. Argon lasers emit at a wavelength of 488 and 514 nm and generate up to a maximum of 20 W. This radiation is mainly absorbed by pigments such as hemoglobin. Absorption is followed by generation of heat, and in this way, a vascular lesion can be photocoagulated by laser irradiation.

Success with argon laser is possible in 80% of cases without complication [14]. Vaporization of tissue is to be avoided because it can augment the bleeding. During treatment the fiber tip should be maintained 0.5–1.0 cm from the lesion. Photocoagulation of small flat lesions with a diameter of less than 4–5 mm is possible with three or four laser pulses. For lesions larger than 5 mm a photocoagulation in a circumferential manner is recommended, moving inwards from the periphery [17]. Raised vascular lesions are most safely treated by photocoagulating a ring at the base of the angiomata, so allowing an edema cuff to form, and then treating the central vascular portion [14]. Large vascular lesions require a great number of laser pulses, and the risk of perforation is increased. Angiomata in these patients generally do not increase gastrointestinal wall thickness [12]. Extensive cecal vascular lesions should be treated cautiously. The colonic vascular lesions should be treated in one session to avoid repeated colonoscopies [17]. In the upper gastrointestinal tract, when large or numerous vascular lesions are present, simultaneous photocoagulation of all of the lesions could produce extensive scars. To prevent large and multiple areas from becoming involved in fibrotic healing processes, repeated lasers sessions are usually performed. The Nd:YAG laser generates up to 100 W of a power output beam at 1.06 μm wavelength. This laser light penetrates more deeply into the tissue than argon laser, causing more extensive coagulation; this may be an advantage in treating large angiomata with extensive submucosal vascular networks, but is associated with increased risks, especially in colonic and small intestinal lesions, since the wall of the human colon is only half as thick as that of the stomach [17] and cecum and right colon are thinner than left colon [14]. For the treatment of vascular lesions localized in the cecum and right colon, the use of argon laser is safer due to the low penetration of this radiation in comparison with Nd:YAG laser.

Endoscopy can be performed again 1 month after laser treatment in order to check that all vascular lesions have been treated. Often the lesion does not disappear completely with the first course of treatment and angiomatous malformation may persist at the rim of the lesion, necessitating a second treatment session [17]. After photocoagulation of the vascular lesions, the mucosa sloughs off, leaving an ulcer of varying depth in place of angiomata [14]; to avoid complications such as perforation or bleeding, the second treatment should be delayed for several days after the first treatment. Ulcers on gastric folds are frequently irregular in shape while ulcers in the antrum, duodenum, and colon are round or oval after 1 week. These ulcers will reepithelialized over the course of a few days to 2 weeks, leaving normal-appearing mucosa or scar fibrous tissue [14]. Sometimes, a "photocoagulation syndrome" may be present. It consists of prolonged pain, fever, and ileus, representing transmural burn without free perforation [14]. In the experience of Rutgeerts et al. [17], 10% of 28 patients developed serious complications, including severe pain during treatment, chronic duodenal ulcer, delayed severe bleeding, and perforation. Rebleeding is more frequent in Osler-Weber-Rendu syndrome because the exact diffusion of this disease is rarely accurately assessed, and in patients with Von Willebrand disease probably as a result of coagulation disorders [17].

FAP can be associated with various phenotypically distinct syndromes such as Gardner´s syndrome, Oldfield´s syndrome, multiple endocrine adenomatosis, Turcot´s syndrome, Canada-Cronkhite syndrome, and Zanca´s syndrome (Table 2). In FAP, more than 100 adenomatous polyps must be present in the colon. The disease is transmitted as an autosomal-dominant inheritance, with up to 90% penetrance. Polyps are not present at birth, but they appear between the age of 4 months and 74 years [18] with a mean age of 22 years [19]. Most of

Table 2.   Familial adenomatous polyposis and associated syndromes

---

Familial adenomatous polyposis (FAP)
- Histology: more than 100 adenomas
- Distribution: colon and rectum more than small intestine and stomach

Gardner´s syndrome
- Histology: multiple adenomas
- Distribution: colon and rectum more than small intestine and stomach
- Associated alterations: epidermoid cysts, fibromas, desmoids, dental and osseus abnormalities, osteomi, retroperitoneal fibrosis

Oldfield´s syndrome
- Histology: multiple adenomas
- Distribution: colon
- Associated alterations: multiple sebaceous cysts

Multiple adenomas
- Histology: five to 50 adenomas, sometimes up to 100
- Distribution: colon and rectum
- Associated alterations: occasionally, breast and endometrial cancer

Turcot´s syndrome
- Histology: multiple adenomas
- Distribution: colon and rectum more than small intestine and stomach
- Associated alterations: central nervous system involvement

Canada-Cronkhite syndrome (not hereditary)
- Histology: inflammatory juvenile polyps
- Distribution: stomach, small intestine, colon, and esophagus
- Associated alterations: alopecia, nail dystrophy, hyperpigmentation, protein-losing enteropathy, multiple myeloma

Zanca´s syndrome
- Histology: multiple adenomas
- Distribution: colon
- Associated alterations: cartilaginous exostoses

---

the young patients are asymptomatic; generally, symptoms appear in the fourth decade and include rectal bleeding, abdominal pain, diarrhea, and mucous discharge. Most of the polyps are sessile, measuring less than 1 cm in diameter. The presence of large sessile lesions is distinctly unusual [1]. Endoscopically, the polyps show the typical raspberry like configuration. Total proctocolectomy or total colectomy with ileorectal anastomosis are recommended by the age of 20–25 years [20]. When a total colectomy has been performed, the follow-up of these patients should include a periodic endoscopic examination of the rectal stump and, possibly, treatment of all new polyps to maintain a rectum free of polyps. The use of argon laser is safer than Nd:YAG laser, but the latter speeds treatment and decreases the number of treatment sessions [21]; however, it causes a deeper injury of the wall with a higher risk of perforation. The ELT is initiated centrally, and care is taken not to irradiate areas of normal-appearing colon [21]. The first endoscopic control should be performed 2–3 months after the surgical resection to allow an eventual early regression of the polyps. The most common complications are ampulla fibrosis, which can require a proctectomy, and late hemorrhage, which probably occurs because laser irradiation determines a central defect with a surrounding coagulation zone [22]; some days after treatment, this area sloughs off, causing hemorrhage in a few cases. In our experience this was observed in one of 35 laser sessions.

In conclusion, laser photocoagulation in our experience proved to be effective in the treatment of gastrointestinal vascular lesions. Regarding patients with FAP, in spite of a single case of severe hemorrhage, periodic endoscopic laser treatments allowed the control of the disease in the rectal stump by decreasing the number of polyps at this level.

References

1. Fenoglio-Preiser CM, Lantz PE, Listrom MB, Davis M, Rilke FO (1989) Polyposis. In: Fenoglio-Preiser CM et al (eds) Gastrointestinal pathology – an atlas and text. Raven, New York, pp 485–508
2. Gallo SH, McClave SA (1992) Blue rubber bleb nevus syndrome: gastrointestinal involvement and its endoscopic presentation. Gastrointest Endosc 38: 72–76
3. Langleben D, Wolkove N, Srolovitz H et al (1989) Hemothorax and hemopericardium in a patient with Bean´s blue rubber bleb nevus syndrome. Chest 95: 1352–1353
4. Smart RH, Newton DE (1975) Hemangioma of the penis with blue-rubber-bleb nevus-syndrome. J Urol 113: 570–571
5. Sandhu KS, Cohen H, Radin R, Buck FS (1987) Blue-rubber-bleb-nevus-syndrome presenting with recurrences. Dig Dis Sci 32: 214–219
6. Wong SH, Lau WY (1982) Blue rubber bleb nevus syndrome. Dis Colon Rectum 25: 371–374
7. Fine RM, Derbes VJ, Clark Jr WH (1961) Blue rubber bleb nevus. Arch Dermatol 84: 802–805
8. Berlyne GM, Berlyne N (1960) Anaemia due to "blue rubber bleb" naevus disease. Lancet 2: 1275–1277
9. Satya-Murti S, Navada S, Eames F (1986) Central nervous system involvement in blue-rubber-bleb-nevus syndrome. Arch Neurol 43: 1184–1186
10. McCarthy JC, Goldberg MJ, Zimbler S (1982) Orthopaedic dysfunction in the blue rubber bleb nevus syndrome. J Bone Joint Surg 64: 280–283
11. Machicado GA, Jensen DM (1991) Upper gastrointestinal angiomata: diagnosis and treatment. Surg Clin North Am 1–2: 241–262

12. Jensen DM, Bown S (1983) Gastrointestinal angiomata: diagnosis and treatment with laser therapy and other endoscopic modalities. In: Fleischer D, Jensen DM, Bright-Asare P (eds) Therapeutic laser endoscopy in gastrointestinal disease. Nijhoff, Boston, pp 151–160
13. Waitman AM, Grant DZ, Chateau F (1982) Pitfalls and aides in the diagnosis of telangiectasia as a cause of recurrent gastrointestinal bleeding. Gastrointest Endosc 28: 153 (abstr)
14. Buchi KN (1992) Vascular malformations of the gastrointestinal tract. Surg Clin North Am 72: 559–570
15. Foutch PG, Sawyer R, Sanowski RA (1990) Push-enteroscopy for diagnosis of patients with gastrointestinal bleeding of obscure origin. Gastrointest Endosc 36: 337–341
16. Lewis BS, Waye JD (1988) Chronic gastrointestinal bleeding of obscure origin: role of small bowel enteroscopy. Gastroenterology 94: 1117–1120
17. Rutgeerts P, Van Gompel F, Geboes K, Vantrappen G et al (1985) Long term results of treatment of vascular malformations of the gastrointestinal tract by Neodymium-Yag-laser photocoagulation. Gut 26: 586–593
18. Kent TH, Mitros FA (1983) Polyps of the colon and small bowel, polyp syndromes and the polyp cancer sequence. In: Norris HT (ed) Contemporary issue in pathology. Pathology of the colon, small intestine and anus. Churchill Livingstone, New York, pp 167–175
19. Bussey HJR (1975) Familial polyposis coli: family studies, histopathology, differential diagnosis and results of treatment. John Hopkins University Press, Baltimore, pp 43–56
20. Jarvinen HJ (1985) Time and type of prophylactic surgery for familial adenomatosis coli. Ann Surg 202: 93–96
21. Bowers J (1983) Laser therapy of colonic neoplasms. In: Fleischer D, Jensen DM, Brigth-Asare P (eds) Therapeutic laser endoscopy in gastrointestinal disease. Nijhoff, Boston, pp 139–150
22. Hochberger J, Guenter E, Ell CH (1989) In comparison: 1.064 nm–1.318 nm Nd:YAG continuous wave lasers. In vitro and in vivo experiments for endoscopic tumour therapy in the gastrointestinal tract. Lasers Med Sci 4: 25–31

Lasers in Childhood: Laparoscopic Applications

J. WALDSCHMIDT

Introduction

Laparoscopic surgery is becoming increasingly important, and this also holds for children. However, the instruments are still of a very large caliber for application in the neonatal period and early childhood, particularly the clips, clip forceps, ligature loops, and diathermy forceps required for hemostasis: this is obstructive and limits indication.

Laser surgery offers a suitable and, in many respects, superior alternative to clip, ligature, and high frequency (HF) surgery [1, 4, 12, 15, 17, 18]. The light guides needed for energy transfer are only 1/2 mm thick and can be introduced into the abdominal cavity through fine working channels or thin puncture needles. An additional working trocar is not necessary. Flexibility renders the laser fiber easily manageable,so that any laparoscopically visible process in the abdominal cavity can be reached with the "bare fiber" without a decrease in efficiency. Inadvertent tissue damage such as that known to be caused in HF surgery by secondary currents or overly large necrosis zones (stump insufficiency in connection with appendectomy, thermic damage to adjacent organs) has not been observed in the more than 500 laser laparoscopies we have performed.

Further advantages of the laser are the simple handling, cleaning, and sterilization of the laser fiber and the possibility of achieving tissue severance and hemostasis in a single procedure [15]. This obviates not only the complicated and time-consuming exchange of instruments (HF forceps, scissors, dissector) but usually also the use of suction and rinsing, so that a working trocar is eliminated and a great deal of time is gained. Further advantages of laser application in laparoscopic surgery are specified in the following:

1. Elimination of additional working trocar
2. Safe and simple handling, easy cleaning, care and sterilization
3. Optimal viewing conditions in a blood-free operating area because of good hemostasis
4. Elimination of suction and rinsing devices
5. Exact selection of the necrosis zone as desired
6. Tissue severance and hemostasis in a single procedure
7. Sealing effect
8. Precise instrument guidance, accessibility of all laparoscopically visible processes
9. Optional application in contact or noncontact and interstitial lasering

10. Shrinking effect, small wound areas, little exudate, rapid endothelialization, decrease of adhesions
11. Possibility of vaporization with reduction of debris
12. Antimicrobial effects

Technique of Laser Application

We use the neodymium-YAG laser Medilas 40/60. Energy transfer is achieved with the "bare fiber," 600 μ; disposable fibers can also be used with the appropriate coupling device. The fiber is pliant and can be introduced into the abdominal cavity through both the flexible and the rigid cannulas or working channels of the endoscope.

Simple hemostasis (planar capillary), puncture, and fenestration of cysts or vessel dissections are achieved by advancing the fiber through a 16-g cannula. This we insert as close as possible to the affected organ under laparoscopic guidance. In newborns with a low abdominal volume, we seal the cannula cone with bone wax, since even slight gas losses collapse their abdominal cavity because of the low compliance. This is dispensed with in larger children.

In preparing for a cholecystectomy, an appendectomy, or extensive adhesiolyses, we manipulate the laser fiber using a 4-mm-thick flexible probe with a central working channel, through which the "bare fiber" is advanced (Fig. 1).

On insertion, the fiber tip is protected by the applicator. The fiber tip can then be easily managed when the light guide is advanced.

The contact technique is generally preferable. Direct contact with the tissue ensures good energy utilization and prevents scattered radiation. Short impulses (0.3–0.5 s) with adequate cooling intervals keep the fiber tip from melting or burning down. On longer application, the tip has to be periodically cleaned of crusts and tissue remnants. We use 15–35 W for tissue transection.

Prior to the transection, we use a noncontact approach at a higher power (35–40 W) to thrombose larger vessels, such as the appendicular artery, the internal spermatic artery, diverticular vessels or intestinal arcades. Precautions

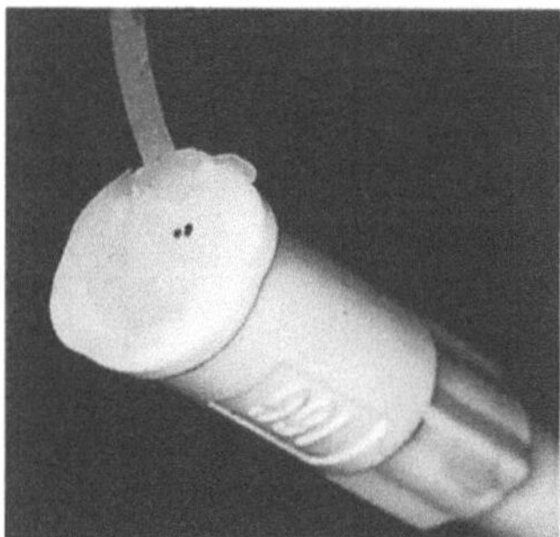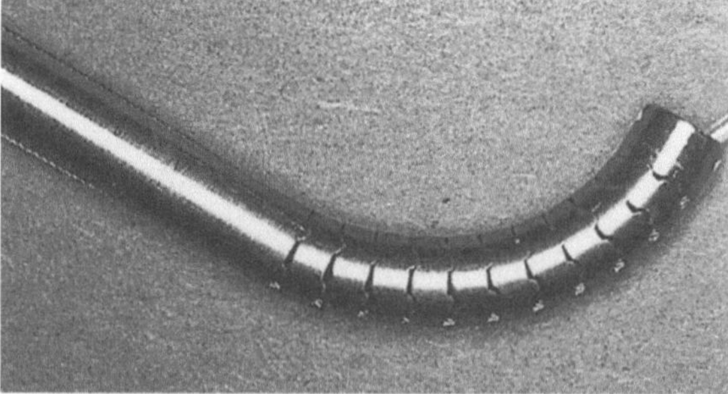

Fig. 1a, b.   **a** The laser beam is transmitted via a bare fibre with a diameter of 0.6 mm by advancing it through a 16-g cannula, sealing with bone wax. **b** In older children we use a flexible probe with a central working channel (Jakoubek, Medizintechnik, Emmingen-Liptingen)

against scattered radiation must be taken here, to avoid undesirable side effects. The possibilities for protecting the abdominal organs against scattering are manifold. It is best to choose the contact technique or interstitial application which does not involve any scattering at all [14].

In applying the noncontact technique, we cover the adjacent intestinal loops or other organs with the greater omentum, which is usually adequate. They can also be kept out of the direct range of the laser fiber by lateral positioning of the children and displacement with the exploring probe.

Table 1. Parameters for laparoscopic laser application in childhood

Application technique	Power (W)	Impulse duration (s)	Impulse interval (s)
Contact	25	0.2	0.3
Noncontact	35–40	0.5	0.3
Interstitial/Intraluminal	5	30	cw

cw, continuous wave.

Long exposure (30–60 s) at low power (5 W) is used in interstitial lasering for devitalization of tumors, regression of angiomas, and intraluminal application in cysts and cavernous hollow spaces. A good volume effect is thus achieved. Large engorged serous cysts are first partially emptied by puncture to shorten the distance from the epithelium of the cyst wall and to somewhat shrink the stretched thin wall. Then intraluminal lasering is done with a freshly broken fiber, followed by fenestration to permit collapse and scarring of the cyst sac (Fig. 2). Vaporization of metastases and other tissue can be achieved by the interstitial technique with the same parameters.

Indications for laparoscopic laser application in childhood are:
- Severance of strongly vascularized tissue: adhesions, cyst wall, mesenteriolum, mesenterium, tube, ovary, liver, and spleen
- Enucleation of cysts and tumors
- Enucleation of the gallbladder
- Hemostasis
- Tissue vaporization
- Devitalization of epithelial linings (cysts, fistulas)
- Incision of compact organ capsules for biopsy
- Vessel dissection: spermatic artery, ovarian artery, appendicular artery, and varicocele
- Cecocolopexy
- Appendectomy
- Resection of Meckel´s diverticulum

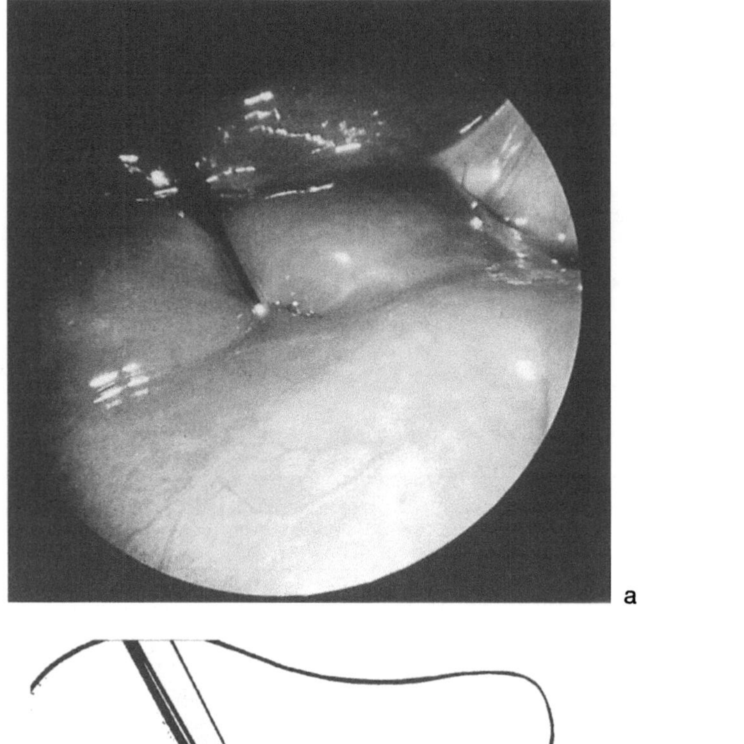

a

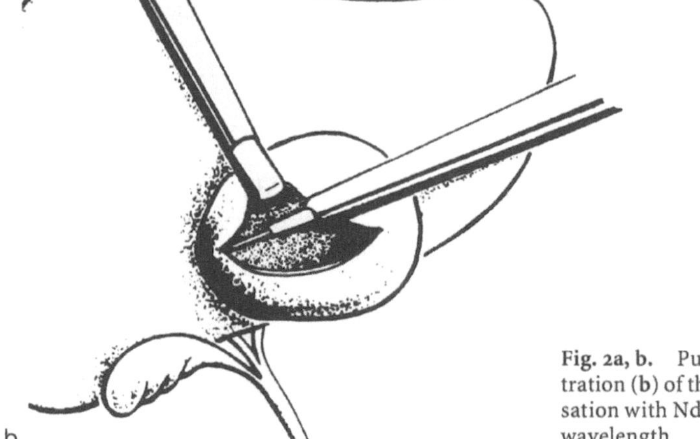

b

Fig. 2a, b.   Puncture (a) and fenestration (b) of the cyst and deepithelisation with Nd-YAG-Laser, 1064-nm wavelength

Fields of Application

Adhesiolysis

Adhesiolysis is performed by applying the contact technique. In the case of cord formations between the omentum and the abdominal wall or an intestinal loop, the tension of the tissue cord due to the pneumoperitoneum can be utilized and the

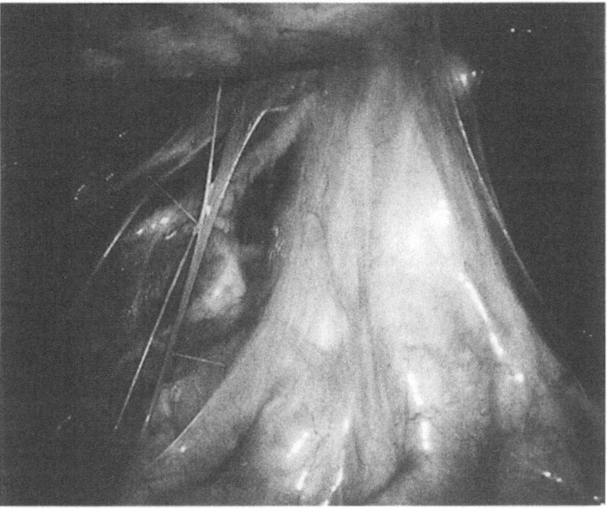

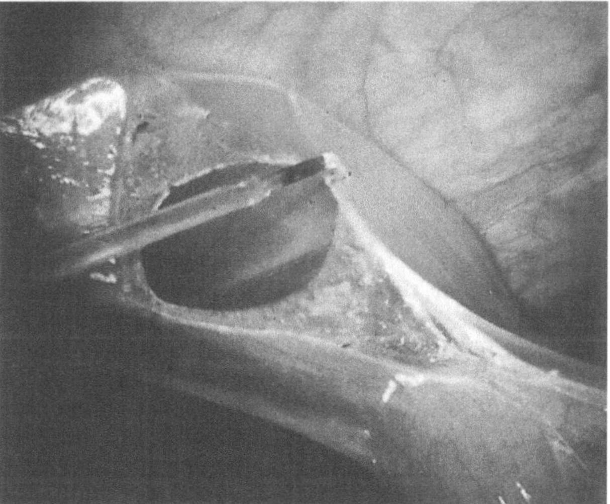

Fig. 3a, b. a Numerous intra abdominal adhesions in a 3-year-old boy. b Laser division without bleeding and exudation of fibrin

separation improved by an increase of pressure (Fig. 3). For massive adhesions between the intestinal loops and for adhesions to the uterine appendages, laser transection should be combined with blunt instrumental adhesiolysis, for which the flexible probe with the central working channel is well suited. Sponges and scissors are rarely needed, and we never apply diathermy together with the laser [10].

Appendectomy

Laparoscopic appendectomy is now a standardized procedure [5, 13]. The skeletization and removal of the vermiform process is performed using HF or clips

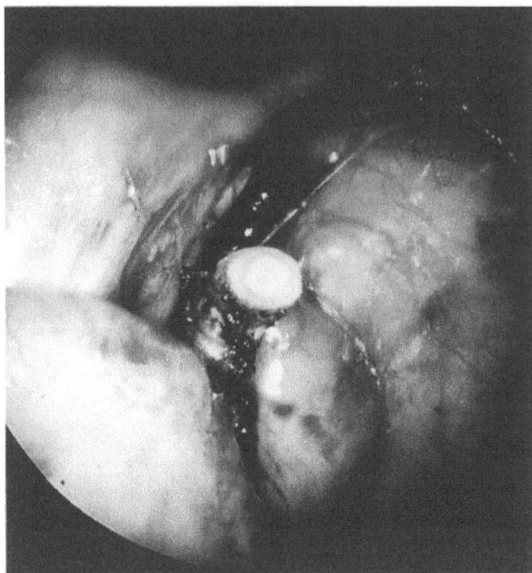

Fig. 4. Dividing the appendix with the Nd YAG-Laser. The cut is sealed and free of bacteria

(Endo-GIA). Nevertheless, the laser offers various advantages. Its application is less traumatic; complications such as stump insufficiency and damage to adjacent structures are unknown. If a laser is available, its utilization is less expensive. Moreover, the 10-mm working trocar for the endo-gia device can be dispensed with. This is particularly advantageous in infants and newborns. Before transecting the appendix, we place a second Roeder loop to prevent the contents of the vermiform process from escaping (Fig. 4). Inflammatory and scarry adhesions as well as congenital adhesions, such as the pathological ileoparietal ligamentum and Jackson´s or Lane´s membrane, are likewise severed with the laser, so that the distorted or kinked intestinal loop can be separated and unfolded. Hemorrhages and fibrin exudation that could lead to renewed adhesion are avoided by applying the laser.

Cecocolopexy

Cecocolopexy can be better performed by laparoscopy than in connection with an open appendectomy. The good overview facilitates the procedure. The pexis can – if necessary – be extended to the right flexure of colon thus drawing tight even a strongly sagging transverse colon. Indications are a common ileocolic mesentary, recurrent cecum torsions, type-I coloptosis, chronically incarcerated pelvic cecum, and the anterior hepatodiaphragmatic colon interposition associated with Chilaiditi syndrome.

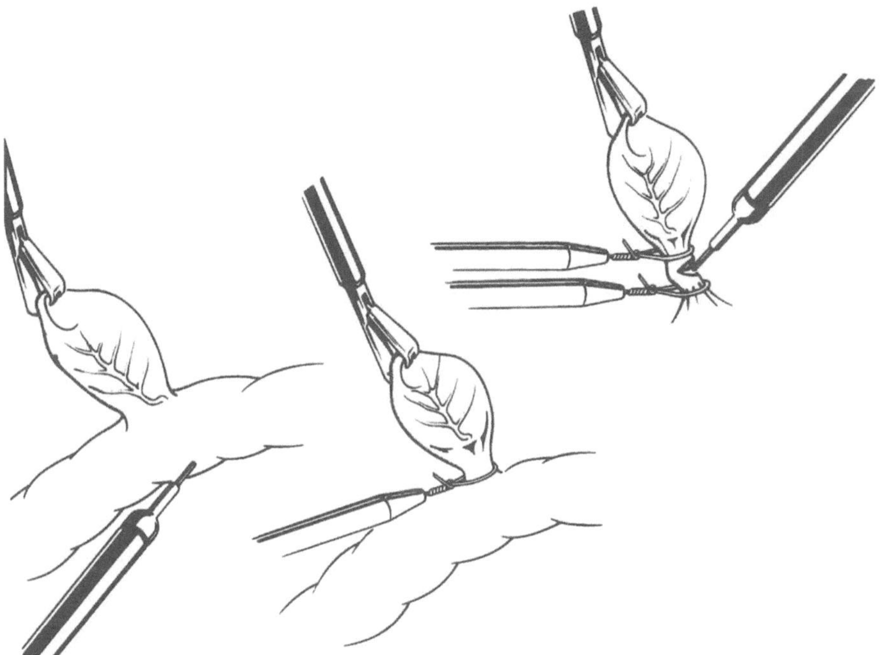

Fig. 5. Laparoscopic laser resection of a Meckel´s diverticulum. The mucosa of the stump is destroyed with the laser, leaving a small scar

The intervention is performed in three steps:
1. Extensive deserosing of the lateral abdominal wall: point-focal deserosing in the course of the taenia libera of the cecum and ascending colon.
2. Coating of the deserosed surfaces with human fibrin tissue glue.
3. Adaptation with an exploring probe and with a decrease in insufflation pressure. The abdominal wall drops and fits better to the colon. Care must be taken that a pocket does not form behind the colon, into which intestinal loops may slip and herniate.

Meckel´s Diverticulum and Other Vestiges of the Ductus Vitellinus

Meckel´s diverticulum is usually detected as a concomitant finding during appendectomies and less frequently in connection with a diverticular complication. The procedure is similar to that applied in laparoscopic appendectomies; no additional instruments are required (Fig. 5).

We grasp the diverticulum tip with the laparoscopy forceps and transect the mesenteriolum with the laser. Now the diverticulum can be stretched and ligated at the base. After placement of the counterligature, the diverticulum is severed between the ligatures; demucosation of the diverticular stump at the

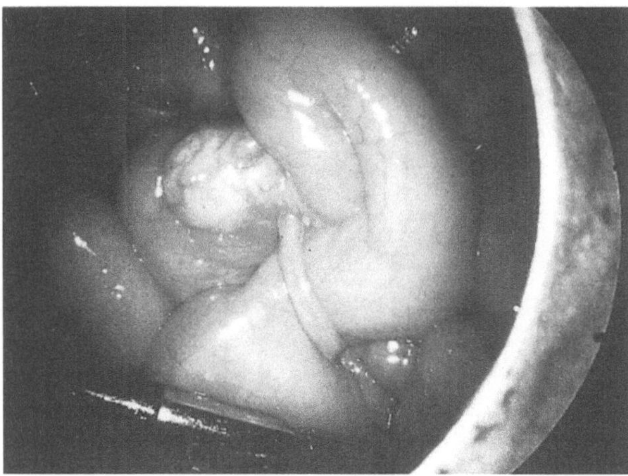

Fig. 6. Meckel´s diverticulum with a remnant of an embryonic ligament, leading to a small bowel obstruction. The ligament has been divided by laser

ileum is performed with the laser. Serosal sutures can thus be dispensed with. Even in the case of broad-based diverticula, the transitional zone to the ileum must also be resected, so that no heterotopic tissue remains. An endo-GIA is occasionally required for this, but only in older children.

Careful attention must be given to a filum terminale or filum enterale and other vestiges of the ductus omphalentericus and the arteria vitellina at the navel and the radix mesenterii (Fig. 6). They always have to be laser-resected in the same session. We also recommend a simultaneous appendectomy in these children if it has not already been performed primarily.

Cholecystectomy

The indication for cholecystectomy is rarer in children than in adults. Sonographically detected concrements usually dissolve spontaneously, particularly in newborns [3, 11, 17]. But even calcareously incrusted, i.e., radiologically recognizable, stones can occasionally dissolve spontaneously. Nevertheless, all complications of stone migration (impaction, obstructive jaundice, chronic dropsy, pancreatitis) and bile-duct infection (cholecystitis, pericholecystitis, empyema, cholangitis, cholangiolitis) may be expected to develop in childhood. Any child with symptomatic cholecystolithiasis should therefore be treated. (Our youngest laparoscopically cholecystectomized child with a symptomatic cholecystolithiasis was 8 months old.)

Indications are thus all complications of gallstone migration, bacterial infection, and local irritation. In cases of chronic hemolysis (spherocytosis, sickle-cell anemia), cholecystectomy of the asymptomatic stone-filled gallbladder should also be considered [3, 7, 11].

The technique of laparoscopic cholecystectomy has been standardized by surgeons for adults. We apply it in older children but have had to make modifications for newborns and infants because of the short working distances and small proportions. Application of the laser plays an important role in this connection. It permits clean dissection in Calot´s triangle without bleeding. The cystic artery and duct can be temporarily occluded with the laser and then transected. The central stumps of the cystic duct and the cystic artery are then ligated with a Roeder loop. The same applies to the neck of the gallbladder. In this way, clips, which are too large and unwieldy for newborns, could be dispensed with. The laser is also used for the further dissection and subserous enucleation of the gallbladder from the liver bed. Advantageous is the good hemostasis and sealing of the liver bed to prevent bile leakage through accessory cystic ducts. We can thus dispense with drainage (Figs. 7, 8).

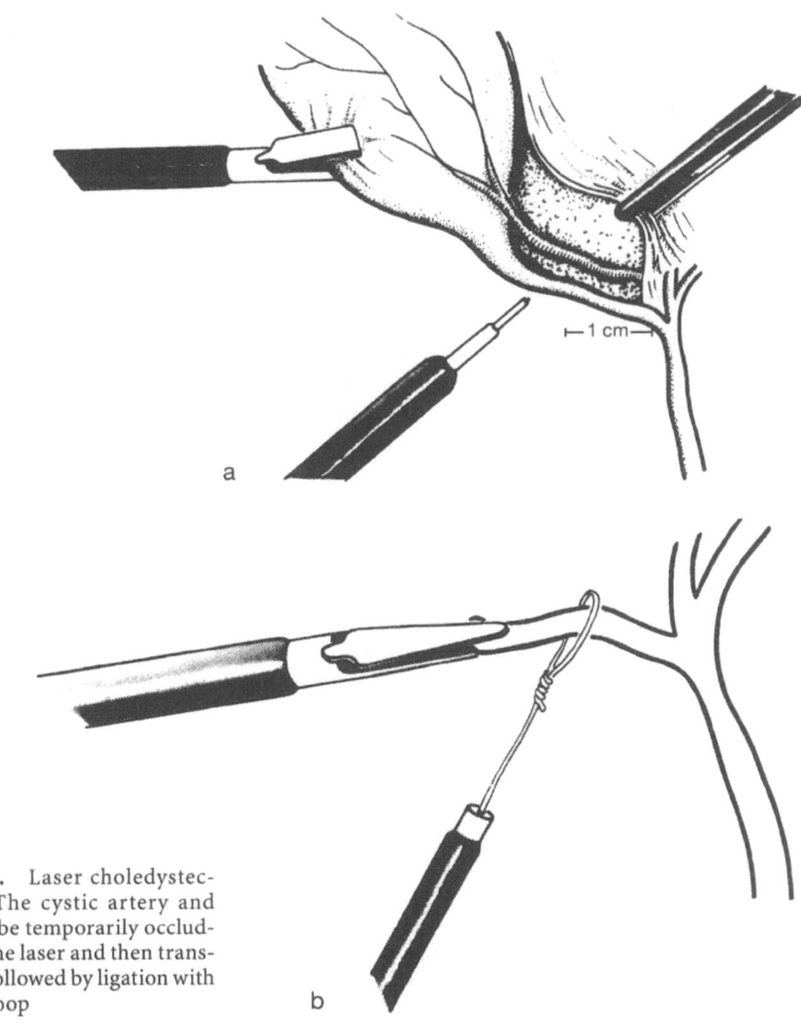

Fig. 7a, b. Laser choledystectomy. **a** The cystic artery and duct can be temporarily occluded with the laser and then transected, **b** followed by ligation with an endoloop

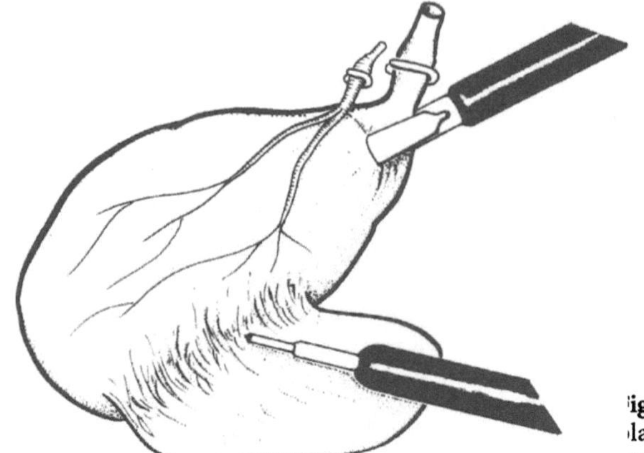

ig. 8. Laser enucleation of the gall-bladder from the liver (Nd-YAG la-er; "contact," 35 W, 0.5/0.3 s)

As in laser-assisted appendectomies, the suction rinsing device is not needed, so that we can manage with 5-mm trocars in newborns and do without the 10-mm trocars. The cystic duct and cystic artery, however, are occluded with clips in older children and transected with the laparoscopy scissors.

Internal Genitals in Girls

We perform the laparoscopy in a Trendelenburg´s position. The optical trocar (5 mm) and working trocar (2 mm) are introduced in the diagonal contralateral quadrants in premature infants and newborns and at the navel in older girls (10-mm trocar). The puncture cannula with the laser fiber is inserted in the hypogastric region near the affected adnexa. This permits a good overview of all sections in the minor pelvis and precise identification through the single lens magnification of the optics. The laser is applied for all of the following indications of gynecological laparoscopy because of its known advantages:
1. Intersexual genitals (hemostasis for biopsy, gonadectomy)
2. Ovarian cysts in newborns (puncture, fenestration, resection)
3. Cyst complications (torsion, rupture, bleeding, knotting)
4. Torsion of ovary, tube, or hydatid (detorsion, resection of the adnexa for necrosis)
5. Salpingolysis and adhesiolysis for the Fitz-Hugh-Curtis syndrome
6. Scarring and tissue reduction for polycystic ovaries, follicle puncture
7. Sterilization in mentally retarded girls

Functional Cysts in Newborns

Laparoscopy or surgery is indicated in cases of further postnatal growth and cyst complications. These cysts generally occupy the entire ovary, so that a cystectomy would involve the loss of the entire ovarian stroma. We therefore punc-

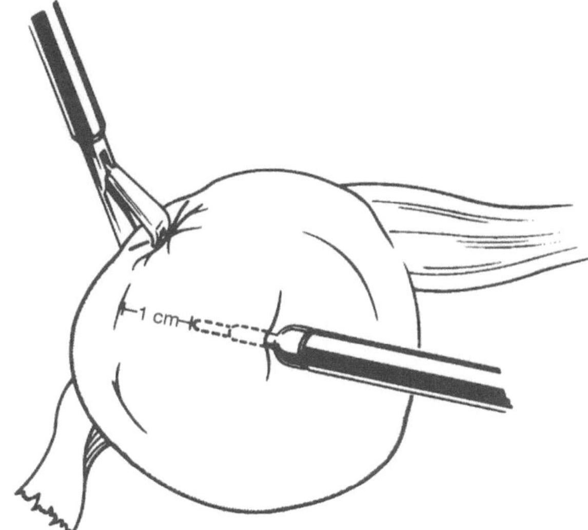

Fig. 9. Puncture of ovarian cyst and emptying of its contants. The inner surface is vaporized with the laser (Nd-YAG laser, intraluminal/interstitial)

ture the cysts and empty them, but only partially (see "Technique of Laser Application"). Then lasing is done intraluminally with 6-W cw, and the remaining fluid is aspirated. The cyst collapses and scars (Fig. 9). The ovarian stroma scattered in the cyst wall can now develop into a new organ.

If the cyst does not collapse, we fenestrate with the laser and devitalize the inner lining with the contact technique. For very large cysts, the bulk must be partially resected and fractionated for easier salvage [8].

Gonadectomy

For a gonadectomy, the suspensory ligament of the ovary is first transected with the internal spermatic artery and vein. This is done by first incising the ligament (contact technique), thrombosing the vessel (noncontact technique), and finally transecting with the contact technique. Then the gonad is lifted with the laparoscopy forceps and stretched and ablated at the mesovarium with the laser. Additional ligatures or clips are not necessary (Fig. 10).

Resections

An adnexectomy becomes necessary for pedicle torsions of cysts and the tube or ovary. In cases of large cysts, the pedicle is doubly ligated and transected between the ligatures.

Salpingotomy and tube transection for sterilization are performed in the same way. The tube lumina are obliterated with the laser, then additionally turned and fixed with a clip or ligature.

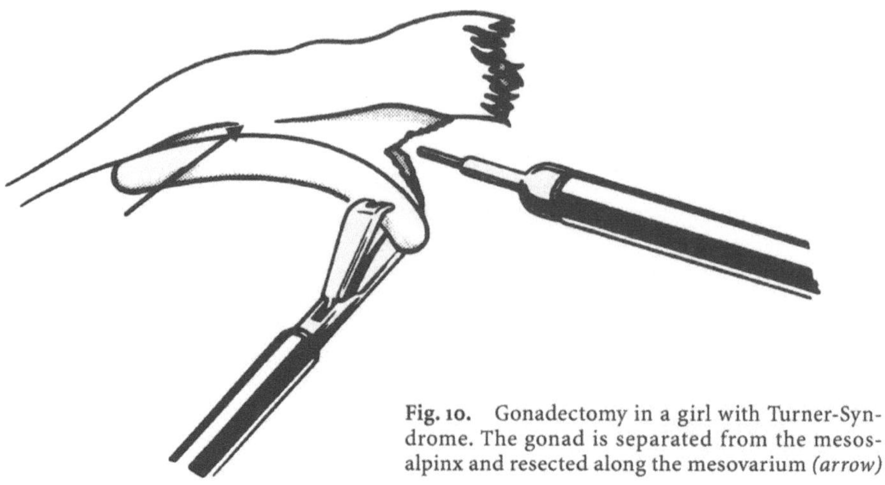

Fig. 10. Gonadectomy in a girl with Turner-Syndrome. The gonad is separated from the mesosalpinx and resected along the mesovarium *(arrow)*

Vessel Dissection in Cryptorchidism

Laparoscopy has long proven effective as a diagnostic measure in cryptorchidism. Reference is made here to testicles evidencing intra-abdominal dystopia and high retroperitoneal retention, the latter usually being associated with an inversion of the epididymis.

Vessel dissection is indicated when the internal spermatic artery and vein are so short that they pass to the gonads stretched out in a straight line and without a loop. An elongation of the vessels with a transfer of the testicle into the scrotum is then no longer possible with conventional techniques.

Alternatives are the free graft, the two-stage procedure according to Corkery and the Fowler technique of vessel dissection [15]. We achieved the best results with respect to testicular atrophy and growth by applying the Fowler technique of vessel dissection. Of the boys, 15% could not be submitted to the Fowler operation, however, since perfusion via collateral vessels was not adequate. This collateral circulation can be improved if tension is relieved on the gubernaculum and its vessels by severing the internal spermatic artery with the laser. After the dissection, the gubernaculum retracts immediately, thus spontaneously drawing the testicle to the internal inguinal ring (Fig. 11). In the further course of time, the testicle even enters into the inguinal canal. At the time of the second session, 4–6 weeks later, the testicle is easy to localize in the inguinal canal. It has increased considerably in size and is very well vascularized by the collateral circulation between the deferential artery, the external spermatic artery, and the gubernacular vessels. The gubernaculum and collateral vessels are spared in the subsequent dissection. The vas deferens is mobilized in the usual manner. The vas deferens is always long enough in the cranially situated testis to permit tension-free transfer into the scrotum and to obviate epigastric-vessel tunneling.

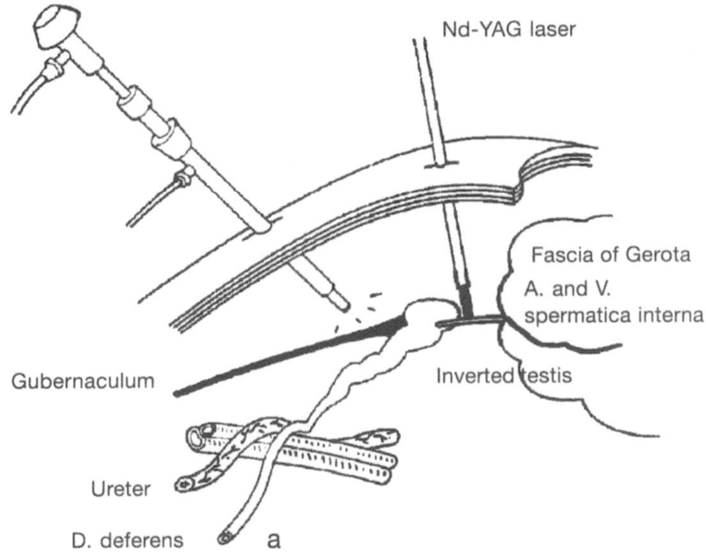

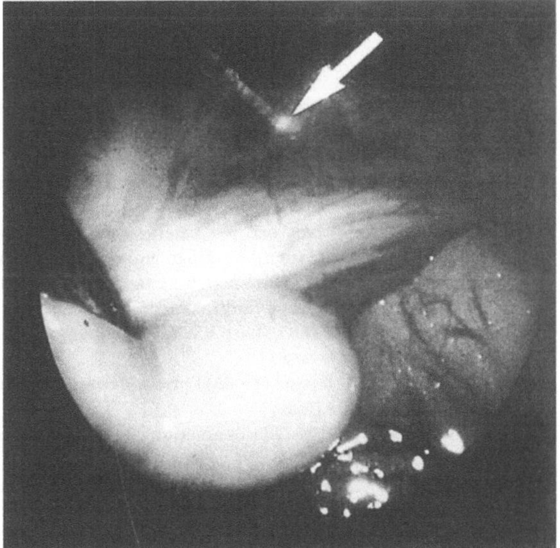

Fig 11a, b. Preliminary laparoscopic-laser dissection of the internal spermatic vessels for cryptorchidism

Varicocele

Operative management of a varicocele is indicated if embolization therapy of extensive collaterals is not adequate or not possible (15% of approximately 250 embolizations in our group of patients). We previously performed high-vein ligature after Paloma in these boys. The laparoscopic technique is better and less traumatic. The overall view is better; even small collateral veins are clearly recognizable by the telescope and video-magnification. The spermatic artery can easily be lifted from the venous plexus with a fine fixation forceps and should therefore be spared. Closure of a thick main vessel is achieved with clips. The collaterals are obliterated with the laser.

Conclusion

The laser is a very good supplement to the instrumentarium for laparoscopic surgery in children. It can be applied both in the contact technique for tissue transection, resection, and fenestration and in the noncontact technique for hemostasis and interstitial/intraluminal lasering. There is thus a broad spectrum of indications. Besides the specific characteristics (such as simultaneous hemostasis and tissue transection, tissue sealing, great precision, and tissue shrinkage), the easy management and small size of the applicators are particularly noteworthy. Thus it is possible to utilize smaller trocars and to dispense with drainages in most cases. The laser is recommendable, especially for laparoscopic surgery in newborns and infants.

References

1. Berlien HP, Müller G, Waldschmidt J (1990) Lasers in pediatric surgery. Progr Pediatr Surg 25: 5–22
2. Bloom DA (1990) Two-step orchiopexy with pelviscopic clip ligation of the spermatic vessels. J Urol 147: 1030–1033
3. Davidoff AM, Branum GD, Murray EA (1992) The technique of laparoscopic cholecystectomy in children. Ann Surg 215: 186–191
4. Feste JR (1989) Laser labaroscopy: A new modality. J Reprod Med 30: 413–417
5. Götz F, Pier A, Bacher C (1990) Modified laparoscopic appendectomy in surgery. Surg Endosc 4: 6–9
6. Hertzmann P (1994) Thermal instrumentation for endoscopic surgery. In: Lobe TE, Schropp KP (eds) Pediatric laparoscopy and thoracoscopy. Saunders, Philadelphia, pp 25–38
7. Holcomb III GW, Olsen DO, Sharp KW (1991) Laparoscopic cholecystectomy in the pediatric patient. J Pediatr Surg 26: 1186–1190
8. Huber JJ, Hosmann J, Spona J (1988) Polycytic ovarian syndrome treated by laser through the laparoscope (letter). Lancet II: 215
9. Lomano JM (1987) Nd:YAG-laser ablation of early pelvic endometriosis: A report of 61 cases. Lasers Surg Med 7: 55–60
10. Mecke H, Freys J, Semm K, Schünke M (1990) Pelviscopic adhesiolysis using the YAG Contact Laser. Laser Med Surg 6: 16–20
11. Newman KD, Marmon LM, Attorri R et al. (1991) Laparoscopic cholecystectomy in pediatric patients. J Pediatr Surg 26: 1184–1185
12. Philipp C, Berlien HP, El Dessouky M, Waldschmidt J (1989) Technik und Problematik bei der laparoskopischen Laseranwendung. Jahresbericht 1987/89, Laser Medicine Center of the Free University, Berlin, pp 251–254
13. Schropp KP, Lobe TE (1993) Laparoscopic appendectomy. In: Holcomb III GW (ed) Pediatric endoscopic surgery. Appleton and Lange, Norwalk, pp 21–27
14. Waldschmidt J (1993) Besonderheiten der Laparoskopie im Neugeborenen- und Säuglingsalter. In: Fahlenkamp D, Loening SA (eds) Laparoskopische Urologie, Blackwell, Berlin, pp 153–162
15. Waldschmidt J, Schier F (1991) Laparoscopical surgery in neonates and infants. Eur J Pediatr Surg 1: 145–150

16. Waldschmidt J, Schier F (1991) Surgical correction of abdominal testes after Fowler-Stephens using the Neodym-YAG-laser for preliminary vessel dissection. Eur J Pediatr Surg 1: 54–57
17. Waldschmidt J, Schier F (1993) Laparoscopic prócedures in neonates and infants. In: Holmcomb III GW (ed) Pediatric endoscopic surgery. Appleton and Lange, Norwalk, pp 67–76
18. Wallwiener D, Pollmann D, Rimbach S, Ganwerky J, Sohn C, Rabe T, Kiesel L, Bastert G (1993) Laser-laparoscopy and GRH agonists: a modern concept in the treatment of endometriosis. Lasermed 9: 94–99
19. Walther H, Woidy L, Filler RD (1995) Die laparoskopische Fenestrierung symptomatischer Leber-zysten. Minimal Invas Chir 4: 177–178

Basics of Laser Resection
in Parenchymatous Organs

C. Philipp, M. Poetke, and H. P. Berlien

Introduction

With the development of modern medical lasers, the role of laser therapy is increasing in the wide spectrum of treatment modalities. In oncology, laser techniques have also become interesting alternatives to radical tumor resection and to palliative tumor treatment methods. Due to the great variability of induced tissue reactions, from microsurgically precise coagulation and cutting to voluminous coagulation or tumor vaporization, the Nd:YAG laser (wavelength 1064 nm) is the most important surgical laser. The possibility of transmitting its light through flexible fibers allows specific application. The longest-term experience exists with all applications of voluminous coagulation for hemostasis and tumor destruction. For the first time, microsurgical preparation with the Nd:YAG laser became possible with the introduction of contact surgery with sapphire tips [1]. The great disadvantages of sapphire tips in practical use led us to introduce bare fiber contact surgery in 1983. Due to the easy handling and low cost of the bare fiber method, this is at present our standard method for all contact applications, especially in endoscopic procedures [2]. Due to the fact that light in the near-infrared range has the greatest penetration depth in tissue, it is also possible to produce homogeneous coagulation during the direct irradiation of the diseased area by the fiber introduced percutaneously into the tissue to be treated. This method, called interstitial laser-induced thermotherapy, was firstly described by Bown [3] and Asher in 1983 [4]. At the same time interstitial laser therapy with the bare fiber was introduced in our center. The first indications were vascular malformations and hemangiomas [5]. We were then able to extend the indications for the Nd:YAG laser therapy to the treatment of benign and malignant tumors and fistulas [6].

Methods

Types of Nd:YAG Laser Application

One can distinguish – independently of medical specialities – between superficial application, open surgery, and intracorporeal application (either with an endoscopic or nonendoscopic approach) such as interstitial or intraluminal application. Particularly in tumor therapy it is sometimes necessary to combine these different methods to obtain the best result.

Four kinds of laser procedures, i.e., cutting and removal, laser-induced thermotherapy (LITT), photochemical reactions, and laser diagnostics are possible in laser medicine. Currently, classical photovaporization and laser-induced thermotherapy are assigned the most important role in laser tumor therapy.

Photovaporization. Due to the absorption of laser radiation by absorbers like chromophores or proteins, a heating of the tissue occurs, followed at 100°C by evaporation of water and at temperatures between 150° and 350°C by tissue dessication and carbonization. The carbonized surfaces will absorb most of the following irradiation and also get vaporized. The typical interaction time of this process ranges from a tenth of a second to several seconds. With longer exposure times, in addition to the penetration depth of the laser irradiation itself, heat conduction in the surrounding tissue occurs and causes thermal effects.

Laser-Induced Thermotherapy. With LITT an in situ coagulation of a defined volume of the tissue due to heating of more than 60°C is possible. Another process is the thermic dynamic reaction. In this case, by a short period of overheating, not an immediate coagulation occurs,, but an inflammatory reaction is induced. This inflammation is followed by an apoptosis with fibrotic repair and can change the structure of the tissue.

Practical Guidelines for Nd:YAG Laser Application

Independently of the specific disease or medical discipline it is possible to give general guidelines for the use of the Nd:YAG laser with different applicators. With an appropriate choice of parameters it is possible to obtain a sufficient result with a low risk of side effects. There is no question that one has to adapt laser parameters to the specific surgical situation.

Focussing Handpiece

Using a focussing handpiece it is possible to induce a wide range of different tissue effects such as a small coagulation seam for preparation, a broad coagulation seam for excellent hemostasis, cutting, or subcutaneous coagulation without any damage to the overlaying tissue. For microsurgical preparation during the operation a handpiece with a small focus diameter of 0.5 mm (which can be achieved with a focal length of 30 mm focussing handpiece) is used. With short exposure times between 0.1 and 0.5 s and a power setting of 30 W one will achieve only small coagulation points for the preparation of tissue. If larger vessels are identified during this procedure, given parameters are not sufficient to perform a coagulation for the purpose of preliminary hemostasis. By defocussing the beam and with longer exposure times (approximately 1–2 s), large vessels can also be coagulated without any risk of vaporization or bleeding. Another possibility is to hold the vessel between the forceps and irradiate the ends of the branches in noncontact with 30 W for a period of 0.5 s or more to achieve the occlusion as with bipolar forceps.

To minimize the risk of a large blood loss in the resection especially of parenchymatous organs or highly perfused tumors, e.g., sarcomas and embryonal tumors one needs a higher power output. With a small focus of 0.5 mm and with a power setting of 60–100 W (depending on the quality of the focussing handpiece) at continuous wave irradiation, one can perform vaporization with a broad coagulation seam after initiating the first carbonization point. By spreading the tissue, especially in partial resection of the liver, one can identify the hepatic veins and arteries and thus reduce the risk of unwanted and inappropriate vaporization and opening of these vessels. Thus, the procedure is comparable to the ultrasound aspirator. However, in contrast to the latter, it has the additional advantage of a coagulated resection surface with a highly reduced risk of immediate or late bleeding or of biliary fistula formation. In case of bleeding, one has to remove the blood by rinsing with saline solution and suction. The water layer causes no absorption of the laser, and one can irradiate with defocussed beam during irrigation for the purpose of coagulation of the bleeding vessel.

For in situ coagulation, for example, of residual tumor either the 30- or 60-mm focussing handpiece can be used with a small coagulation seam. With low power output of about 30 W but with a larger spot diameter as in microsurgical preparation and with short exposure times of 0.2–0.5 s, a small coagulation seam will be achieved. If necessary, one can perform multiple exposures on the same area until blanching occurs. To avoid carbonization and for deep coagulation it is advisable to rinse the surface with saline solution. As the coagulation seam depends widely on the exposure time, longer exposure times should be used for deeper coagulation. Also for coagulation of major bleeding, one has to use 60 W, a large spot diameter and continuous rinsing with saline solution during irradiation. With this saline rinsing, all of the blood that would otherwise absorb most of the irradiation can be removed. In this way one can avoid carbonization and achieve a cooling effect on the surface and additionally a deeper coagulation effect in the tissue.

Bare Fiber Application in Air

Comparable to how the focussing handpiece is used, one can also use a bare fiber in noncontact coagulation. For precise cutting or if only a small coagulation seam is desired, the bare fiber in contact can be used. The main application field is endoscopic surgery but it is also utilized in open surgery. The basic effect of bare fiber contact cutting is a boundary phenomenon. A carbonization layer that absorbs almost all of the Nd:YAG laser irradiation is formed on the border of fiber end and tissue. Thus, in contrast to the typical Nd:YAG laser tissue interaction, no efficient photon penetration into the tissue occurs because most of the photons are absorbed by the carbonization seam. The depth of the coagulation seam depends strongly on the exposure time and heat conduction in tissue.

For procedures in which microsurgical contact vaporization is predominantly required, a fiber with an extremely small diameter should be used. If in addition a broad coagulation seam is desired, it is better to use the 600-µm fiber. With a power setting of more than 30 W especially when using the 200- or the 400-µm fiber, one needs additional gas or water cooling to prevent destruction of the fiber end. The 600-µm fiber used with short exposure times (up to 0.3 s) of the single chopped pulses requires no cooling up to an output of 35 W. Major bleeding requires continuous saline rinsing to remove the blood. In this cases one needs 50–60 W and exposure times of around 0.3 s/pulse in noncontact and continuous wave irradiation. For exposure times longer than 0.5 s an additional cooling of the fiber end is necessary.

The bare fiber offers the significant advantage of working alternatively within contact for cutting and in noncontact for coagulation. For instant contact cutting, the fiber has to be precarbonized. This can be done in advance of the procedure on sterile cork or wooden spatula, or with some exposures in direct tissue contact. If additional noncontact coagulation is to be performed, for example, for the primary coagulation of larger vessels, one has to remove the fiber from the tissue. With the first chopped pulses in the noncontact method the carbonization layer on the surface is removed by pyrolysis and most of the radiation is emitted from the fiber end again. Thus, during a procedure it is not necessary to cut the fiber to change several times between contact and noncontact.

If the fiber tip becomes widely scattered or even shows deformations (curves), the fiber should be broken and freshly prepared by, in the case of PCS-fibers, stripping the outer coating. If an immediate vaporization is desired, a precarbonization should be performed.

This advantage becomes especially evident in endoscopic surgery. With one and the same instrument, one has a precise cutting tool or an effective coagulation instrument simply by changing the kind of application from contact to noncontact.

It is important to remember that the bare fiber in contact surgery is not a mechanical scalpel, so it should not be pressed into the tissue; only the fiber end has to be kept in contact. Furthermore, fiber is not a drill, so the fiber end must constantly be visible in the operation field.

Contact Surgery in Water

The greatest advantage of laser application, especially in endoscopic surgery, over any kind of high frequency application is that there are no limitations to work under saline solution. In principle the application is the same as in air, with only two major differences. Due to the cooling effect of the surrounding water, a noncontact vaporization is nearly impossible and a higher power is required for a contact vaporization. Another effect of the cooling is a smaller coagulation seam, so even more precise microsurgical vaporization is possibly than in air. For vaporization an appropriate power setting between 25 and 50 W can be chosen, depending on the fiber diameter and the desired effect. For coagulation either with a small or broad coagulation seam a higher power setting is necessary, as in air, yet one has less risk of surface carbonization. In the same way as in air or open surgery one has the choice of changing between contact cutting and noncontact coagulation. The cleaning procedure by pyrolysis is also possible in water, but it takes longer exposure times and higher power to start the pyrolysis.

Table 1. Fields of application of laser surgery

Indication	ND:YAG noncontact	Nd:YAG contact	CO_2
Skin/soft tissue:			
Molluscum	++		+(+)
Condylomata acuminatum	+(+)	+	++
Verrucae			
– Palmar	++		+
– Planta			++
Tumors			
– Localized	+		+
– Infiltrating			+
Mouth:			
Tongue tumors		+(+)	(+)
Gingiva hyperplasia			(+)
Airways:			
Polyps		+	
Papillomatosis	++	+	+
Stenosis			
– Larynx		(+)	++
– Trachea		++	(+)
– Bronchii		++	
Thorax:			
Infiltrating tumors	(+)		(+)
Decortication	(+)	+	(+)
Abdominal tumors			
– Preparation	++	++	
– Resection	++		
Liver/spleen	++		
Kidney/pancreas	+	+	
Abscess		+	(+)
fistula			
– Shrinking		++	
– Excision			+
Adhesions (laparoscopic)		++	+
Anal stenosis		++	+
Marisques	+	++	

Interstitial LITT

Interstitial LITT, by which a bare fiber or a special LITT applicator is inserted through a needle or catheter into the tissue to be treated, enables the delivery of Nd:YAG laser light directly into the center of diseased area. Due to photon absorption and heat conduction, both coagulative and hyperthermic effects can be obtained and thus an immediate or delayed tissue destruction is caused. With adequate treatment parameters the effects of LITT can be limited to the diseased area without destruction of the surrounding tissue. The access to the tissue to be treated can be provided percutaneously, endoscopically, or during open surgery. In contrast to the endoscopic application or application during open surgery, in which direct control is possible, during the percutaneous approach indirect methods of process control are needed. If the lesion is not deeper than 3 cm, it is possible to palpate the fiber for precise positioning and control the reaction by a crepitation caused by the outgasing reaction of in-tissue-dissolving gas. Furthermore, one can control the temperature of the overlying tissue, especially the skin, to prevent overheating and unintended coagulation. For deep-seated lesions magnetic resonance imaging (MRI), ultrasonography (US) or color-coded duplex sonography (CCDS) monitoring can be used [7–10].

Interstitial laser-induced hyperthermia (LIHT) requires an output of 2 W and long exposure times. In contrast to hyperthermia, interstitial LIC causes a definite tissue destruction by coagulation necrosis. With a clean newly broken and cleaved bare fiber of 600 or 800 μm one has to use no more than 5 W. The diameter of the coagulation zone depends on power setting and exposure time. The advantages of the bare fiber over special ITT applicators are the lower price and easier handling. Using the power setting of 5 W, there is no risk of destruction of the fiber. Due to its smaller diameter compared to the ITT applicator one can use conventional puncture sets without dilatation. This is especially helpful in the treatment of secondaries with a hard structure. Furthermore, in dependence on the chosen parameter, a well-defined coagulation volume of up to 15 mm in diameter can be achieved. The extent of the damaged area can be enlarged by reposition of a fiber or by a multiple fiber application. Due to the easy handling of the system, longer operation times for larger volumes are not needed as opposed to special ITT applicators (Table 1).

Fields of Application

Superficial Laser Therapy

The therapeutic spectrum includes such diseases as benign and malignant vascular tumors, congenital vascular disorders (e.g., hemangiomas and vascular malformations), virus-induced lesions (e.g., papillomas, verrucae), fibrotic tumors as neurofibromas, and anal stenosis.

Direct transcutaneous coagulation in the noncontact method either with a focussing handpiece or with the newly broken air-cooled bare fiber was performed most often. For larger exophytic growing tumors we use a tangential circumferential irradiation of the base of the tumor with a defocussed beam. The irradiation is stopped when the base is blanched. Sometimes it is necessary to keep the surface wet to avoid carbonization. Smaller tumors with a diameter of up to 2 mm are coagulated with the defocussed beam in a rectangular direction.

If the tumor is localized subcutaneously, it is neccesary to expand therapy to an interstitial application.

Endoscopic Application

Due to the small diameter of the fibers, they can be employed in nearly all endoscopic procedures. We use laser treatment for the recanalization of laryngeal, bronchial, and esophageal stenosis (benign/malignant) as well as for the treatment of benign urethra or ureter stenosis. The palliative ablation of tumor masses and the treatment of benign and malignant stenosis are mostly performed using a flexible bare fiber either for a noncontact coagulation or subsequent contact vaporization. Furthermore, in the treatment of complications after conventional surgical therapy of tumors such as esophagotracheal fistulas, we use the bare fiber technique in endoscopic application. After introducing the fiber into the fistula under endoscopic control, the coagulation of the mucosa is performed, followed by a shrinking and occlusion of the fistula [11].

Peritoneal Cavity Laparoscopic Surgery. One of the greatest advantages of laser application is the use of endoscopy especially in laparoscopic surgery. Here the Nd:YAG laser is very successful due to the possibility of using the bare fiber to work either in noncontact for coagulation or in contact for cutting, or even alternately. When using the bare fiber, the fiber end must be visible all the time. During the chopped exposure one can observe the white light at the fiber end during the cutting process. This light is used by automatically controlled laser systems to adjust laser power for fiber protection purposes. As the power is automatically reduced an immediate change between cutting and coagulation only by changing the application from contact to noncontact is not possible. These syptens offer only limited advantage, since in the chopped mode, with any Nd:YAG laser, one has precise control over the coagulation seam, cutting efficiency, and fiber wear.

Gastrointestinal Tract. For the treatment of colorectal tumors a primary noncontact application for homogenous coagulation of the tumor and hemostasis and a subsequend contact cutting or evaporization to remove the tumor masses is used. With this combined technique the risk of perforation and postoperative bleeding is reduced.

For the treatment of angiodysplasia within an interval, one can coagulate the vessel malformations with about 20 W. In acute bleeding, in the case of larger vessels or in angiodysplasia, flushing with saline is needed to remove the blood, and more power output of approximately 50 W is used. Angiodysplasias of the esophagus should not be treated with Nd:YAG lasers, because of the risk of perforation.

Open Surgery

Thorax.   In open surgery, for atypical segmental resection of the lung we prefer the noncontact method with a power output of 60 W and a focussing handpiece. In this way not only hemostasis is achieved but also complete sealing of the alveoli, so no sutures are necessary.

For tumor resection the use of the Nd:YAG laser in thoracic surgery also provides a great advantage. A nearly bloodless removal of tumor is possible and furthermore – and this is very importent in tumor surgery – one can coagulate the tumor bed to destroy possible tumor rests. Thus the radicalness of tumor removal can be increased and at the same time important anatomical structures can be saved.

Peritoneal Cavity Abdominal Surgery.   In open surgery of tumors in parenchymatous organs the same techniques are used as in endoscopic surgery for preparation, coagulation, and removal. With the Nd:YAG laser and the use of a bare fiber the resection of tumors of liver, pancreas, and spleen can be performed if little coagulation is desired. Equipped with a maximum power output of 60 W and by the use of the focussing handpiece, parenchymatous organs and tumors can be resected with very good results. In liver surgery in particular the use of the Nd:YAG laser is more successful than the ultrasound aspirator. The ultrasound aspirator is merely able to identify the vessels and remove only the parenchymatous tissue. However, it offers no possibility of occlusion of capillary vessels. This is not only important for hemostasis, but in liver surgery one great postoperative risk is biliary leakage postoperatively of intra-abdominal abscesses. Using the laser one achieves a sealed surface of the resection margin which not only closes smaller veins and arteries but also smaller biliary ducts. Only veins with a diameter of more than 3 mm and arteries of more than 1.5 mm require ligature. For practical use it is helpful to spread the tissue. Due to the earlier onset of vaporization in the parenchymatous tissue than the vessels, they resist irradiation longer if perfused and can be identified easily, and a preliminary ligature can be performed. Thus, the procedure is comparable to the ultrasound aspirator but with the additional advantage of laser-induced hemostasis. The coagulation seam is approximately 5 mm wide as can be seen in the specimen of an intrahepatic angioma with recurrent hematobilia. The ultrasound aspirator in spleen and pancreatic surgery is not an alternative. With the Nd:YAG laser a hemisplenectomy is also possible with a minimized risk of bleeding. As in general, during the resection no preliminary turniquet was necessary here either and only he central vessel required a ligature. In pancreatic surgery an additional advantage over hemostasis is the sealing of the parenchymatous surfaces, so the risk of loss of pancreatic fluid is minimized. This technique requires no additional pancreaticojejunostomy. No laser-related complications could be observed and hospitalization time could be reduced [6, 7].

Interstitial Laser-Induced Thermotherapy

A predominant field in our therapeutic program is interstitial LITT of benign vascular tumors, deep-seated primary and secondary liver tumors, and subcutaneous metastases of breast carcinoma.

Since 1983 we have performed over 1000 interstitial treatments. For an exact guidance of the coagulation process there is the need and the possibility of process control. Since 1992 color-coded duplex sonography has been used for the on-line control of this procedure. After preoperative diagnostics and puncture of the lesion to be treated a newly broken and cleaved bare fiber was inserted. Using a power setting of 4–5 W the coagulation of tumors was performed. The changes in CCDS signal were observed and provided information about the intensity of tissue reaction. The area of coagulation was visible in a B scan several minutes after laser exposure.

Magnetic resonance imaging (MRI) enables the monitoring of temperature changes; and its three-dimensional resolution is by far the best among all monitoring methods for interstitial laser therapy. Therefore it is absolutely necessary in the stereotactic treatment of brain tumors. Disadvantages of this technique, such as the artifacts caused by movements of the patient, limited direct access to the patient and the high costs of this method limit the use of MRI for on-line monitoring of interstitial LITT in other body regions. Furthermore, it cannot be used either in open or endoscopic surgery at present.

In contrast, CCDS is a reliable and simple technique which enables control and steering of tissue changes during interstitial laser therapy without great strain for the patient. This simple technique provides complete information, such as the determination of the precise puncture route, the control of fiber position, the visualization of tissue changes during the procedure, as well as the depiction of the reduction of tumor vascularization and coagulated volume. In combination with the techniques of endoscopic laser application one has a wide range of techniques for minimally invasive surgery which make a number of open surgical procedures unnecessary.

Discussion

To our experience the Nd:YAG laser is a very useful tool in tumor surgery. Owing to the high optical penetration depth in tissue, the ability to control tissue effects by the use of certain application parameters (e.g., contact 1/N noncontact), and the possibility of transmitting its radiation through optical fibers, the Nd:YAG laser can be applied universally. With either flexible or rigid endoscopes one can use it for coagulation of hemorrhages and tumors and for recanalization of benign or malignant stenoses. With either a handpiece or a bare fiber and corresponding high energy densities the resection of tumors in parenchymatous organs with simultaneous hemostasis is possible. Especially with a bare fiber which is inexpensive and easy to handle one has the possibility of working alternately in noncontact for coagulation or in contact for cutting, even in endoscopic procedures. This results in the effectivity of laser application and in diminished operation time [8].

The sapphire tips sometimes used in contact laser surgery [8–10] are not recommended. Because of the reflection from the connecting surfaces between fiber and sapphire as well as high absorption within the sapphire tip itself, an efficient cooling of the surfaces is required. Therefore, a relatively large diameter of the fiber connector is needed. Furthermore, there is a high risk of gas embolism due to the cooling gas, especially in endoscopic or interstitial application [10]. Sculptured fibers permit a better cutting efficiency than bare fiber initially, but they change their quality during the procedure and one is not able to cut in contact and to coagulate in noncontact such as with the simple bare fiber [12]. For fine preparations, small fiber diameters should be used instead.

For the resection of tumors in parenchymatous organs and bloody, invasive tumors, the Nd:YAG laser has proved to be a very effective instrument. The ultrasound aspirator (CUSA) which is comparable with non contact surgery in liver resection can cut the parenchyma, so that all the vessels are saved and can be ligated by clamping [13, 14]. The subsequent repair of the resection area requires fibrin glue with the risk of bleeding beneath the glue layer. Besides this the CUSA is not suitable for resection of other parenchymatous organs such as lung, is spleen, kidney, and pancreas. High frequency electrocautery may also be used for cutting and coagulation, but its penetration depth in tissue is limited [15]. In comparison to the electrocautery, bare fiber contact surgery is a safer and more effective device for both cutting and coagulation. Thus, it is possible to carry out resection of tumors in parenchymatous organs and bloody tumors, even under difficult conditions. Due to a bloodless and hermetically sealed resection field obtained during laser resection of intrapulmonary metastases, the danger of pneumothorax and hydrothorax can be reduced. Even the extirpation of infiltrating malignant tumors in the abdomen and thorax with protection of important structures can be performed [8]. Yet care has to be taken as late effects of coagulation, especially in the intestine, should be avoided.

The advantages of Nd:YAG laser application for tumor removal can be summarized as follows:
- Hemostasis
- High precision
- Reduced instrumentation at the treatment site
- Minimalization of the risk of infection
- Minimal trauma of the surrounding tissue.

Summary

In the past 20 years laser techniques have become interesting alternatives to standard therapeutic methods in all medical fields. Due to the wide variability of tissue interactions and the possibility of specific applications, Nd:YAG laser is the most important surgical laser. With the adequate choice of application mode and relationship between interaction time and power density it can be used for precise cutting, specific coagulation, and homogeneous coagulation. Thus, the field of laser application in tumor therapy ranges from treatment of superficial tumors to endoscopic tumor ablation and resection of neoplastic tissue in parenchymatous organs as well as interstitial coagulation of deep-seated primary and secondary malignancies.

References

1. Daikuzono N, Joffe SN (1985) Artificial sapphire probe for contact photocoagulation and tissue vaporization with the Nd:YAG laser. Med Instrum 19: 173–178
2. Berlien H-P, Biewald W, Waldschmidt J, Müller G (1988) Laser application in pediatric urology. In: Waidelich R, Waidelich W (eds) Laser. Optoelectronics in medicine. Springer, Berlin Heidelberg New York, pp 341–344
3. Bown SG (1983) Phototherapy of tumors. World J Surg 7: 700-709
4. Ascher P (1983) Verhandlungsbericht der DGLM-Tagung, Graz. EBM Erdmann-Brengar, Munich
5. Berlien H-P, Waldschmidt J, Müller G (1988) Laser treatment of cutan and deep vessel anomalies. In: Waidelich R, Waidelich W (eds) Laser. Optoelectronics in medicine. Springer, Berlin Heidelberg New York, pp 526–528
6. Berlien H-P, Philipp C, Waldschmidt J (1990) Tumor ablation by laser in general surgery. In: Trelles MA (ed) Laser tumor therapy. Madrid: Illustre Colegio Oficial Medicos 3: 67–77
7. Berlien H-P, Müller G, Waldschmidt J (1990) Lasers in pediatric surgery. Prog Pediatr Surg 25: 6–22
8. Schneider PD (1992) Liver resection and laser hyperthermia. Surg Clin North Am 72 (3): 623–639
9. Landau ST, Wood TW, Smith JA (1987) Evaluation of sapphire tip Nd:YAG laser fibers in partial nephrectomy. Lasers Surg Med 7: 426–428
10. Baggish MS, Daniell JF (1989) Catastrophic injury secondary to the use of coaxial gas-cooled fibers and artificial sapphire tips for intrauterine surgery: a report of five cases. Lasers Surg Med 9: 581–584
11. Hess M, Gross M, Berlien H-P (1994) Ösophagotrachealer Fistelverschluß mit NEODYM:YAG Laser. Eur Arch Otorhinolaryngol 341 Suppl
12. Shirk GJ, Gimpelson RJ, Krewer K (1991) Comparison of tissue effects with sculptured fiberoptic cables and other Nd:YAG laser and argon laser treatments. Lasers Surg Med 11: 563–568
13. Schröder T, Hasselgren P-O, Brackett KA, Joffe N (1987) Techniques of liver resection. Comparison of suction knife, ultrasonic dissector, and contact neodymium-YAG laser. Arch Surg 122: 1166–1169
14. Tranberg K-G, Rigotti P, Brackett KA et al (1986) Liver resection. A comparison using the Nd-YAG laser, an ultrasonic surgical aspirator, or blut dissection. Am J Surg 151: 368–373
15. Schröder T, Brackett KA, Joffe SN (1987) An experimental study of the effects of electrocautery and various lasers on gastrointestinal tissue. Surgery 101: 691–697

Tumor Removal by Laser

S. L. GANS

Introduction

Although the use of lasers in children for treatment of tumors provides important advantages, it must be stressed at the outset that traditional concepts of tumor surgery must be maintained: knowledge of anatomy, respect for tissue viability, adequate exposure, and skillful and gentle technique. Furthermore, it must be added that since we have been using lasers, we have not removed any conventional instruments from our operating theater. The laser is an important and useful *adjunct* to traditional methods of tumor surgery.

In general, what advantages does the laser provide? It has been well established that the laser seals blood vessels and lymphatics during surgery. This hemostatic effect often enables the surgeon to distinguish between normal and pathologic tissues. It also reduces the amount of blood loss, and serosanguineous collections of fluid in the postoperative period are diminished.

It is also well accepted that the surgery of neoplasms should be performed with minimal opening of blood vessels and lymphatics, minimal manipulation of involved tissues and maximal visualization.

The combination of the above-stated laser effects and the above-stated optimal conditions is the hypothesis upon which the use of lasers in tumor surgery is based. We do not have the numbers of cases, and the complexity of follow-up does not permit us at this time to provide statistics and conclusions as to the ultimate results. The following material is derived from personal experience and observations. Having the laser always at hand and available in the operating theater provides opportunities for creative use and expansion of the indications and advantages of laser surgery.

Liver Tumors

Liver Biopsy.   Excision of a piece of liver tissue provides an excellent sample of tissue and leaves a clean, dry and secure bed.

Small Tumors or Metastasis.   The ability to carve out a small tumor or metastasis is advantageous for the same reasons. It is also possible to destroy or evaporate such multiple lesions quickly and bloodlessly with the laser used outside of the focussed or cutting mode.

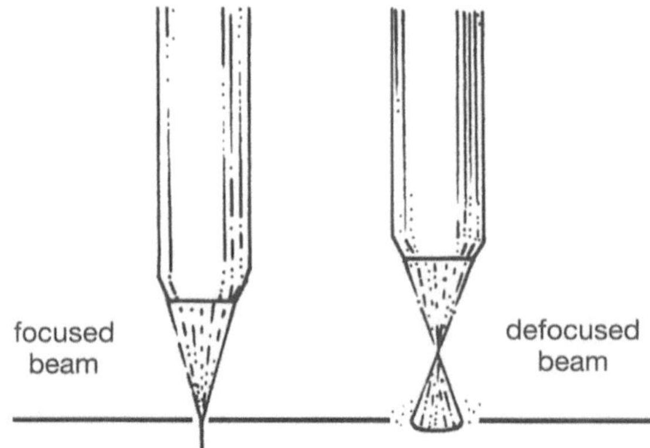

Fig. 1. Focused CO_2 laser beam for incision and fine dissection. Defocused beam for hemostasis

Liver Resection.   The same strict attention to anatomic principles of exposure, dissection and ligation must be applied. However, ultimately liver tissue must be divided. For this purpose CO_2 lasers, Nd:YAG lasers, and combinations and variations of these lasers have been used. Our own modest experience indicates that the combination of conventional methods with the addition of lasers provides the best results. It is important to compress that portion of the liver to be transected, which is much more easily done in children than in adults. This can be done with hepatic clamps, padded sponges or with the fingers in the smaller and softer livers of infants. Accurate visualization and control of the larger vessels and bile ducts with ligatures and clips is accomplished as the laser cuts through compressed liver tissue in a more or less dry field. Mattress sutures may be applied and this severed surface of the liver is "painted" with a defocussed laser beam (Fig. 1). This results in liver resection with a minimum of destruction of tissue and a maximum of safety from postoperative bleeding, bile drainage and necrosis.

Adrenal Tumors

One of our earliest and most impressive cases was that of a 4-year-old child with symptoms of Cushing's syndrome due to a very large malignant tumor of the left adrenal gland (Fig. 2). Through a large thoracoabdominal incision (Figs. 1, 2), the tumor was completely removed with a combination of conventional instruments and CO_2 laser dissection (Fig. 2) with a minimal loss of blood.

Neuroblastomas

Neuroblastomas spread by direct extension, lymphatic involvement or blood-borne metastasis. Regional and distant lymph nodes, liver, bone marrow and bone cortex are often involved. Conventional treatment is unchanged at this time, but lasers may be useful as described below.

Encapsulated tumors in very young patients have excellent results with complete excision by either conventional methods or with the laser.

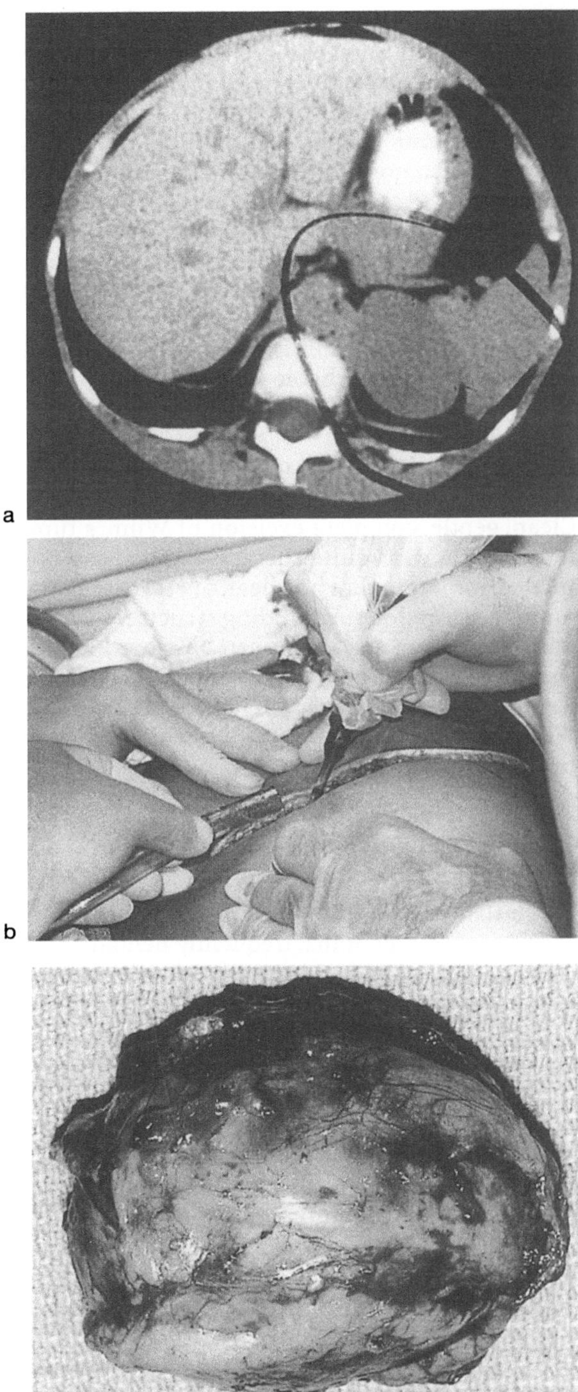

Fig. 2a–c. a Scan showing a huge mass in the left adrenal area due to a very vascular malignant tumor. b Almost bloodless long thoracoabdominal incision made with a CO_2 laser. c Specimen completely removed

In patients with large primary tumors of the retroperitoneum, the operation is carried out through a large transverse transperitoneal incision, and in some cases a thoracoabdominal incision may be required. Use of the laser for the incision will result in less bleeding and postoperative drainage. In situations in which the tumor margin is not clear, laser application may be useful to distinguish between normal and pathologic tissue in the course of the dissection and to seal blood vessels and lymphatics in the periphery.

Furthermore, unresectable tumors may be evaporated and removed and large tumors debulked with less bleeding and trauma, adding a safety factor in preventing overzealous surgical excision and destruction of neighboring important structures and organs.

Tumors more difficult to reach because of location, such as presacral lesions, may be more approachable with the laser.

Wilms' Tumor

Clean, gentle, complete excision of Wilm's tumor with dissection by conventional methods is quite successful. The laser is helpful, however, in dissection where the margins are not clear, in very large tumors, and particularly where the tumor has invaded surrounding structures such as the liver, diaphragm or abdominal wall. Such extensions can be carved out or destroyed more or less bloodlessly and without further spreading the malignant cells.

In instances in which part of a kidney is to be preserved, such as bilateral Wilms' tumor, transection of the renal tissue can be done advantageously with the laser.

Teratomas

Two instances of laser dissection and removal of teratomas are herein described. Sacrococcygeal teratoma, frequently benign at birth, has a great tendency to become malignant and to spread locally. Furthermore, it is usually a very vascular tumor and blood loss must be anticipated in its removal. For these reasons, early surgery is recommended and the use of lasers is considered important in preventing spread and limiting blood loss (Fig. 3). Preliminary ligation of major vessels is carried out before the remaining dissection can be safely accomplished.

Our single case of gastric teratoma occurred in a neonate with omphalocele and the Beckwith-Wiedemann-syndrome (Fig. 4). The laser was particularly useful in the deep posterior dissection and in transection of the gastric and esophageal ends preliminary to anastomosis.

Photodynamic Therapy

Photodynamic therapy has great promise and is undergoing intensive as well as extensive investigation. Certain exogenous photosensitizers, i.e., hematopor-

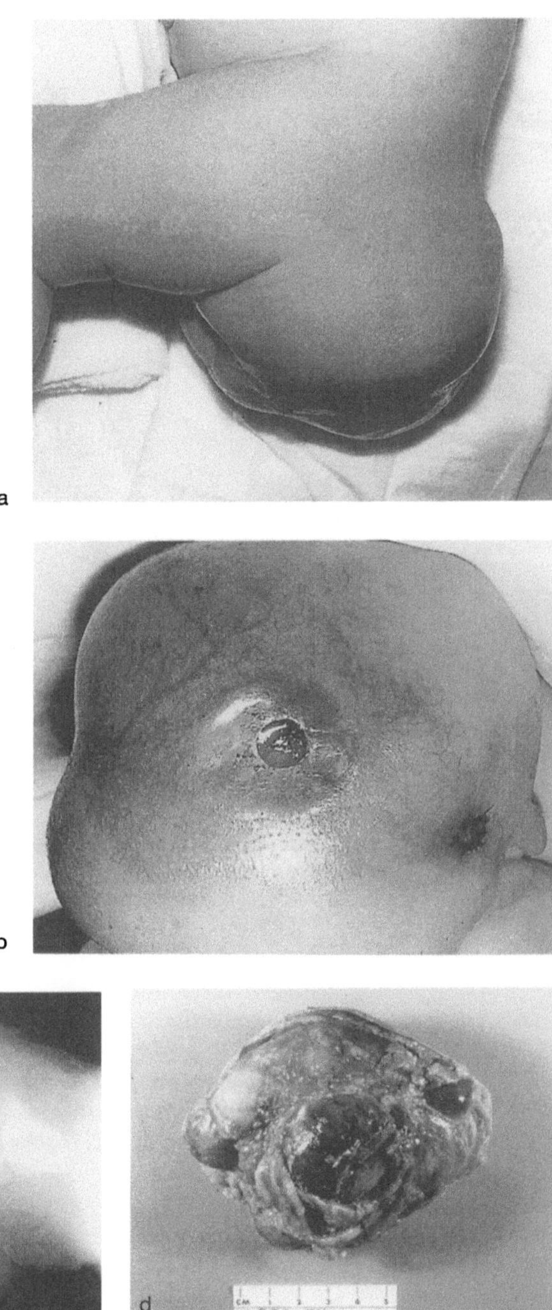

Fig. 3a-d. **a** Large neonatal sacrococcygeal teratoma. **b** Necrosis is already present at birth. **c** Roentgenogram demonstrates vascularity and calcification. **d** Specimen completely removed with minimum blood loss

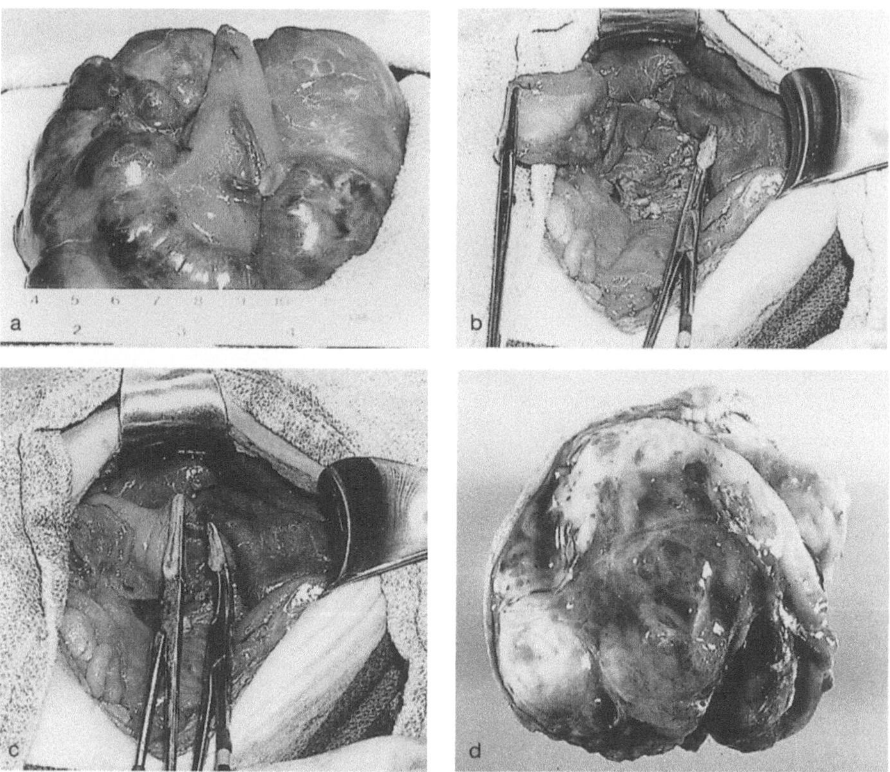

Fig. 4a–d.   Neonate with large gastric teratoma. **a** The pylorus is stretched over the tumor.
b The tumor has been bloodlessly dissected and removed. **c** The remaining pylorus and the lower
end of the esophagus are prepared for anastomosis. **d** The completely removed tumor

phyrin derivatives, when injected into the blood stream, have the capability of
localizing in specific malignant tissues, thereby "marking" them, while passing
through and out of surrounding normal tissues. This characteristic trait sub-
jects the marked tissue to destruction by some wavelengths. The surrounding
unmarked tissue is not affected. Already successful in some superficial tumors,
we are looking forward to progress in this method for use in other lesions.

Summary

We have discussed the reasons for using lasers in tumor removal from children
and the apparent advantages of this method. Specifically outlined are tumors of
the liver, adrenal and kidney (Wilms´ tumor), neuroblastomas and teratomas.
Briefly mentioned is the interesting and promising subject of photodynamic
therapy.

The Use of Lasers in Pediatric Neurosurgery

M. L. WALKER

Introduction

The use of lasers in neurosurgery dates back approximately one and a half decades [1, 12, 27], and the experience in pediatric neurosurgery goes back almost as far [4, 6, 8, 32]. Pediatric neurosurgeons became interested in surgical lasers in the early 1980s and rapidly explored their use for the various lesions encountered in the subspecialty of pediatric neurosurgery. Over this period of time experience has led to a much more clear understanding of where lasers are useful, where they are specifically indicated and where their use is essentially not helpful.

It should be pointed out that surgical ultrasonic aspirators are in essence competing tools with surgical lasers [9]. Most neurosurgeons have access to both tools. For the majority of tumors the ultrasonic aspirator is probably preferred as the surgical instrument of choice by the majority of neurosurgeons. However, there are specific tumors where the laser adds an increased dimension and can be very helpful in tumor removal.

The advantages of surgical lasers include the concept of minimal surgical trauma and the very precise way in which they can be applied [28]. Pediatric neurosurgeons are concerned with minimizing trauma when working with the immature and developing central nervous system. The developing nervous system is especially vulnerable. The traumatic effects of surgery, radiation therapy and/or chemotherapy can be additive to the developing nervous system. Any surgical modality that limits the trauma in these circumstances is welcomed. It is for this reason that surgical lasers have found such favor in the practice of pediatric neurosurgeons.

In the first few years of experience with lasers in pediatric neurosurgery the carbon dioxide laser was essentially the only surgical laser tool available [1, 8, 17, 29]. However, experience over the past 7 or 8 years has grown to include the Nd:YAG laser, KTP laser and argon laser [23, 24, 33, 34]. These different wavelengths have added new dimensions to the armamentarium of pediatric neurosurgeons. Already we see approaches and techniques used that were simply not available with the carbon dioxide laser alone. This chapter will look at the experience of pediatric neurosurgeons using the various surgical laser modalities. The chapter will be divided into considerations for the use of laser in lesions on the brain and the spine.

Minimal Surgical Trauma

One of the great benefits for the use of lasers in pediatric neurosurgery is the limitation of surgical trauma [28]. This, as noted above, can be extremely important in the developing nervous system. Minimization of trauma is especially significant in an infant in whom the developing brain is rapidly undergoing the maturation process. Trauma can have a significant and lasting effect on the developing nervous system, especially in the child under 2 years of age. The young child's brain is considerably less firm, poorly myelinated, and has a higher water content than the adult counterpart. The use of lasers can allow for less retraction and manipulation during surgery and thus decreased trauma. In addition, the atraumatic vaporization of tissue is of significant benefit.

Decreased blood loss can also be a secondary benefit to the use of lasers. Minimization of blood loss is especially important in an infant. A blood loss of 100 cc in an infant weighing 10 kg can be significant. Any surgical modality that can help to minimize blood loss should be considered important in the small child.

The surgical precision of lasers becomes important when they are used in vital or eloquent brain regions. The control of the depth of penetration of surgical lasers and the minimization of the surrounding trauma are all significantly important in these regions. Thus, lasers have become increasingly useful as a part of the overall microsurgical armamentarium of the neurosurgeon.

Use of Surgical Lasers on the Brain

Supratentorial Tumor

The majority of tumors occurring in the supratentorial region in children are amenable to excision with either a laser or a surgical ultrasonic aspirator [9, 30]. The vast majority of neurosurgeons prefer the ultrasonic aspirator. It can debulk a tumor faster than a laser and thus is often the surgical instrument of choice in these lesions. However, lasers may be useful in debulking supratentorial tumors for several reasons (Fig. 1). Depending upon the location of the tumor and the size of blood vessels involved, decreased blood loss may be significantly lessened by the use of laser. We have found this to be especially true in chorioid plexus papillomas. Although these are usually quite vascular lesions, the majority of them are easily vaporized using either CO_2 or contact Nd:YAG lasers. Blood loss is usually kept to a minimum with laser technology. This, of course, varies from case to case. Often the surgeon who is fortunate to have both lasers and ultrasonic aspirators available will experiment to find out which is more useful in removing a given tumor.

When very precise control of the amount of tumor removal is required, the laser is often far superior to the ultrasonic aspirator. This could be especially important in the region of the visual pathway and the hypothalamus. Not surprisingly then, lasers are often much more useful in this area. It should also be noted that the ultrasonic aspirator is generally a very large instrument and the ability

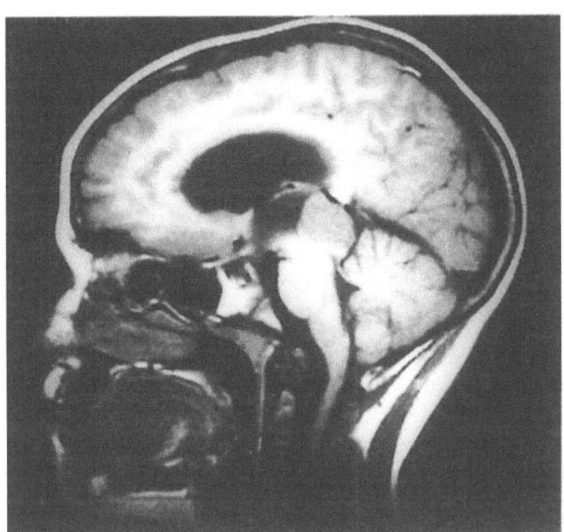

Fig. 1. Sagittal magnetic resonance image showing a tumor of the pineal region. Because of the depth of this lesion and the relatively small opening, laser technology is often useful

to get that instrument into an area deep within the brain or beneath the brain may be limited, cumbersome and difficult whereas the delivery of laser energy to this same area may be much more easily accomplished.

We have found the contact Nd:YAG to be especially useful in critical areas. The amount of energy delivered can be controlled very precisely. The penetration into the tissue is minimal and, in essence, the same effect occurs as with CO_2. The contact Nd:YAG is delivered through a fiber system and held by means of a hand tool that is very similar to a pencil. The surgeon thus retains the usual touch and feel that can often be very important when very precise control of tumor removal is required. For this reason our own experience over the past 5 years has leaned much more heavily toward the contact Nd:YAG. We have especially enjoyed the SLT-contact Nd:YAG fibers (Surgical Laser Technologies, Oaks, PA, USA). Their crystal-tipped technology allows for extremely precise delivery of Nd:YAG laser energy.

Infratentorial Tumors

Tumors within the posterior fossa, by their very nature, are located in vital brain areas. The majority of these lesions have some effect upon the brain stem and thus careful consideration as to the surgical approach and the instrumentation for tumor removal is important. Although the ultrasonic aspirator is still the most commonly used instrument for debulking tumors within the posterior fossa, the surgical laser is importunat if very small amounts of tumor are located adjacent to or within the brain stem, and precise control over removal of tumors in this location is required.

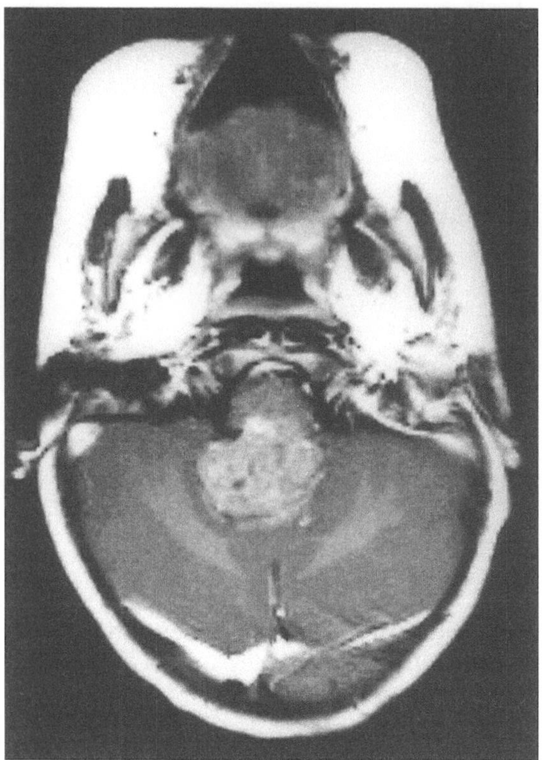

Fig. 2. Gadolinium-enhanced magnetic resonance image showing a medulloblastoma filling the vermis of the cerebellum and possibly invading the floor of the 4th ventricle. Laser surgery is helpful to remove the portion of the tumor that is adjacent to or adherent to the brain stem

The most common use of lasers in posterior fossa surgery in children is in removal of tumors that originate within the cerebellum or 4th ventricle but invade the floor of the 4th ventricle into the brain stem [28] (Fig. 2). The portion of the tumor invading the brain stem can often be removed using surgical lasers. Both the CO_2 and contact Nd:YAG are appropriate for this particular use. It should be pointed out that it is not always necessary to try to excise the portion of the tumor invading the brain stem, but, when the decision is made to try to remove these tumors, laser technology is extremely valuable.

Laser technology has allowed surgeons to be much more aggressive with tumors arising within the brain stem. As a result, a vast experience has accrued over the past 17 years such that the surgical approach to tumors of the brain stem has changed dramatically [10, 11, 13, 31]. In the early 1980s surgery on lesions within the brain stem was considered unwise. Now essentially all areas of the brain stem can be approached surgically (Fig. 3). The only tumor that is considered definitely not surgically treatable is the diffuse infiltrating glioma. However, focal tumors of the medulla and the mesencephalon can be approached and often excised. For these lesions surgical lasers have proved to be extremely valuable.

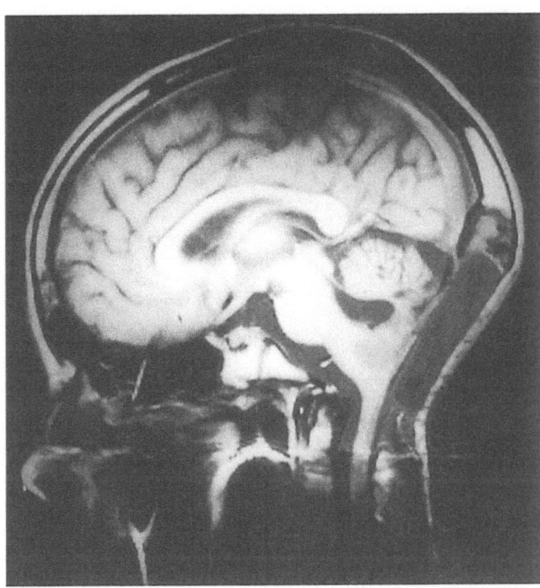

Fig. 3. Sagittal plane magnetic resonance image showing a tumor within the medulla oblongata at the level of the obex. Lasers are used to open the dorsal portion of the medulla and to vaporize the tumor within

In approaching brain stem lesions the laser is used to make an opening overlying the tumor. This is generally accomplished through the portion of the brain stem that is the thinnest, where the tumor is closest to the surface. In the typical tumor of the medulla oblongata the approach is a midline posterior incision into the brain stem with exposure of the tumor immediately beneath this area. Tumors of the cerebellar peduncle are often approached through subtemporal transtentorial routes [26], allowing for a direct exposure of tumors within the peduncle.

Focal tumors in the pons and tumors on the anterior portion of the medulla oblongata often require a parapetrosal transtentorial approach through the skull base [20] (Fig. 4). This allows for excellent exposure of tumors in this region. Lasers can then be used to incise the brain stem and vaporize the tumor within. The minimization of surgical trauma has thus allowed a more aggressive approach to tumors within the brain stem, as well as an understanding of those lesions which should and should not be considered surgical candidates.

Ventriculoscopy

Many neurosurgeons have begun to use endoscopes [2, 14, 22]. This technology has been especially useful in pediatric neurosurgery. However, most neurosurgeons have not been trained in endoscopy and this field has been one in which rapid progress has taken place as neurosurgeons have learned the various brain anomalies and lesions that are amenable to endoscopic surgery. As experience and technology progresses, the use of endoscopes in neurological surgery will increase.

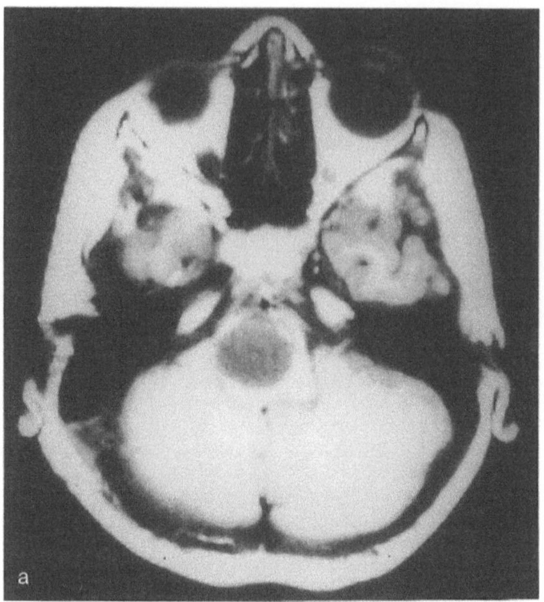

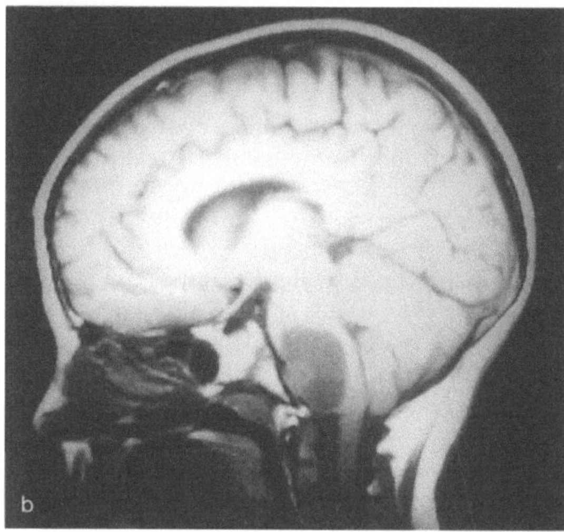

Fig. 4a, b. Axial (a) and sagittal (b) magnetic resonance images showing a focal tumor of the lower pons. Focal lesions within the pons are often benign and amenable to excision with laser technology

Endoscopes lend themselves to the use of laser technology quite easily. This does require, however, that laser be able to be delivered through an optical fiber, thus eliminating the CO_2 laser as a part of this technology. Contact Nd:YAG fibers can be delivered through the endoscope, as can KTP and argon laser wavelengths. This allows for a very precise way of opening cyst walls and gliotic membranes, fenestrating the septum pellucidum, etc. The use of lasers for tumor removal through endoscopy is only in its infancy. This technology will rapidly progress, but up to this point in time experience has been limited.

Children who have had intraventricular bleeding secondary to prematurity or neonatal meningitis are at high risk to develop either isolated lateral ventricles (the two ventricles do not communicate together through the foramen of Monro) or loculated ventricles secondary to scarring [25]. In addition, some congenital anomalies present with multiloculated ventricles and/or a failure of communication between the two lateral ventricles. Laser technology in conjunction with endoscopy has allowed treatment of these conditions through small burr hole openings. This has proven highly successful in the majority of cases. Instead of having to do a formal craniotomy to lyse adhesions and open pathways between the ventricles, minimal surgery is required. As experience has been broadened, smaller and smaller endoscopes have been found to be useful. The delivery of laser energy through small fiberoptic fibers is an integral part of this surgical technology. Both KTP and Nd:YAG laser energy have been used for this purpose and both are highly successful. Argon laser energy has been used only by a few in pediatric neurosurgery; however, one of the advantages of argon is the very small fibers that can be used. Fibers 300 µm in diameter are available. As endoscopes become smaller and smaller, the fiber size becomes much more critical. Argon energy through a fiberoptic fiber can fenestrate cyst walls just as easily as Nd:YAG or KTP; thus we may see an increasing use of argon in neuroendoscopy.

It has been our approach to try to avoid adding a second shunt when children present with an isolated lateral ventricle or scarring and cyst formation within the ventricular system. If additional shunt systems are required, the management of these patients becomes increasingly complex. These patients are, by their very nature, sometimes difficult to assess because of the underlying insult which has resulted in loculation of the ventricles. If they present with

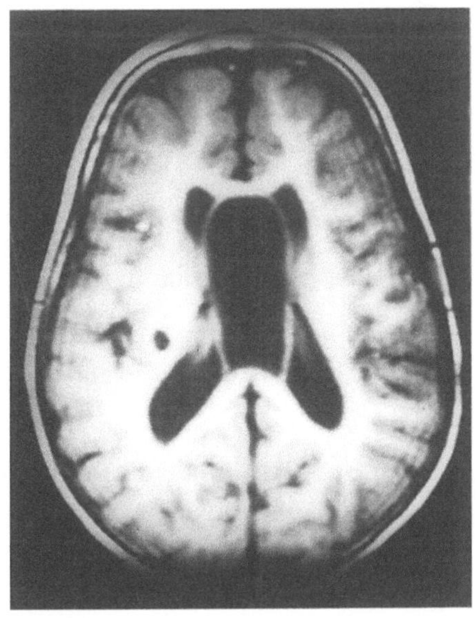

Fig. 5. Axial magnetic resonance image showing a large cavum septum pallucidum cyst with early hydrocephalus. This cystic area is easily opened with laser energy delivered through a fiberoptic fiber and an endoscope

signs and symptoms of increased intracranial pressure, it is often difficult to assess which of their several shunt systems may be malfunctioning. It thus becomes increasingly important to try to limit the number of shunt systems needed by a given patient. Laser technology and endoscopy have provided an avenue for treatment of these children and it has been done with great success. Although not always successful, the chances of success in these patients is quite high when using laser technology combined with endoscopy. Fenestrations across the septum pellucidum are easily made, thus allowing the two ventricular systems to once again communicate and allowing one shunt system to drain both sides (Fig. 5). Likewise, fenestration of cysts within the ventricle can communicate the cyst into the ventricular system and thus one shunt may drain everything instead of having to add a second shunt system.

Many pediatric neurosurgeons approach the patient with the new onset of hydrocephalus in a completely different manner since endoscopy has become available. The question always arises as to whether the patient could be made shunt independent by performing a third ventriculostomy. Although the exact ideal candidate for this procedure has not yet been completely identified, it appears the patients who present with findings of aqueduct stenosis, either congenitally or secondary to tumors or other lesions, may be the best candidates [16, 21]. It has been our practice to attempt third ventriculostomy in all of these patients to see which ones may be able to be shunt independent.

Some have written that lasers can be used to perform third ventriculostomy [5]. At present, with the state of technology that is available, we strongly disagree that lasers should be used to make the opening in the floor of the third ventricle. The vasculature immediately external to the floor of the third ventricle is extremely important. Even the small perforating vessels from the basilar artery and the posterior communicating arteries are vital. Injury to these vessels can result in serious and permanent neurologic dysfunction. Laser energy delivered through the floor of the third ventricle, in our opinion, cannot be delivered with enough safety to assure that no penetration beyond the arachnoid membrane of the third ventricular floor will occur; thus, the potential for injury immediately external to the floor of the third ventricle is high. Although we initially used laser energy to fenestrate the floor of the third ventricle in several patients, it became apparent that use of the laser fibers through endoscopes on the floor of the third ventricle lacks sufficient touch and feel to be sure that penetration through the floor was not too deep. Our personal preference is to use a laser fiber to make an opening in the floor of the third ventricle, but we do not use laser energy. The laser fiber is stiff, easily penetrates the floor of the third ventricle and then allows the use of either the scope itself or a Fogarty catheter to dilate the opening to a sufficient size.

Use of Surgical Lasers on the Spine

Tumors.   Tumors in the spinal cord have been extremely amenable to laser use (Fig. 6). Intrinsic astrocytomas within the spinal cord are easily exposed by opening the dorsal midline of the cord, using either CO_2 [7–9] or contact

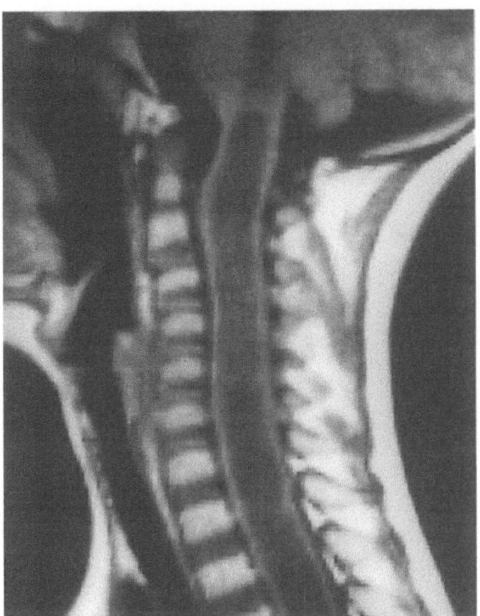

Fig. 6. Sagittal magnetic resonance image showing a large intrinsic astrocytoma of the cervical spinal cord extending up to the medulla oblongata. Lasers are used to open the dorsal cord and to debulk the tumor

Nd:YAG lasers. Once the dorsal midline has been opened, the tumor is usually immediately exposed. The pie can then be retracted by means of tack up sutures giving a wide exposure to the intrinsic tumor. The use of the surgical ultrasonic aspirator and laser technology has proven very valuable in these lesions [9]. We often use the ultrasonic aspirator to remove the gross portion of the tumor and use either the CO_2 or contact Nd:YAG laser for the final removal around the edges of the tumor. Most of these children can be expected to be improved neurologically following tumor excision. Likewise, excision of ependymomas within the cord have proven to be amenable to laser therapy. A dorsal incision in the midline allows exposure and the tumor itself can be easily vaporized.

Syringomyelia.   Lasers have been shown to be useful in the treatment of syringomyelia [3] (Fig. 7). An opening into the syrinx by the laser allows for a small minimally traumatic exposure into the syringomyelic cavity. This can either be done at the level of the dorsal root entry or in the midline, depending upon the extent and location of the syringomyelia. The laser has thus proven to be extremely valuable in this type of surgery.

Lipomyelomeningoceles.   The removal of lipomyelomeningoceles (spinal lipomas) from the spinal cord is an area where laser surgery is essentially indispensable [4, 15, 17, 18] (Fig. 8). Removal of these lesions by standard bipolar and suction technique is much more traumatic and frustrating than with the use of lasers. Likewise, the ultrasonic aspirator has proven to be much less useful in these lesions. The ultrasonic aspirator usually leaves a stroma after the fat has been debulked that still requires a traumatic removal if not done using laser technology.

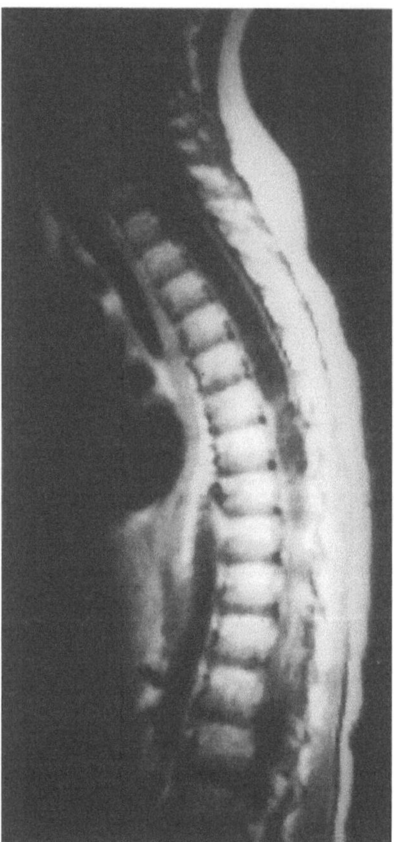

Fig. 7. Sagittal magnetic resonance image showing a large syringomyelia. A laser is used to open the cord to allow communication of the syringomyelic fluid into the subarachnoid space or to allow for the placement of a shunt tube into the syringomyelic cavity

Fig. 8. Sagittal magnetic resonance image showing a large lipomyelomeningocele tethering the spinal cord into the sacral region. Lasers have allowed essentially complete removal of the lipoma without injury to the surrounding normal neural tissue

Both the CO_2 and contact Nd:YAG lasers have been extremely useful with lipomyelomeningoceles. The fat can be vaporized away gently, easily and precisely. Identification of the surrounding normal and abnormal anatomy is obviously important and the use of lasers has allowed the gradual debulking of these lesions with the increasing recognition of the surrounding anatomy as it becomes more apparent after the removal of the fatty mass (Fig. 9). Without question, laser technology has allowed a much more aggressive approach to these lesions and in our opinion a much more successful long-term outcome.

Tethered Cord Release. Another area where laser technology has proven to be extremely valuable is in the release of the tethered cord, especially the recurrent

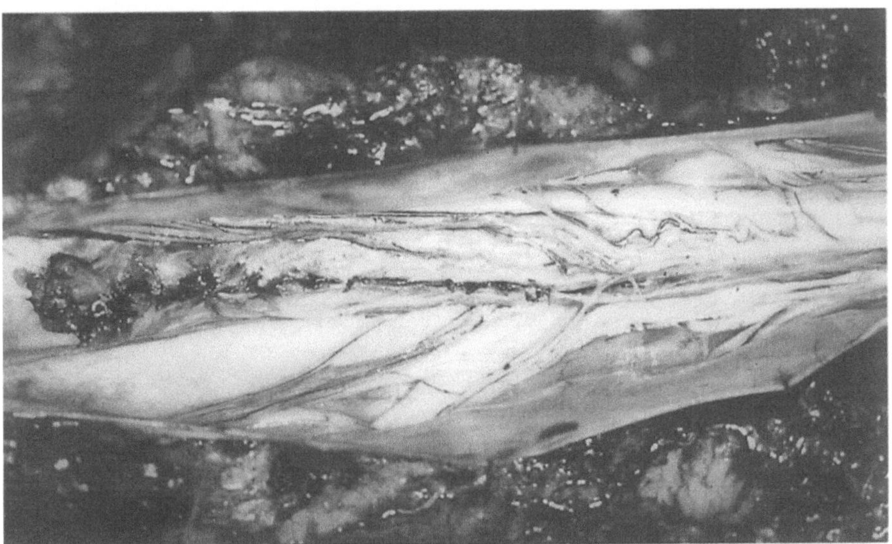

Fig. 9.   Operative photograph of a spinal cord that has been untethered from a distal lipo-myelomeningocele. All of the lipoma has been vaporized. The cord now has a normal anatomical appearance and is able to be closed within the dura

tethered cord. This is most commonly seen in pediatric neurosurgical practice in the child with myelomeningocele [19]. Because of scarring that occurs surrounding the area of the placode as the child grows in height, stretching of the spinal cord becomes problematic. These patients typically show deterioration of neurological function and if not untethered will continue to deteriorate. Because the scarring that they experience is immediately surrounding the area of the neural placode, the chance for increasing neurological deficit is high. Thus, the use of laser for taking down the surrounding scar tissue and exposing the normal neural tissue beneath has become important.

We prefer the contact Nd:YAG laser for tethered cord release. The contact fiber delivers a very precise amount of energy and the touch of the laser allows the surgeon the touch and feel that is necessary to precisely dissect away this scarring. We have found that the scar can be easily vaporized, exposing the normal neural tissue beneath with minimal or no trauma to the adjacent neural tissue in the vast majority of patients.

Conclusion

Surgical lasers have an important part in the armamentarium of pediatric neurosurgeons. Their use in both brain and spinal tumors is well established. In addition, more recently lasers have been found to be extremely valuable in conjunction with endoscopy in the treatment of both congenital and acquired lesions, especially lesions causing hydrocephalus. Lasers are also valuable in treatment of syringomyelia, lipomyelomeningoceles and release of the tethered spinal cord.

Contact Nd:YAG, CO_2, KTP and argon lasers all have various indications in pediatric neurosurgery. As experience with these and other laser wavelengths increases and as experience with endoscopy increases, more and more applications of laser energy to pediatric neurosurgical problems will be found.

References

1. Asher P (1987) The use of CO_2 laser in neurosurgery. In: Kaplan I (eds) Laser surgery II. Jerusalem Academic Jerusalem, pp 76–78
2. Auer L, Holzer P, Asher P, Heppner F (1988) Endoscopic neurosurgery. Acta Neurochir (Wien) 90: 1–14
3. Brown J (1988) Neuroablative procedures. In: Cerullo L (ed) Application of lasers in neurosurgery. Year Book Medical Publishers, Chicago, pp 115–128
4. Chapman P, KR D (1983) Surgical treatment of spinal lipomas. Concepts Pediatr Neurosurg 3: 178–190
5. Cohen A (1993) Endoscopic neurosurgery. In: Rengachary S, Wilkins R (eds) Neurosurgical operative atlas. Williams and Wilkins, Baltimore, pp 435–447
6. Edwards M, Boggan J (1984) Argon laser surgery of pediatric neural neoplasms. Childs Brain 11: 171–175
7. Epstein F (1983) Surgical treatment of extensive spinal cord astrocytomas of childhood. Concepts Pediatr Neurosurg 3: 157–169
8. Epstein F, Epstein N (1982) Surgical treatment of spinal cord astrocytoma in children. J Neurosurg 157: 685–689
9. Epstein F, Farmer J (1991) Trends in surgery: laser surgery, use of the cavitron, and debulking surgery. Neurol Clin 9 (2): 307–315
10. Epstein F, McCleary E (1986) Intrinsic brainstem tumors of childhood: surgical indications. J Neurosurg 64: 11–15
11. Epstein F, Wisoff J (1989) Brainstem tumors in childhood: surgical indications. In: McLaurin R, Schut L, Venes J (eds) Pediatric neurosurgery. Surgery of the developing nervous system. Saunders, Philadelpha, pp 357–365
12. Heppner F (1978) The laser scalpel on the nervous system. In: Kaplan I (ed) Laser surgery II. Jerusalem Academic, Jerusalem, pp 79–80
13. Hoffman H, Stroink A, Davidson G (1987) Pediatric brainstem gliomas: evaluation of biopsy. Concepts Pediatr Neurosurg 7: 105–116
14. Hor F, Desgeorges M, Rosseau G (1992) Tumour resection by stereotactic laser endoscopy. Acta Neurochir (Wien) 54: 77–82
15. James H, Williams J, Brock W et al (1984) Radical removal of lipomas of the conus and cauda equine with laser microsurgery. Neurosurgery 15: 340–343
16. Jones R, Stering W, Brydon M (1990) Endoscopic third ventriculoscopy. Neurosurgery 26: 86–92
17. McLone D, Naidich T (1986) Laser resection of fifty spinal lipomas. Neurosurgery 18: 611–615
18. McLone D, Hayashida S, Caldarelli M (1985) Surgical resection of lipomyelomeningoceles in 18 asymptomatic infants. J Pediatr Neurosci 12: 239–242
19. McLone D, Herman J, Gabrieli A, Dias L (1990) Tethered cord as a cause of scoliosis in children with a myelomeningocele. Pediatr Neurosurg 16: 8–13
20. Miller C, van Loveren H, Keller J, Pensak M, El-Kalliny M, Tew J (1993) Transpetrosal approach: surgical anatomy and technique. Neurosurgery 33: 461–469
21. Pierre-Kahn A, Renier D, Bombois B (1975) Place de la ventriculocisternostomie dans le traitement des hydrocéphalus non communicates. Neurochirurgie 21: 557–569
22. Powers S (1992) Fenestration of intraventricular cysts using a flexible, steerable endoscope. Acta Neurochir (Wien) 54: 42–46
23. Powers S, Edwards M, Boggan J, Pitts L, Gutin P, Hosobuchi Y, Adams J, Wilson C (1984) Use of the argon surgical laser in neurosurgery. J Neurosurg 60: 523–530

24. Roux F, Mordon S, Faller-Bianco C, Merienne L, Devaux B, Chodkiewicz J (1990) Effects of 1.32 μm Nd:YAG laser on brain thermal and histological experimental data. Surg Neurol 34: 402–407
25. Shultz P, Leeds N (1973) Intraventricular septations complicating neonatal meningitis. J Neurosurg 38: 620–626
26. Symon L (1982) Surgical approaches to the tentorial hiatus. In: Krayenbuhl H (ed) Advances and technical standards in neurosurgery. Springer, New York, pp 69–112
27. Takizawa T, Yamazaki T, Miura N (1980) Laser surgery of basal, orbital, and ventricular meningiomas which are difficult to extirpate by conventional methods. Neurol Med Chir 20: 729–737
28. Walker M (1988) Using lasers in pediatric neurosurgery. In: Robertson J, Clark W (eds) Lasers in neurosurgery. Kluwer, Dordrecht, pp 101–114
29. Walker M, McLone D (1988) Lasers in pediatric neurosurgery. In: Cerullo L (ed) Applications of lasers in neurosurgery. Year Book Medical Publishers, Chicago, pp 60–81
30. Walker M, Storrs B (1985) Lasers in pediatric neurosurgery. Pediatr Neurosci 12: 23–30
31. Walker M, Storrs B (1985) Surgical therapy for intrinsic brainstem gliomas. Concepts Pediatr Neurosurg 5: 178–186
32. Walker M, Storrs B, Goodman S (1983) Use of the CO_2 laser for surgical excision of primary brain tumors in children. Concepts Pediatr Neurosurg 3: 297–315
33. Wharen R, Anderson R, Sundt T (1984) The Nd:YAG laser in neurosurgery. J Neurosurg 60: 540–547
34. Wirth F, Downing E, Cannon C Jr, Baker R (1987) Experience with the neodymium: yttrium-aluminum-garnet laser in forty-two cases. Neurosurgery 21: 867–871